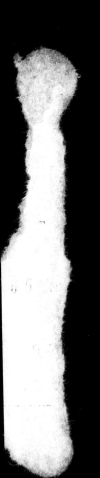

The Scourging Angel

The Black Death in the British Isles

THE
SCOURGING
ANGEL

The Black Death
in the British Isles

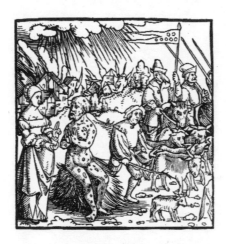

BENEDICT GUMMER

THE BODLEY HEAD
LONDON

Published by The Bodley Head 2009

2 4 6 8 10 9 7 5 3 1

Copyright © Benedict Gummer 2009

First published in Great Britain in 2009 by
The Bodley Head
Random House, 20 Vauxhall Bridge Road,
London SW1V 2SA

www.bodleyhead.co.uk
www.rbooks.co.uk

Addresses for companies within The Random House Group Limited can be found at:
www.randomhouse.co.uk/offices.htm

The Random House Group Limited Reg. No. 954009

A CIP catalogue record for this book
is available from the British Library

ISBN 9780224077675

The Random House Group Limited supports The Forest Stewardship
Council (FSC), the leading international forest certification organisation. All our titles
that are printed on Greenpeace approved FSC certified paper carry the FSC logo. Our
paper procurement policy can be found at www.rbooks.co.uk/environment

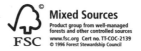

Mixed Sources
Product group from well-managed
forests and other controlled sources
www.fsc.org Cert no. TT-COC-2139
© 1996 Forest Stewardship Council

FSC

Typeset in Dante MT by Palimpsest Book Production Limited,
Grangemouth, Stirlingshire
Printed and bound in Great Britain by
Clays Ltd, St Ives plc

To my mother with admiration and love

Remember, O Lord, your covenant, and say to the the scourging angel,
'Now hold your hand', so that the earth is not left desolate and you do
not lose every living soul.

Missa Recordare Domini,
written and issued by Pope Clement VI
during the time of the pestilence.[1]

Contents

Illustrations and Maps

Effigy (alabaster) of Philippa of Hainault by Jean de Liège (fl.1361–81) (© *The Dean and Chapter of Westminster Abbey/The Bridgeman Art Library*); Funeral effigy of Edward III (© *The Dean and Chapter of Westminster Abbey*); Effigy (alabaster) of William Edington (© *Dr John Crook FSA*); Coin, obverse, half groat, reign of David II (© *National Museums of Scotland*); Reconstruction of a medieval cruck house, Wharram Percy (© *Peter Dunn/English Heritage*); Reconstruction of medieval Faccombe Netherton (© *The Trustees of the British Museum*); Scenes from the Luttrell Psalter, *c.*1325–35 (vellum), English School, Add. 42130 f.170, f.171v and f.172v (© *British Library Board/The Bridgeman Art Library*); Scourging angels, from Le Chroniche di Giovanni Sercambi (© *Archivio di Stato di Luca/Ministero per i Beni e le Attività Culturali*); Black Death in Tournai, Gilles de Muisit (1279–1352), after 1349 (vellum) (© *Bibliotheque Royale de Belgique/The Bridgeman Art Library*); Burials in East Smithfield (© *Museum of London Archaeology*); Extreme Unction, French School, Ms 137/1687 f.87v (© *Musée Condé, Chantilly/ Giraudon/The Bridgeman Art Library*); William of Wykeham and New College, English School, Ms New Coll 258 f.3v (© *Warden and Scholars of New College, Oxford/The Bridgeman Art Library*); Choir and east window of Gloucester Cathedral (© *Alamy/Alamy*); Edington Church (© *Christopher Jones*); Chaplet from the Colmar Treasure (© *RMN/ Jean-Gilles Berizzi*); Ashwell graffiti (© *Adams Picture Library t/a apl/Alamy*).

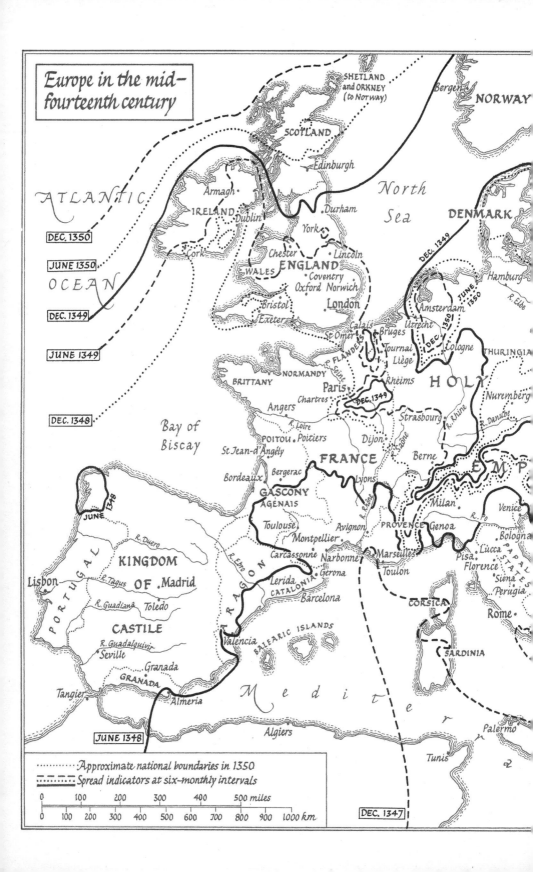

Europe in the mid-fourteenth century

SHETLAND
AND ORKNEY
(to Norway)

NORWAY

Bergen

SCOTLAND

Edinburgh

ATLANTIC

North
Sea

DENMARK

DEC. 1350

Armagh

IRELAND

Dublin

Durham

York

Hamburg

JUNE 1350

Cork

Chester

Lincoln

WALES

ENGLAND

Coventry

Oxford Norwich

Amsterdam

Cologne

OCEAN

DEC. 1349

London

THURINGIA

Bristol

Exeter

Calais

St Omer

Bruges

Utrecht

Liège

HOLY

JUNE 1349

R. Elbe

DEC. 1350

JUNE 1350

DEC. 1349

R. FLANDERS

Tournai

Saint

BRITTANY

NORMANDY

Rheims

Paris

Nuremberg

DEC. 1348

Angers

Chartres

DEC. 1349

Strasbourg

*Bay of
Biscay*

R. Loire

POITOU

Poitiers

Dijon

R. Rhine

R. Danube

St Jean-d'Angély

Berne

EMP

Bordeaux

Bergerac

FRANCE

Lyons

Milan

Venice

JUNE 1348

GASCONY

AGENAIS

Avignon

PROVENCE

Genoa

R. Po

Bologna

Toulouse

Montpellier

Marseilles

Lucca

Florence

PAPAL

STATES

Lisbon

PORTUGAL

R. Duero

KINGDOM

OF .Madrid

Carcassonne

Narbonne

Toulon

Pisa

Siena

Perugia

R. Tagus

Lerida

CATALONIA

Gerona

CORSICA

Rome

R. Guadiana

Toledo

Barcelona

CASTILE

ARAGON

R. Ebro

Valencia

BALEARIC ISLANDS

SARDINIA

R. Guadalquivir

Seville

Granada

GRANADA

Medi

Tangier

Almeria

JUNE 1348

ter

Palermo

Algiers

r

Tunis

a

.... Approximate national boundaries in 1350
------ Spread indicators at six-monthly intervals

0   100   200   300   400   500 miles
0 100 200 300 400 500 600 700 800 900 1000 km

DEC. 1347

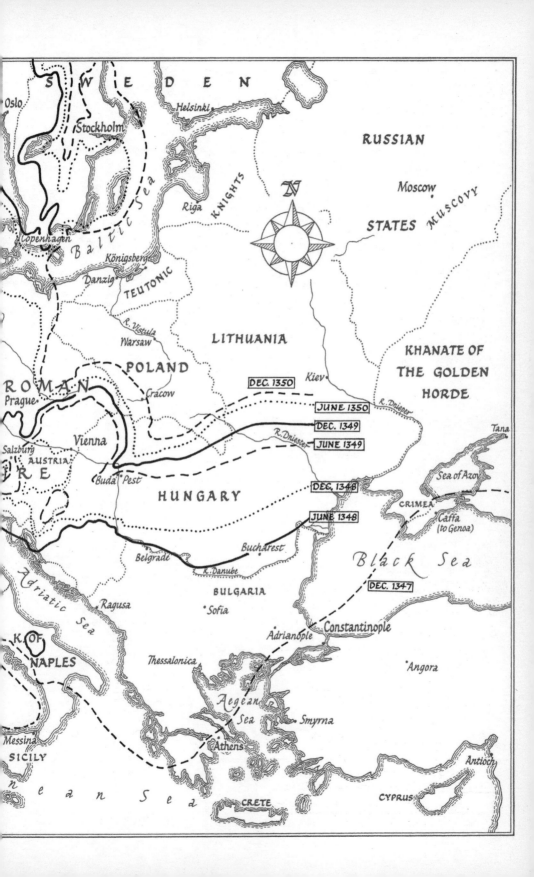

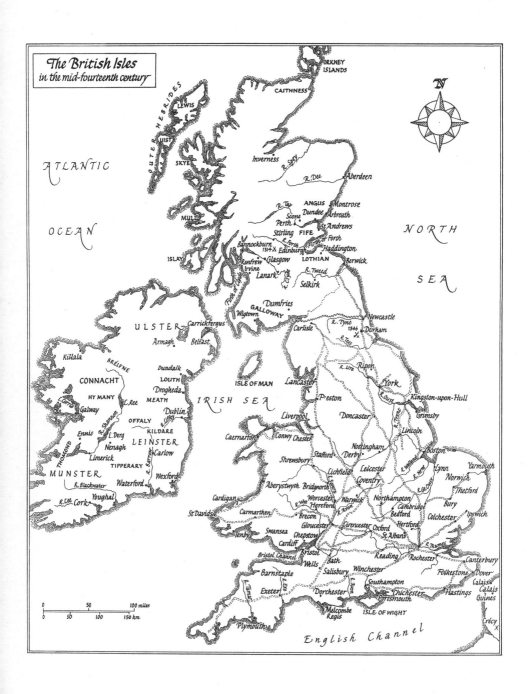

The British Isles
in the mid-fourteenth century

ATLANTIC

OCEAN

NORTH

SEA

ORKNEY
ISLANDS

CAITHNESS

OUTER HEBRIDES

LEWIS

UIST

SKYE

MULL

ISLAY

Inverness

R. Spey

R. Dee

Aberdeen

ANGUS Montrose
R. Tay Dundee Arbroath
Scone
Perth St Andrews
Stirling FIFE
Bannockburn Firth of Forth
1314-X Edinburgh Haddington
R. Forth Firth of Forth
Glasgow LOTHIAN
Renfrew Irvine R. Clyde Berwick
Lanark R. Tweed
Selkirk

Dumfries
Wigtown GALLOWAY

Firth of Clyde

ULSTER Carrickfergus
Armagh Belfast

Carlisle

Newcastle
R. Tyne 1346 Durham
R. Tees

Killala
BRÉIFNE
CONNACHT
HY MANY
Galway L. Corrib
L. Ree
R. Shannon
OFFALY
Ennis L. Derg
Nenagh
THOMOND Limerick
MUNSTER TIPPERARY
R. Blackwater
R. Lee Cork Youghal

Dundalk
LOUTH
Drogheda
MEATH
Dublin
R. Liffey
KILDARE
LEINSTER Carlow
R. Barrow
Wexford
Waterford

ISLE OF MAN

IRISH SEA

Ripon
R. Ure
Lancaster
Preston York
R. Ouse
Liverpool Doncaster Kingston-upon-Hull
Grimsby
Caernarfon Conwy Chester
Lincoln
Shrewsbury Stafford
Nottingham Derby Boston
Lichfield Leicester R. Witham Lynn
Aberystwyth Bridgnorth Coventry R. Nene Norwich Yarmouth
Worcester Warwick Northampton R. Gt. Ouse Thetford
St Davids Cardigan Hereford R. Avon Cambridge Bury
Carmarthen Brecon Cirencester Bedford Colchester Ipswich
Swansea Gloucester Oxford Hertford
Tenby Chepstow St Albans
Cardiff R. Thames
Bristol Channel Bristol Bath Reading Rochester Canterbury
Wells Salisbury Winchester Folkestone Dover
Barnstaple Southampton Chichester Hastings Calais
R. Taw R. Exe Dorchester Portsmouth Guines
Exeter R. Avon
Melcombe ISLE OF WIGHT
Regis Crécy
Plymouth

English Channel

0   50   100 miles
0   50   100   150 km

Preface

The purpose of this book is straightforward: to give a description of the British Isles on the eve of the Black Death; to provide an account of the progress of the epidemic through those islands; and to survey England, Wales, Scotland and Ireland as they were left after the pandemic had ceased.

The narrative starts in 1346 and ends in 1381. These dates require some explanation. It was in 1346 that the first chapter of England's armed dispute with France, later to be called the Hundred Years War, came to an end, on the field of Crécy. At the same time the Scots' war of independence was brought to an abrupt halt by the capture of King David II at the Battle of Neville's Cross. These events provide a natural caesura in the political history of the British Isles and an appropriate place to begin the account of the horrors that would shortly follow. For it was also in 1346 that the first European contracted an unknown disease that soon swept across the Continent, killing millions as it went. The pandemic reached British and Irish shores by mid-1348 and was gone within two years, leaving perhaps half the population dead. So great a mortality, incurred in so short a space of time, had a profound effect on the survivors that remained; yet even the youngest were reaching late middle age by the 1380s, by which point it is increasingly difficult to untangle the influence of this and succeeding plagues from other, more immediate matters – political crisis, schism in the church, wildly erratic weather and the unsettling alternation of bounty and dearth. It is here, therefore, that the narrative of this book comes to an end.

The compass of this book also requires explanation, for there was none of the modern political unity in the medieval British Isles; indeed, England in these years had a closer political relationship with

Gascony and Calais than it did with the Highlands of Scotland. Yet it would be an even greater contrivance to extend the scope of this book to these places without drawing in France and Flanders and much of western Europe at the same time. So this book concerns itself largely with what happened north of the English Channel. It was a limitation that would have been understood by medieval as well as modern audiences – for the English, Welsh, Scots, Anglo-Irish and Gaelic Irish peoples of the Middle Ages inhabited islands that both they and outsiders considered to have a degree of geographical and historical unity. There are a number of benefits to considering these nations together. For while the odd collection of peoples that inhabited the British Isles were divided among themselves, into kingdoms and nations, they rubbed up against one another along indistinct and shifting frontiers. The study of an epidemic that swept through the British Isles, crossing these boundaries almost as if they did not exist, tells us something about how these peoples related to each other. Furthermore, the extraordinary diversity of the peoples of the British Isles – their differing degrees of commercialization, governmental competence, bureaucratic sophistication, agricultural development, and cultural distinctiveness – provide a useful means by which differing reactions and varying results of the pestilence might be compared.

Although this book aims to present as balanced a picture of these times as is possible, five specific caveats should be given. First, England was not only the largest country by size and population but it also produced far more written material than Scotland, Wales and every part of Ireland, all added together; indeed, the extent of English record-keeping was unparalleled across Europe. The experience of this country predominates, therefore. Secondly, the voice of the literate, especially the clergy, was far louder than that of the great mass of people, whose evidence it is sometimes very difficult to hear. Consequently, this account (like many others) relies on the evidence of bishops and monks while the descriptions of villages and rural life are drawn from the records of their owners rather than the recollections of their inhabitants. Thirdly, while a thematic treatment of the story of the Black Death has been firmly rejected, the material falls naturally into discrete accounts, such as those relating to medicine or architecture. Fourthly, there is a necessary concentration on the key events of the Black Death itself, so whereas those chapters concerned with the pestilence may cover only a few months, the later chapters that deal with the aftermath of the plague cover years and decades at a time. Finally, while the book is organized in a strictly chronological order, for the purposes of comprehension and continuity there is in places some degree of overlap between chapters. On occasion, the text may also refer to events outside the timeframe of the chapter or book. It is hoped, despite these necessary imbalances and divisions, that the reader will draw from the narrative those subtleties, complexities and finely balanced conclusions that might, in a more systematized history, be obscured.

The book covers the same ground oft-ploughed by historians. Broadly speaking, arguments about the Black Death and its effects have centred on three key issues: the extent to which the advent and progress of the pandemic was predetermined by the structure, state and population density of European society; a corresponding discussion concerning the effects of the epidemic and its mortality on every aspect of European life; and a largely separate controversy about the nature of the disease and the manner in which it was spread. While this book offers an opinion on the first two of these debates, it does not seek to identify the pathogen that caused the disease. The reasons for this are twofold. In the last twenty years, very considerable and detailed analysis has led to the assumptions on which the long-standing diagnosis of medieval pestilence as bubonic plague being questioned. While the arguments against this diagnosis are persuasive, no serious alternative has emerged, other than the suggestion that the pestilence bore a likeness to one of the more virulent haemorrhagic fevers currently found in central Africa. Until there is a significant advance in archaeological science, it is unlikely that the precise cause of the Black Death will be positively identified. To speculate any more would not only be futile but would be to risk precisely the same problems caused by the interpolation of the epidemiology of modern bubonic plague into so many histories of the period. The intention of this book is not, therefore, to rehearse the arguments about what caused the Black Death and how it spread, or to construct the narrative around any one of the theories about what the disease might have been. Instead, the pestilence is described only as it was seen by people at the time and the extent of the mortality is judged only by its enumeration in contemporary records. Readers might prefer to approach the book from this standpoint, viewing the unfolding terror with something of the bewilderment suffered by those who experienced it first-hand. However, those who wish to be briefed on the current state of the debate before they embark on the book should first read Appendix 1, which provides a summary of current scholarship on the epidemiology of the Black Death. It should be stated here that when the text refers to 'plague', it is referring to the generic word used at the time (*plaga*) and not to any modern definition, and that 'contagion' and 'infection' are used loosely, not according to their strict epidemiological meaning.

A few more points require explanation. A remarkable amount has been achieved in the discovery and interpretation of fourteenth-century records over the last hundred years. This book draws on that work and does not bring any new source material to bear. For ease of reading, I have, therefore, taken a minimal view of annotating the text, and no citations – except in the case of direct quotations – are given. The Julian calendar has been used throughout, although unless otherwise stated the new year is taken to be 1st January. In some of the longer descriptions, I have endeavoured to choose those places that are open to the public. Most names, especially when they derive from a place, have been modernized, and Gaelic Irish names have been anglicized (although the proper form is given in a footnote). Full maps are provided, including a new representation of the progress of the disease across Europe and the British Isles, a short explanation of which is given in the second appendix. Technical terms are explained at their first mention. Finally, it should be made clear that the artificial insertion of great hordes of rats and their ravenous fleas into the history of the Black Death is not the only anachronism to have entered most popular histories of the period: another is the common name for the pandemic, the 'Black Death', which was an invention of the early nineteenth century. I have opted not to use that term at all in the text and instead prefer those translations of the words used at the time: pestilence, plague, and the Great Death.

I

Galling the Gleaned Land

October 1346–July 1347

It was a sight the garrison soldiers of Liddel Strength had hoped never to see. As they scanned the flat-bottomed Liddel valley from their redoubt, they observed Scottish troops, making their way across the river. Scotland began on one bank, England the other. This was no mere raiding party, however, which would have been all too familiar, but a great army, perhaps 12,000 strong, advancing behind a fluttering banner that bore the arms of the young Scots king, David II.

Not in a generation had Scottish soldiers marched on England with such confidence. Every one of them knew that the English king, Edward III, was detained in France, laying siege to Calais. Only six weeks previously he had routed the French at Crécy, a defeat so absolute that Philip VI of France had been forced to plead with the Scots to invade just so as to distract Edward on his northern frontier. Although David felt his obligation to Philip keenly, he knew perfectly well that Edward would not have left England without making provision for a Scots attack. So David chose to cross the border in the west, where an incursion was least expected. It was Saturday, 7th October 1346.

By midday the Scots had laid siege to the fortress, which was defended bravely by its garrison under the command of the Constable of the North, Sir William Selby. It took until Monday for the Scots to force their way inside. There the soldiers butchered Selby's two sons in front of their father and the Scottish king, before beheading Sir William himself. Keen to avoid a similar fate, the burghers of Carlisle, eleven miles to the south, bought the Scots off, thereby avoiding an assault they could not hope to resist. Its rear now protected, the Scots army marched east, down the valley that ran eventually to Tynemouth and the North Sea. Unleashing his men over the countryside, David and his host came first upon Lanercost Priory which, forty years earlier, Edward I had used as a campaigning base against Scotland. Unsurprisingly, the place excited little piety in the Scots: they strode into the holy sanctuary, seized what jewels they could find and destroyed that which they could not take with them. As David struck south to Hexham Priory, where he spent a full three days piling up loot, his able lieutenant William Douglas rode east, towards the farms of the bishop and priory of Durham which had for centuries offered the Scots an easy source of plunder. Douglas's rapid progress brought him, on Sunday, 15th October, to Tynemouth Priory, where finally he found his thieving checked: on ordering the prior, Thomas de la Mare, to pay him tribute money, Douglas was given nothing but a refusal, point blank. Conscious that he had to return to the main force, Douglas had time only to threaten the prior with a quip: de la Mare should be ready with breakfast for him in two days, the Scot declared, as by then he would be back to seize what, for now, he could not win simply by demand.

De la Mare's defiance excepted, the Scots' raid had gone unchallenged. It had not, however, gone unnoticed. Although the larger part of the English nobility was in France, Edward had ensured that two Northern barons, Ralph Neville and Henry Percy, remained in England in order to counter any Scottish invasion, and appointed the archbishop of York, William Zouche, warden of the north-eastern March, to co-ordinate the English defence. So when eventually that invasion came, the English reaction was rapid: by Saturday, 14th October, only a week after the Scots had crossed the border, an advance English army numbering as many as 4,000 troops had already mustered at Barnard Castle in County Durham, with a reserve army, sixty-five miles to the south-east, cobbled together out of the criminal fugitives of Beverley (who made use of the sanctuary that by ancient tradition was provided there) and a band of sword-toting priests. That Saturday evening, the prelate and Northern barons dined in the timber-vaulted great hall of Barnard Castle, with Sir Thomas Rokeby, the sheriff of Yorkshire, and Edward Balliol, the pretender to the Scottish throne. They ate venison from the castle estates and fish from the Tees, which wound its way round the foot of the castle wall below. Their army was encamped on the opposite bank, passing the night in flare-lit gloom.

Unaware of the English gathering just to the south, David pursued his casual plunder, making for the greatest prize of the North – the cathedral priory of St Cuthbert in Durham. This massive Norman church stood sentinel over a loop in the River Wear, proclaiming the power of its prince-bishop and the wealth of its Benedictine monks. It was little surprise, therefore, that the priory had presented so attractive a target for so many Scottish armies; indeed, it was a mere five years since the Scots had last pillaged Durham, leaving the town burning as they went. With nine days of profitable raiding behind him, David swaggered this way once again, Douglas rejoining him *en route*. The Scots had, by now, crossed almost the breadth of the country, a journey that, by virtue of the diagonal border, brought them deep into northern England, as far south from Berwick as they had come east from Carlisle. By Monday, 16th October, the Scots troops had reached the prior of Durham's estate at Bear Park, just within sight of the great cathedral in the east. There they made camp, while David pondered his next move.

The Scots king's quandary was this: he could bank his winnings and return to Scotland, crossing the eastern border so that he might have a shot at retaking the fortified town of Berwick (the loss of which thirteen years before had forced him into exile in France, whence he had returned in 1341); or he could strike south, and attempt something far greater than the glorified cattle raid he had achieved thus far. True fidelity to the alliance with France, cemented by his father at Corbeil in 1326, dictated that David should take the latter course; it had been for that purpose, after all, that the French had encouraged the invasion and equipped David with men and armour. If he were able to deliver York, then he would secure most of England north of the River Trent and force Edward's return from France. But for all David's enthusiasm as a marauder, he was a reluctant conqueror: indeed, the relaxed pace of the Scottish advance betrayed their king's hesitation in taking on the larger challenge. Something bode ill for the invasion. Perhaps it was the ominous murder of the highland chieftain Ranald MacRuairi, by William, earl of Ross at the army's muster in Perth. Maybe the whole raid had proved just too easy. Most likely David simply doubted his own strength. His dithering was to cost him any choice he might have had in the matter.

Whilst David prevaricated, the rag-tag Beverley reserve, under the command of Thomas, Lord Lucy, had been urgently making its way north. They passed through the town of Northallerton, where in 1138 Archbishop Thurstan had led an English army into battle against the Scots beneath the standard of St Cuthbert and the Northern saints. A former Balliol had fought under this holy standard, as had an earlier Bruce. Now their two descendants were to face each other as opponents: a Balliol again with England, challenging a Bruce king of Scotland. Archbishop Zouche, meanwhile, had moved the main army twelve and a half miles north-east to Bishop Auckland, the better to join with Lucy's troops as they approached Durham. Early the next day, Tuesday, 17th October, Zouche sent out scouts to locate these reinforcements; instead, they ran into a Scottish reconnaissance party. The Scots, led by Douglas, turned heel and were chased almost to Durham; now aware of just how close the invaders were, Zouche set out straight to meet them, not even waiting for Lucy's reserve.

Douglas delivered the bad news to David back at the Scots' camp: the English were but eight miles away. Desperate to retain a fraction of the initiative he had once wholly possessed, David moved his army out of the Bear Park onto the ridge that lay to the west of Durham. It was not long before he could see English soldiers mount the same ridge to the south and march towards him, stopping about 500 metres short of his front line. Both sides disposed their forces: the Scots straggled awkwardly over the ridge, their right flank hemmed in by the river Browney, and the English before an ancient marker – Neville's Cross. The opposing armies glared and yelled at each other whilst final adjustments were made to their ranks; then, with their lines complete, the Scots and English began walking towards each other – the determined prelude to the wild charge that would bring them together. But as they neared the ground which would very soon be filled with the bloody mangle of battle, an extraordinary sight interrupted their closing advance. The soldiers on the cathedral side of the ridge saw one, then several tonsured heads rising up the hill from the Wear. Soon everyone could share in the spectacle: a band of monks, making their way towards the two massed ranks of men-at-arms, carrying the holy cloth of St Cuthbert on a spear, just as it had been carried above Thurstan's army two centuries earlier. David decided to move forward before the monks got in his way. As the Scots stampeded towards the English line, the Durham monks dropped to their knees in prayer. Their brothers, meanwhile, had just ascended the western towers of the cathedral, where they would have a grand-stand view of the terrible drama about to unfold.

Down by the Browney River, the Scots struggled over hedges and marshy ground, leaving them all the more vulnerable to the English arrows that fell like rain from the sky above. On higher ground things were going better: David pressed into the English line while Robert Stewart fought hard on the eastern flank, nearest the cathedral. The Scots bravely held their own until Neville brought forward the small squadron of cavalry that had, for the first hour of the battle, been stomping the soil behind the English lines. The charging knights separated King David from Stewart, splitting the Scots' main formation in two. Stewart fled the confusion, just escaping the English knights, who had wheeled round to attack his ward from the rear.

In a losing battle, the king's heir had good incentive to flee. David stuck his ground, however, despite being struck by an arrow through his nose. Yet no amount of bravery could save him now. Just as his commanders deserted him and his men gave way, the English were receiving reinforcements: Lucy's reserve of priests and thugs, who had marched the better part of a day, now arrived on the scene. They quickly took the places of exhausted Durham men, whom Neville was still leading against what remained of King David's line. Only the day before, these replacements had been reminded of Thurstan's holy standard; now they saw Cuthbert's holy cloth for themselves, held aloft by the Durham monks who still knelt in prayer by the side of the battlefield. On the western towers of the cathedral the spectator monks saw that more English had come and burst into song. Legend has it that even amid the clattering swords, shouts of action and yells of dying men, their *Te Deum* could be heard on the battle-ridge, spurring the Northerners on to finish the job. So Lucy's reserve joined the fray, as did Percy's Northumberland men and Rokeby's troops, both now released from their respective flanks on the west and the east. The balance of the battle was now irrevocably tipped. Those Scots still standing turned and fled the field, followed by jubilant Englishmen keen to get their hands on a noble prisoner. In that afternoon at Neville's Cross, more than fifty Scots nobles, the greater part of Scotland's governing class, were killed or captured. It was a most terrible defeat.

As the light faded, the monks returned to the priory with their miraculous shroud, which had (at least for now) protected them from financial ruin. Survivors rifled through the remains of the fallen, whilst prisoners were led away. Among them was King David, found hiding in the River Browney, under a bridge, by a Northumbrian yeoman named John Copeland. (Pugnacious to the last, David knocked out two of Copeland's front teeth in a final effort to avoid capture.) William Douglas, too, had been apprehended, seized while trying to escape back north. It was left to Henry Percy to find safe captivity for this prize prisoner. The best he could do was to haul him off to Tynemouth Priory, arriving well after dark, where Henry was assured a good welcome: the Percys had given generously to the monastery and Prior Thomas was Henry's confessor. Greeting the weary band in person, Thomas de la Mare cut a handsome figure against Douglas's gashed, muddy and exhausted frame. Prior Thomas took them all inside, where a table had been prepared. Two days earlier the Scot had ordered de la Mare to have breakfast ready for him: Douglas was a little late but the prior delighted in serving the vanquished Scot nonetheless, telling him that he could not have come in more desirable a manner. Douglas could be forgiven for his grudging response, for how the Englishman's sarcasm must have stuck in the proud Scot's throat.

Victorious, the bulk of Zouche's army turned south towards home, leaving behind them the wild borderlands of the North, whose inhabitants were now inured to the violence of frontier life. It was not long before they were in more peaceful climes, through lowland villages surrounded by recently harvested fields and over hills and moors where sheep were reared for wool and meat. One or two of the army's number may well have split *en route* to Beverley and returned home to Wharram Percy, whose owner (or 'lord') was a cousin of Henry Percy. Subsequently deserted, the site of Wharram Percy has retained valuable evidence about how the vast majority of fourteenth-century English men and women lived.

There was nothing remarkable about Wharram Percy: it is all the more important, therefore, for it was in many ways typical of the thousands of villages that spread across England's countryside, within and around which over 90 per cent of England's population lived. Wharram sat on the rising left bank of a brook that meandered, eventually, into the River Derwent. The stream's small valley cut through flat, open farmland, which was divided into strips worked through the year by the villagers. It was a functional, unmanicured sight. A street ran parallel with the brook, with peasant cottages on either side, number-ing perhaps forty in all; some had a garden, a few had small barns, most had some chickens and geese. At either end of the street were the twin symbols of authority within the community: the church and vicarage to the south, and the manor house and farm buildings to the north. The manor house, the church, the many peasant cottages: these were the components of almost every village in medieval England.

By 1346 there were between a hundred and two hundred people living in Wharram, some in families of five or more, some on their own. A few villagers lived in comparatively large buildings, with separate barns and maybe even a kitchen, whilst others made do with a single room. Most houses were longhouses built from a number of 'A' frame timber 'crucks' placed on stone footings. Walls were made of insulating wattle and daub; the roofs were thatched. Doors were sturdy (some even had locks) and the windows, even though they were not glazed, had shutters which could keep out the cold. Inside, the long-house was divided into three parts. A hall filled most of the space: here the family warmed themselves, cooked and ate around a central hearth where a fire burned, smoke wafting up into the rafters from which meat was hung, out of the way of any mice. Earthenware pots held dry stores; food was served on wooden plates with basic metal utensils. At one end of the hall, separated by a partition or perhaps a curtain, was where the family slept; at the other, there was a storage space which in winter accommodated livestock. During the coldest months of the year the family's animals were taken into the longhouse itself – not only to protect precious assets but to help heat the building. Nothing, not even warmth, was wasted. Rubbish, night soil and manure were collected daily and scattered as fertilizer on the fields nearby. This was not luxurious living, but neither was it especially uncom-fortable. There was warmth enough except on the most bitter of nights and when it was dark tallow candles provided a modicum of light. The men would pass the evenings drinking ale and playing dice, the women weaving clothes, and the children might spin a top. Almost without exception the longhouses were kept scrupulously clean, both inside and in the yard without. It was an unfurnished existence but one no more simple than that lived by a large part of the world's population today.

The church at Wharram Percy was built of stone and had, over the previous two hundred years, been extended beyond its Norman nave. It was a modest contribution to the many thousands of medieval parish churches that still survive, which today give such scant indication of the richness that once lay within. Candles illuminated mural-covered walls. A rood screen, brightly painted in gold, green and red, separated the nave from the chancel, where the stone altar was draped in coloured cloth and behind which stood a processional cross. Side altars, in the body of the church, were reserved for private devotion and the remembrance of the dead. It was in this vivid space that every villager, no matter who they were, marked the key moments of their life: baptism in the same font, marriage before the same altar and burial in the same graveyard.

If the church spoke of an equality before God, the manor house was evidence of a more obvious, temporal, hierarchy. There is little evidence of what this building looked like at Wharram, but far more is known about the manor house at Faccombe Netherton, a village in east Hampshire that, in most respects, differed little from Wharram Percy. At Faccombe a gatehouse gave entry to the manor house complex, with the main house at its centre. The walls of this building were built in flint; the roof was tiled and crowned with a decorated ridge, with miniature clay figures coming together in a hunting scene that rode the crest of the gable. Although the windows were shuttered and unglazed like those in Wharram, the walls inside were plastered and painted. Around the manor house lay the stables, bakehouse, separate kitchen, dovecote, vegetable garden and fishpond, all enclosed – with the manor house itself – within a boundary wall. As an assembly of buildings, it had much in common with a common peasant dwelling, with its cottage, yard and odd barn or two; only in the manor complex, everything was on a far grander scale. The same was true of the division and use of the manor house itself, which was in several respects analogous to the simple peasant longhouse. As in the longhouse, the inside space was arranged in three parts. There was a central hall, with a hearth, fire, benches and tables. Beyond was a two-storey 'solar', with a bed chamber reached by an internal stair. This was where the family slept, with a garderobe providing a lavatory which could be emptied for use on the land. Two thirds of the manor house, therefore, was arranged and used precisely as was the far simpler dwelling lived in by the peasant villager. It was at the storage end where the difference lay, for in this part, which in the peasant building doubled as a pen in which to keep livestock, was in the manor house used not for animals but the accommodation of servants. The very arrangement of the manor house, therefore, as with the peasant long-house, the church and the village itself, revealed much about the basic hierarchies of medieval society and the ties that bound its various elements together.

Both of these villages – Wharram Percy and Faccombe Netherton – were, in the bureaucratic lexicon of medieval clerks, called a 'manor': an agglomeration of land, normally surrounding a settlement, which was cultivated for the benefit of its owner, or 'lord'. The lord of the manor might be a minor noble (as at Wharram, where the lord since 1321 had been Eustachia Percy, a cousin of Henry Percy, and at Faccombe, which was the property of Oliver Punchardon, who was both lord of the manor and also the village rector), a great magnate, or possibly even the king. About a quarter of all the manors in England were in the possession of the church, the majority the ancient prop-erty of bishoprics and the older monastic foundations. The separate estates of the bishop and prior of Durham that constituted the greater part of the county palatine of Durham had been put together follow-ing the Norman Conquest. Some estates, such as that of Glastonbury Abbey in Somerset, were older still, accumulated in Saxon and even earlier times.

The seasons ordered the routine of the manor. The long wait of winter was brought to an end when 'the weather of nature with winter contends', in late March.[1] April showers loosened the hardened ground, allowing the winter-rested land to be prepared by the plough. Barley and oats were sown by broadcast, peas and beans painstakingly dibbled into the ground by hand. Children protected the seeds from birds, spending days in their parents' fields with a sling and a pile of stones. Early summer was for making hay, which would feed the animals through the cold winter months to come. Sheep were grazed on the fallow, their manure folded back into the earth later in the year. The back-breaking work of weeding the fields of ripening crop was continued through July, and everyone prayed for gentle rain and regular sunshine. August was spent reaping the wheat and rye that had been sown the previous autumn, September the crops planted in the spring – barley, oats and legumes. These were the most onerous months: reaping with scythe and sickle, threshing and winnowing, all crammed into the eight weeks of late summer. By October it was all over, and the ploughmen set to work, turning the fallow a final time in preparation for the sowing of winter wheat and rye, while women and children collected what nuts, berries and other fruits the woods still had to offer. Martinmas on 11th November was the traditional day for slaughtering pigs which, salted down, would provide meat through the cold days to come. Winter was endured rather than used to any advantage: as the preservation of heat was so important, villagers moved from their homes only when necessary. Besides, the ground was hard and there was little to be achieved in the fields. Even for the families huddled together (not to speak of the poor labourer or widow left on their own), this was a solitary time, broken only by the great celebration of Christmas. The first portent of spring came with February lambing and by the end of March the ploughmen were out in the fields again. The year had come full-circle, completing the cycle of growth, fruition and decay.

The agricultural and calendar years began on 25th March – Lady Day, which marked the angel Gabriel's Annunciation to Mary and normally corresponded with the final weeks of the great fast of Lent. Lady Day was, therefore, a potent symbol of new life. It was no coincidence that this should be so, for the church had long framed the liturgical year around the turn of the seasons, just as it dignified agricultural work as an expression of faith. The peasant was told that his labour was not just for food but for the better cultivation – actual and spiritual – of God's garden. This then was God-given work, an ideal in which, as the fourteenth-century poet William Langland would have it, 'men worked eagerly, each in his manner finding something useful to do.'[2] His was a sentiment derived in part from a common understanding of the correct ordering of society and the universe; it was also a reflection of a widespread belief in the redemptive value of work, a belief that was given its classic definition in the monastic Rule of St Benedict, which provided for a life lived by the best use of the hours of the day, employing every moment in fruitful endeavour. To this end, St Benedict's maxim that 'idleness is the enemy of the soul' was as applicable to the peasant as it was to the monk, both of whom laboured daily in the hope of salvation.

For many peasants, this simple notion was the means by which meaning could be found in a life of monotony and graft. Only the infant found temporary reprieve from this sentence. Children were expected to work from a young age, achieve self-sufficiency in their mid-teens and, if they reached adulthood, would be fortunate to live beyond their mid-forties. By this age, the peasant was old beyond his years – a leathery face, bent back and work-worn hands all proofs of the effort to subsist from year to year. A typical working man had to labour for at least two thirds of the year just to ensure that his family was fed. Much of the cash-generating surplus he made in the remaining third had to be reinvested in tools, used to honour debts, or paid over to his lord in dues or to the king in taxes. Work, therefore, was an exercise in survival, not occupation, in which the drudgery of hard labour was given meaning by the church, communal focus by its feast days, and purpose by the needs and very modest ambitions of the individual and his family.

A pair of villages along the River Wylye in the hills of west Wiltshire offer some suitable examples of peasant life. Peter Boket was a land-less labourer in Monkton Deverill, an ancient manor long held by Glastonbury Abbey. He was one of that half of all the villagers who had no land and relied upon the wages they got from hired work. Boket may have had to live with his parents, hardly able to make ends meet. He might just have earned sufficient income, with a little illicit brewing on the side, to afford a small cottage. His neighbours, the Peter family, were more fortunate. They were comparatively wealthy. Robert, Stephen, Agnes and Alice Peter all lived separately and each had at least fifteen acres to their name. Their father, John, who by 1346 was well into his sixties, had thirty acres, which made him one of the more well-off – and long-lived – villagers. At times he had grazed as many as a hundred sheep on the downs. It is likely that John Peter and most of his children lived in the more comfortable long-house that befitted their comparative wealth. Like Boket, John Peter supplemented his income by brewing ale for sale. Brewing was a common occupation, especially among widows. One such was Agnes

Panel, who lived nearby in Longbridge Deverill. Although she had lost her husband Robert in 1340, Agnes had taken on his thirty acres of land – a sizeable holding – which she would have had farmed by a son or son-in-law, or even by directly employed labour. As with many widows, it is likely that she kept a room in her old house, if indeed it was now occupied by relatives, through a formal retirement agreement.

All of these people – Peter Boket, the Peter family, Agnes Panel – held their lands and houses for life, paying rent in cash and in kind to Glastonbury Abbey, which was the lord of the Deverill manors. It was a relationship arising from their common status as 'villein' tenants – a derivation of the system of feudal landholding introduced by William the Conqueror – and was, in reality, an elevated form of serfdom. Typically, the lord would cultivate only a small area of his manor himself (his 'demesne'), the rest of the manor being tilled by the villein tenants. To hold a house and any amount of land, the villein was required to work a certain number of days a year on the lord's demesne – work that was defined by long-standing and hereditary custom and was therefore referred to as 'customary works' or *opera*.[i] The lord gave out the right to cultivate a small portion of land and in return for that he received the labour he needed to cultivate his demesne.

The theory was neat; inevitably the practice was more complex. For some time, many lords had found it preferable to sell tenants' customary works back to them for cash, in effect charging rent in money rather than labour. The practice was known as 'commutation'. John Peter had made a one-off payment to Glastonbury Abbey of 20s.[ii] in 1319 to be relieved of some of his autumn works, a privilege he retained through an additional annual payment of 2s.[iii] So the abbey, instead of having use of John's labour for a set number of days in the autumn, received a cash payment. Glastonbury would then pay for a hired labourer, like Peter Boket, to do the work in John Peter's place. John could use his extra time to cultivate his tenement more effectively, work for wages elsewhere or set up his own small business (in

---

[i] This being the origin of the word 'job', i.e. one 'work' (*unum opus*) written in the medieval accountant's shorthand as 'i.op', the 'p' being a Middle English long 'p', thus mutilated in English as 'jobbe'. The sense remains: 'I have a job to do' being directly task-related.

[ii] £1.00.

[iii] £0.10.

his case, brewing). Nonetheless, although John had bought the freedom to dispose of his time as he wished, he remained a villein of the abbey. Indeed, despite the gradual shift to cash rent, the vast majority of peasants – even those who were relatively well-off like John Peter and Agnes Panel – were bound in a feudal relationship of villeinage, whether they held land or not. From birth, they were the lord's property; only he could free them from that bond. The few peasants that did enjoy the privilege of holding land by free tenure, paying only rent and owing nothing in customary works, were known as 'freemen'. Their status had come about by historical accident: they were the heirs of peasants who had escaped the service of the first Norman lords after the Conquest. A small minority had bought their manumission since. There were few freemen in the Deverills or elsewhere in Wiltshire, or indeed over much of England. However, in East Anglia, freemen were more numerous and in Kent they may well have been in the majority.

All peasants, whether free or unfree, had feudal obligations – one of which was to attend the lord's court. This would usually be held after Easter and after Michaelmas, 29th September – the end of the financial year. In most manors, including Longbridge and Monkton, each was in fact two courts, sitting in one session: the halmoot, which dealt with land transactions, and a 'hundred' law court, which dealt with disputes, communal dues and feudal fines. Where the lord had a hall, as at Wharram and Faccombe, the court would assemble there; where there was none, as at Longbridge or Monkton, the village would meet in the nave of the church or simply in the open. In the Deverill villages, on the same day, courts would sit in the morning at Longbridge and in the afternoon at Monkton (or vice versa). A table would be erected, at which sat the abbey's bailiff, who represented its interests across a number of its manors. His responsibilities were legally binding and he was liable to imprisonment if his accounts failed their audit. With him was the reeve, a villein elected by his neighbours to help plan crop rotations and oversee labourers on the abbey's demesne. The reeve was remitted part or all of his customary works in return for his service but he was personally liable for any shortfall in the manorial accounts. A certain John Cutel held this important position at Longbridge in 1346, as he had done with only one year's interruption since 1330. (In Monkton, John Peter had been reeve between 1330 and 1336, and it was in this term of office that his sons bought their land, a fact that leads one to suspect that, like Chaucer's Reeve Oswald, he was not beyond getting one over the bailiff!) With the reeve were his assistants, the hayward (who oversaw sowing and meadows) and the woodward (responsible for the maintenance and protection of woodland). Sitting together, the officers would hear presentations from villagers, take pledges on behalf of newcomers or visitors and refer disputes to juries of villein men for judgement. Even capital crimes such as theft and robbery would be heard first in the hundred court, where usually the offender would be ordered to be detained and then sent for trial at the next session of the King's Bench. Thus, the manorial court was much more than a chance to see village affairs aired in public: it was where the first appeal to justice could be made, the only means by which property could be conveyed, and the sole forum where the seasonal planting strategy was discussed.

This last function was crucial. The good management of land was key to the success of the manor, for villein and lord alike. The distribution of land itself was, therefore, of great importance. Where arable farming predominated, as it did in much of central, southern and eastern England, strips of land, each measuring an acre, were divided into rows. Each strip was held by a freeman, by the lord, or by one of his tenants. Individuals tended not to hold a number of strips as a block: there was a deliberate policy to scatter holdings, no matter who held the land. This arrangement not only ensured that the good land was shared around fairly but, importantly, it facilitated the three-field crop rotation system that was, by the fourteenth century, usual in areas of intensive agriculture. Strips would be organized into common fields, each field being treated as a single unit of cultivation, which would be left fallow for one year out of every three. Through the organized rotation of these dispersed landholdings, there was a more efficient use of the plough, a more consistent sowing of seed and a better concentration of labour at harvest time.

The three-field system was just one of many innovations adopted by lords and their tenants in their joint effort to increase the productivity and profitability of the land. It was an endeavour that had brought considerable wealth to Glastonbury Abbey. Indeed, in these very years, the abbot was building a new kitchen in the monastery precinct, with four huge fireplaces to cook the food required by the abbey community and its many guests. Every brick of this new building was in part paid for by the villein tenants of Longbridge and Monkton, just as their ancestors had contributed to the construction of the great abbey church itself. It was through the labours of countless men and women like these – whether in lowland arable manors or upland pastoral estates – that the wealth was generated to pay for the Punchardon manor house at Faccombe, the Percy church at Wharram, the treasures of the Border abbeys, and the gold of Durham Cathedral, over which the Scots had recently cast so avaricious an eye. The persistence of feudalism in all these places was evidence of the solidity of medieval lordship, yet this appearance of ancient stability belied ever-present change. For the neat hierarchy and ordered economy of Anglo-Norman feudalism had to respond to the powerful forces – natural, chaotic and human – that acted upon it. Some were exogenous, like the weather and disease; others – the most potent – were the consequence of men and women living together in community: conflict, population growth, the challenge of subsistence, and the irrepressible desire of the individual to improve his life.

Thus, far from being static and immobile, feudal England was in fact vital and dynamic. Although the great buildings of Glastonbury and Durham spoke of continuity, the manors that funded them had changed beyond all recognition since the Norman Conquest that had brought feudalism to England 280 years earlier. The great paradox of late-medieval feudalism was, therefore, that in spite of its inherent conservatism, it was forced to accommodate, and indeed contribute to, the constant evolution of the very society it sought to contain and control. Nor did this amount only to imperceptible changes. Major innovations such as three-field crop rotation were the result of the conscious effort of villeins, manorial managers and their lords to improve their livelihood. For whilst medieval people were intensely conscious of those things that they could not change, they were not without the simple human ambition to better themselves. The cumulative effect of these many modest aspirations was transformative. For people like the Peters, Agnes Panel and Peter Boket, the motivation to improve their lot reinterpreted, slowly but very surely, the daily challenge of survival and increase. In so doing, it changed the world in which they lived.

*   *   *

The peasants of Durham must have been cheered by the news of Zouche's victory at Neville's Cross, for the victory promised a respite from the frequent raids with which they had to contend. Beyond the hardy border region, however – in Wharram, Faccombe, the Deverills and across the rest of England – the news, if it was heard at all, can have excited little interest. The Scots wars meant almost nothing to these villagers; as they stored away what they had made from the lean harvest of 1346, they were more likely concerned with the prospect of a winter of want. None of them were to know, however, that far, far away, another battle had just taken place, which would soon make its outcome felt in every part of England, from the fields of Durham to the lee of the West Wiltshire Downs.

In Caffa,[iv] a port in the eastern corner of the Crimea, the third siege in as many years had come to an unexpected end. Caffa was a colony of the Italian city-state of Genoa and the origin of the furs, slaves and grain merchants brought to markets in the Middle East and European West. Most of these commodities came from the southern Russian steppes, via trading agents at Tana[v] on the mouth of the River Don. From here small ships followed the eastern coast of the Sea of Azov to the isthmus which gave entry to the Black Sea, before making their way west to Caffa where the goods were moved to larger vessels for distribution around the Mediterranean. It was a tiny European encampment in a great Mongol plain: this was the land of the Kipchak Khanate, which for a century had been the westernmost extension of the now fractured empire once built by Jinghiz Khan. The population, largely Turkic and Mongol, was mainly nomadic; indeed, it was the golden tents of the khans which earned their territory the name of the Golden Horde. The Venetians and Genoese, Marco Polo among them, had traded with the Kipchak khans almost since their arrival on the Steppes, a tradition that continued during the reign of the great khan Özbeg, who established Islam across this swathe of central Asia. However, Özbeg's son, Janibeg, took a less indulgent attitude towards his Genoese guests. In 1343 he ejected the Europeans from Tana following a street brawl and chased the refugees back to Caffa, where he laid siege. He abandoned and

---

[iv] Modern-day Feodosiya.
[v] Modern-day Azov.

picked up the siege twice more but his efforts were largely ineffective, since the port could be strongly defended on land whilst still being supplied from the sea. It was by now a small city, where two concentric walls enclosed more than a thousand houses. By the time of Janibeg's third attempt in 1346, the Genoese had mounted a blockade of the isthmus, ensuring that no trade whatsoever could pass back to the Khanate. Thus the besiegers had become the besieged and Janibeg's attempt to trade without foreign intermediaries seemed to be doomed.

The khan must have hoped that attrition would, in the end, win him the day. Yet suddenly his men, stationed behind the palisades he had erected around Caffa's walls, dropped – one by one – dead. The doctors could do nothing. A soldier would find a swelling in his groin or armpit, quickly succumb to fever and, just as soon as these symptoms appeared, die. Janibeg was stupefied. Within weeks he had lost most of his army. Unable to continue the siege of Caffa, he made one last gamble. The Mongols were using siege engines in their attempts to break into the city, just as Edward III was doing several thousand miles away in Calais. The most potent of these was a trebuchet, a great wooden arm placed over a pivot, weighted at one end, with a scoop lashed to the ground at the other. Huge rocks could be placed into the scoop, the arm released and the rock thus launched at the city walls. Janibeg moved the trebuchets a little closer, substituted the rotting corpses of his dead men for the rocks and lobbed them over the walls and into the streets and market places of Caffa. The Genoese rushed to throw the bodies into the sea but the relentless barrage from Janibeg's siege engines made it impossible to avoid the stench of death that now poisoned the air. The khan's desperate strategy worked: the Genoese quickly started dropping just as their Mongol assailants had done. Whatever caused such sudden death seemed to pass from one person to the next, from neighbourhood to neighbourhood, as if by the terrified glances of men and women. As Janibeg had found that he no longer had an army to besiege Caffa, the Genoese soon lacked a garrison to defend it. Realising they had so few left to defend, the survivors made for the harbour, where Genoese boats were landing their crucial supplies. They scrambled aboard and fled, leaving behind them streets strewn with the corpses of Mongols and Europeans alike. With a macabre army of the dead, Janibeg had finally taken what he could not capture with the living.

The fleeing ships crossed the Black Sea and many put in at Pera, the Genoese colony on the Bosphorus. Across the Golden Horn was Constantinople, now no more than a collection of ruins – the tiny rump of the once great Byzantine empire. The city had just emerged from one of its regular bouts of civil war, in which the boy-emperor John V Palaiologus had been supplanted by the courtier John Kantakouzenos, who had been crowned John VI. Kantakouzenos had succeeded only with the support of the Ottoman bey, Orhan I, to whom Kantakouzenos had given his daughter in marriage. As Orhan had conquered what remained of Byzantine Anatolia in the preceding decades, it was judged by Christian contemporaries to have been a shameful pact.

The threat to Constantinople in 1347, however, came neither from the Turks, nor from internal feuding, but from a hitherto unknown enemy. Across the water in Pera, the Genoese had brought whatever had killed their comrades in Caffa to the shores of the Golden Horn. An epidemic broke out amongst the Genoese of Pera; by July it had crossed the short stretch of water to Constantinople. Writing a few years later, John VI Kantakouzenos recalled that this 'plague', as he called it, had come from the southern Russian Steppe.[vi] 'So incurable was the evil', Kantakouzenos continued, that nothing could resist it. The symptoms were horrifying. Some suffered a terrible fever, which rendered the victim senseless and speechless until death. In others the lungs were affected: 'Sputum suffused with blood was brought up and disgusting and stinking breath from within. The throat and tongue, parched from the heat, were black and congested with blood.' On others 'great abscesses were formed on the legs or the arms, from which when cut, a large quantity of foul-smelling pus flowed.' Other symptoms appeared also: 'some people broke out with black spots all over their bodies.' What did not vary was the promise of death, as Kantakouzenos dryly reported: 'everyone died the same from these symptoms.' 'There was no hope from anywhere', nothing that doctors could do to bring relief to the afflicted. Indeed, trying to

[vi] John Kantakouzenos abdicated in 1355 and retired to a monastery, where he wrote a history of the Byzantine Empire from 1320 to 1356, in which the following account is included.

give assistance was often counter-productive: hinting at how death
was passed from one person to the next, John lamented that 'some
by treating others, became infected with the disease'.[3]

The epidemic gripped Constantinople just as it had taken hold at
Caffa and at Pera. It defied explanation. Kantakouzenos gave up his
description of the 'plague', concluding that 'no words could express
the nature of the disease. All that can be pointed out is that it had
nothing in common with the everyday evils to which the nature of
man is subject.' It was beyond the 'normal' and by implication, therefore, divine. This was the natural conclusion to which a Christian
commentator should arrive, since plague was a recurrent punishment
in the Old Testament. God had inflicted Ten Plagues on the Egyp-
tians,[vii] the fifth being a murrain of cattle, the sixth a plague of boils,
and the last being the slaying of every firstborn Egyptian and their
cattle.[4] The Old Testament God did not reserve plague for Israel's
enemies, however. King David, in his hubris, undertook a census of
the tribes of Israel, counting on the force he had to hand rather than
relying on the power of God. Angered, God gave David a choice of
punishments: seven years of famine, three months of pursuit by his
enemies or three days pestilence. David submitted himself to God's
mercy rather than fall into the hands of his enemies, whose mercies
were less certain. God proceeded to inflict pestilence, an expression
of His absolute and unconstrained power.[5] It was in this tradition that
St John freely adapted the plagues of Egypt into the seven plagues of
the Apocalypse, poured from vials onto the world to bring humanity
to repentance.[6] The end-time was presaged by the arrival of the Four
Horsemen of the Apocalypse, representing Victory, War, Famine and
Death. This last Horseman, Death, rode a pallid horse which was
commonly understood to signify pestilence.[7]

For Byzantine Christians eager to find a cause for their suffering,
there was thus much biblical evidence of God's use of plague to
chastise His enemies, punish His chosen people for their errors and

---

[vii] The Ten Plagues being 1. Blood; 2. Frogs; 3. Lice; 4. Flies; 5. Murrain of Cattle; 6.
Boils; 7. Hail; 8. Locusts; 9. Darkness; 10. Death of First Born. Later, the Ark of the
Covenant, which held the Ten Commandments given down to the Israelites after
their exodus from Egypt, brought plague to the Philistines after they carried it off
following their victory over Israel at Ebenezer-Aphek, inflicting 'very great destruction' to the Philistine cities of Ashdod, Gath and Ekron, killing 'small and great' alike.

– ominously – inaugurate the end of the world.[viii] There was also a historical precedent which was easily recalled. Eight hundred years earlier, in happier times, Constantinople had been the centre of an empire that stretched from Italy to the Levant, ruled by its greatest ever emperor, Justinian. In 542 the city had been struck by a great epidemic that killed many thousands and then spread around its Mediterranean dominions to kill countless more. Given the travesty of his own rule, any mention of the Justinian era was too dangerous for John VI Kantakouzenos. He chose, therefore, to refer in his account to an even earlier epidemic, that of Athens, in 429 BC, described by Thucydides in his history of the Peloponnesian wars. Although Kantakouzenos apes some of the Greek's language (and flatters himself in his implicit parallel with Pericles: they both lost their sons in the respective epidemics), the classical references are merely tangential. This is the account of a Christian man and a Christian commentator. Kantakouzenos, one of the first in Europe to witness this terrible new disease, arrived at the only explanation that was open to him: this plague was a punishment from God and was a reason to be fearful of His Judgement. It was a conclusion that would be repeated, across the Christian world, innumerable times in the years to come.

[viii] This final apocalyptic vision will have had a special relevance for the citizens of Constantinople. The Book of the Apocalypse is addressed to seven churches, amongst them the church of Smyrna (modern-day İzmir). In this, the angel sent to the church of Smyrna (Rev. 2:8–11) proclaimed 'I know thy works, and tribulation, and poverty, . . .' (Rev. 2:9). Later in the revelation, plague arrives. To Byzantine Christians, the striking immediacy of this statement will have been clear: Smyrna, an ancient western Anatolian city, had long been reduced to ruin, largely in the course of its frequent change of hands between Byzantines and Turks. The Ottoman Turks had recently been ejected but the Christians' hold on the city was precarious. In the light of the problems at Smyrna and the coming of the epidemic to Constantinople, there must have been an added piquancy to St John's eschatological vaticinations.

2

The Fruits of Peace

August 1347–June 1348

Dim moon-eyed fishes near
Gaze at the gilded gear
And query: 'What does this vaingloriousness down here?' . . .

Well: while was fashioning
This creature of cleaving wing,
The Immanent Will that stirs and urges everything

Prepared a sinister mate
Thomas Hardy, 'The Convergence of the Twain'[1]

Some years after the Scots' defeat at Neville's Cross, the English court poet Laurence Minot claimed that David II had boasted as he set out on his campaign that he would 'ride through all England' in order that 'at the Westminster Hall should his steeds stand, whilst our king Edward made war out of the land'.[2] After recuperating from his injuries at Bamburgh Castle, tended by physicians sent from York, David had indeed travelled south: not in triumph but under heavy guard and the watchful eye of Edward's queen, Philippa of Hainault, who had been in York at the time of the battle and had helped rouse the troops. She now accompanied her royal charge back to London, from where she sailed for Calais, joining her husband for Christmas in the makeshift royal palace that had been built under the walls of the besieged town.[3] As the people of Calais shivered and starved within, the English without toasted their triumphs, and those they hoped to come. David, meanwhile, was incarcerated in the Tower of London with all the other prisoners captured after the battle.[i] On 6th January 1347 the Scots king was led through the capital on a large black charger, displayed as a trophy of war to the finely liveried city worthies and guild grandees who lined the streets. To one who had hoped to ride his horse into Westminster Hall, this was more than a great humiliation. The Scots had been told to expect no resistance other than 'shepherds' with 'staves'; instead they had lost a battle in which many of their great barons had been either captured or killed, leaving the way clear for Edward Balliol to claim a throne left vacant by an imprisoned king.

Londoners were treated to yet more good news on the return of Henry of Grosmont, earl of Lancaster, fresh from a remarkable armed dash through south-west France.[4] The earl had taken Bergerac, recovered much of Périgord and the Agenais, freed the warrior Sir Walter Manny and his party from captivity in St Jean-d'Angély and then stormed the city of Poitiers. In under two years Lancaster had recovered every inch of territory that England had lost to France in the war. Having rested in London at his palace of the Savoy, the earl joined the king in early summer outside Calais, which was still stubbornly holding out in the hope of being saved by Philip VI. In vain the burghers of Calais implored the French king for deliverance: they had been reduced to eating the town's dogs and cats. Philip, despite their pleas, turned his back on Calais and hurried back to Paris: the risk of taking on Edward's huge army was just too great. Failed by their king, the brave townsmen had no alternative but to submit themselves to the mercy of the English monarch. Angered at having to wait a full seven months for this submission, Edward was far from inclined to leniency and ordered the execution of the six leading burghers, who had presented themselves with the town's keys. Sir Walter Manny implored the king to show clemency but Edward was unmoved. It was only when Queen Philippa made her famous intercession, weeping before the king on her knees, appealing in the name of his love for her to spare the lives of the six burghers, that, after a long silence, Edward agreed.[ii] It was either a genuine change of heart or a brilliantly

---

[i] The earls of Fife and Menteith, who had previously sworn allegiance to Edward, were executed.
[ii] On Saturday, 4th August 1347.

conceived piece of chivalric theatre. The king's intention was not the issue, however, for the message was all: Edward was a monarch terrible in war but just in peace.

Staying only to sign a truce with the French,[iii] Edward returned home as soon as he was able, arriving in Sandwich on 12th October 1347. Two days later he was in London, where he was received by enthusiastic crowds. It was the first time since the beginning of the war, in 1337, that Edward had been able to return from France with the victor's laurels. Better still, he returned to a realm that had been ably managed in his absence, even though he had been abroad from England for nearly sixteen months.[iv] Although it was not this feat that the crowds cheered, it must nonetheless have been of great satisfaction to the king. His exploits abroad had previously been hampered by difficulties at home, forcing him on one occasion to make a premature return: in late 1340, Edward had had to rush back to London from Flanders on reports of maladministration by his ministers in his absence. His over-reaction (five royal judges and two leading merchants – including the great London draper John Pulteney – were arrested, while the archbishop of Canterbury and chancellor, John Stratford, was dismissed amid an exchange of insults not seen between monarch and primate since the days of Thomas Becket) precipitated a near revolt, which was settled only when Edward made peace with his opponents. Not yet thirty, Edward had demonstrated his political acumen and an ability to attract support even in a crisis of his own making, qualities that his father, Edward II, had never possessed. It had been a dangerous moment for the young king, one that he was determined to ensure would never happen again.

Following the crisis of 1340–41, Edward had taken care to mould a new administration that was more suited to his foreign ambitions. For he now claimed the French throne itself, a pretension that possessed neither his father, nor his grandfather Edward I, nor his great-grandfather Henry III – nor even Henry II, who had ruled more of France than any English monarch before or since. For Edward, the claim to the title may always have been a bargaining chip; the claim to territory, however, was non-negotiable. The pursuit of this

---

[iii] Mid-September 1347.
[iv] 28th June 1346–12th October 1347.

tremendous enterprise required not only the king's extended absence from England but the expenditure of truly extraordinary sums. The total cost of the three years of the war to 1340 had been £500,000, far in advance of the king's annual income, the difference largely being made up with loans from Italian bankers. Edward came to understand that the necessary precondition of victory on the field of battle was an administration that could both keep the peace at home and raise the revenues to fund his exploits abroad. That he was able to return in 1347 to a nation well-governed and peaceful was confirmation of his success.

Like Henry II and Henry I before him, Edward had turned to capable men who relied solely on him for their promotion. Foremost among them were two clerics: John Ufford[v] and William Edington. Ufford was a career diplomat who, as Keeper of the Privy Seal, had already been entrusted with the king's private instructions and correspondence after the debacle of 1340–41. In 1345, having proved himself to be both biddable and reliable, Ufford had been made chancellor, the chief of the king's ministers. William Edington, whose modest Wiltshire background did not prevent him from rising fast through the crown service, showed an early appetite for difficult jobs – notably responsibility for the hugely unpopular tax of the 'ninth',[vi] levied by parliament in 1341 to pay for the war. In the same year he was appointed Keeper of the King's Wardrobe, which gave him responsibility for expenditure on the king's campaigns. Very quickly Edington showed a prodigious ability as both accountant and administrator: budgeting was introduced and as a consequence the costs of war started to fall. Edward made him treasurer in 1344, the second most important ministerial post after the chancellorship, with overall responsibility for the finances of royal government. Edington immediately set about reforming his department. Thus, when Edward sailed for France in the summer of 1346, he entrusted England to a rejuvenated administration, staffed by loyal and able civil servants, who could be relied upon to provide both the money and the security that he needed in order to wage war on Europe's

[v] Probably born in Ufford in Cambridgeshire. His name is often rendered as 'Offord'.
[vi] Because it was for a payment of a ninth of all produce, which could be paid – unusually – in kind.

most powerful monarch. This careful preparation of his regent government ensured that when Edward arrived in London on 14th October 1347, he could immediately turn to celebrating his victories in an untroubled and appreciative realm.

The royal family enjoyed an extravagant Christmas in Guildford, so much different from the camping Christmas they endured the previous year in Calais. The celebrations, with great feasts and masked plays, were in large part public affairs. Display was a crucial element of the exercise of kingship, a fact that Edward knew well: it was a necessary part of the creation and confirmation of regalian power, vital in times of turmoil as much as in moments of victory. During the crisis of 1340–41, for example, Edward had performed – in a time-honoured affirmation of kingship – 355 ritual healings for scrofula; now, in the afterglow of triumphs in Normandy, Poitou, Scotland and also Brittany, he promised his subjects a season of festivities and tournaments the like of which had never been seen before. The Christmas extravaganza was merely the prelude: nineteen tournaments were to take place before May 1348 alone, the majority in Westminster but many in provincial towns and cities such as Reading, Bury St Edmunds, Lichfield and Berwick. These jousts between mounted knights competing for the favour of noblewomen spectators were more than chivalric charades. As stylized re-enactments of feats achieved on foreign fields, tournaments afforded a wide audience the opportunity of seeing the king and his barons in action. For added realism, the king's prisoners – the Count of Eu, Constable of France, Charles of Blois, captured in Brittany, and David II – also attended as honoured 'guests'. It was a show, a vehicle and a celebration; but, crucially, it was also a mechanism to retain the enthusiastic loyalty of his fighting captains, the *esprit de corps* that would otherwise evaporate in the anti-climax of a return to wet and windy England.

Edward's tournaments gave his noble warriors the chance to display their booty, newly won from France. Their wives and mistresses were also there, wearing the latest fashions, some of which, not long before, had been hanging in the closets of French noble families. It was only recently that tailors and dressmakers had started cutting cloth on the bias, hugely extending what they could do for their well-dressed customers. The short 'cote-hardie' was now all the rage – a fitted sleeved tunic running from just above the knee, tightly buttoned and with streamers hanging from the cuffs. Tight clothes encouraged greater exposure: for the first time in centuries, women's hair was now uncovered, bound in gold fretwork buns to leave the neck naked. Inevitably, the new style drew criticism from censorious quarters – one Westminster monk, John of Reading, described with a degree of mock-horror how some noblewomen wore clothes 'that were so tight that they wore a fox tail hanging down inside their skirts at the back, to hide their arses'.[5] John would have been far more shocked with the goings-on behind the tournament stands. About thirty years later, the Leicester canon Henry Knighton related how a troop of forty damsels, dressed in men's clothes, attended these tournaments. They were, apparently, all 'very eye-catching and beautiful', with daggers (in a none-too-subtle priapic suggestion) slung low across their hips. Thus, 'with disgraceful lasciviousness', they 'encouraged the relaxation of matrimonial restraint'.[6] John of Reading thought this exhibitionism would 'surely bring down misfortune in the future',[7] although Knighton claimed that God's remedy was more immediate – casting storms over the tournaments. It must have been punishment enough for Edward's French prisoners, forced to traipse around England on this rain-lashed chivalric circus, obliged to look as if they were having fun. No doubt they too bridled at the unabashed vulgarity of the English, who flaunted their ill-worn loot in celebration of conquest. It was not an attractive sight and, to the shrewd observer, it may well have betrayed the evanescence of Edward's success.

The celebrations did not distract Edward from his most pressing concern: to secure a new grant of taxation from parliament. The Lords and Commons were summoned to Westminster, meeting through January and February 1348, and reconvening for another month in April. Edward received due praise for his victories and in return sought to flatter his audience by consulting them on the terms of the truce he had made with France. Sweet victories did not make the costs of war any less bitter, however, and the Commons politely refused the opportunity to offer their opinion. These were, after all, the first tangible fruits of fully ten years of war taxation. Many were not only irritated with the bill but resentful at the continuing disputes that accompanied the crown's collection of revenue. The Commons, made up of county gentry and city burghers, complained at the forced loan of 20,000 sacks of wool imposed the previous year and at the ongoing malpractice of the king's purveyors, who purchased supplies, by compulsion, on behalf of the crown. Finally, the Commons returned to a previous charge, all the more pressing for its closeness to home, that the crown was proving impotent in the face of increasing disorder and lawlessness in the shires.

The king and his ministers were well aware of this last problem. In Worcester, for example, William Carter and his two sons William and John led a criminal gang that successfully thumbed their noses at royal authority, in large part because of the complicity of local officials. In 1345 the gang assaulted a royal justice and his servants. The next year the two sons were indicted for stealing from Robert Rivers at Little Malvern a horse worth 1 mark, two robes worth 2 marks, 60s. in cash, a harness worth 20s. and a seal, a girdle and a pouch, worth together 40s.[vii] This was a significant haul – a considerable amount even for a rich man and beyond the dreams of a common labourer. The king's justices made no headway against them: the thieves, they said, were being protected by local people, who had rioted and thus prevented them holding their sessions.

Cases like these were currently tried by justices employed by the crown, making their rounds, county by county. In parliament, landowners claimed that they would be better equipped to deal, in the first instance at least, with these criminal investigations: the crown justices had no local knowledge and only came irregularly, the Commons argued; not so the landowners, who were local and had their ear to the ground. Moreover, the Commons averred that the royal judges were corrupt, unlike the local gentry, who had an interest in seeing that lawlessness was punished. The king was nonetheless extremely reluctant to hand even limited judicial powers to landowners: the revenues of justice were useful to a monarch with pressing financial needs; the display of royal power was inherent in the distribution of justice; and in providing justice to the wronged and aggrieved, the king honoured his duty to uphold the law and judge with fairness – all of which he had promised in his coronation oath.[viii] Through his anointing, the king became God's coadjutor in

---

[vii] i.e. a horse worth £0.67 (a mark being equal to two thirds of a pound sterling, or 13s. 4d.), two robes worth £1.33, £3.00 in cash, a harness worth £1.00 and a seal, girdle and pouch valued in total at £2.00.

[viii] The form of the coronation oath imposed on Edward II in 1308 which became the basis of the oath used since.

the earthly realm. Thus, just as the prosecution of war and regalian display were central to Edward's kingship, so too was the distribution of justice. Any devolution of these judicial powers would be an inappropriate encroachment on his royal authority. Edward did not in fact consider the situation serious enough to merit action, so he made bland promises to rein in his purveyors and improve the performance of his judges. Doubtless less than satisfied, parliament had little more they could say. So, with rumours reaching Westminster that French officials were assessing towns and villages across France for infantry service in anticipation of an invasion attempt in the summer,[ix] parliament reluctantly granted Edward a subsidy to be collected each year for the next three years.[x] It was a holding compromise: both king and parliament fully expected that events would force the reopening of discussions on tax and local justice.

With the business of parliamentary consent out of the way, Edward was free to return to jousting. In May, Philippa bore Edward a sixth son, William of Windsor, and the following month the entire royal family was brought together for a lavish tournament to celebrate this birth – all except the fourteen-year-old Princess Joan, who, in a concordat negotiated by Henry of Lancaster and the chancellor, John Ufford, with Alfonso XI of Castile, had been promised as bride to the infante Pedro. Alfonso's ambassadors had arrived in England in April to complete the deal and the young princess had already departed (with Ufford's brother, Andrew, and the former chancellor, Robert Bourchier) for Castile by early June.[xi] The journey, which would take

---

[ix] Indeed, the chronicler Robert of Avesbury claims that a French invasion 'plan' was read out in parliament. If so, it clearly demonstrated the lengths to which Edward was prepared to go in order to secure taxation and parliamentary approbation for his expeditions abroad.

[x] An annual tax (for the duration of the grant – in this case three years) equivalent to the value of a tenth (10 per cent) of all movable goods from eligible taxpayers in the boroughs and a fifteenth (6.66 per cent) of all movable goods from eligible taxpayers in the countryside. Each subsidy required the assent of parliament, although since 1332 the format of the tax – a tenth and fifteenth – rarely varied. Similarly, the actual tax assessment continued to be based on a survey of taxable communities carried out in 1334, whereby each town or village had a fixed tax liability and it was left to each community to work out how they raised that amount. The clergy largely paid subsidies of a tenth (10 per cent).

[xi] See Ch. 3, n. 7.

her down the western French seaboard to the shores of north Spain, carried no more than the usual degree of risk, or at least that is what Edward thought. For although news of a mysterious disease was coming back from France, for which reason the kings had only just agreed an extension to their truce, Joan's party would be many leagues from the cities of Provence, from where the latest word of the strange epidemic had come. There was no reason, therefore, for Edward to doubt the safety of his precious daughter.

Joan's anticipated marriage brought another of Edward's long-conceived plans – a pact with Castile – close to fruition. Another was the king's royal chapel of St Stephen in Westminster, where the scaffolding was coming down at last. Begun by Edward I in 1292 in imitation and rivalry of St Louis's magnificent Sainte-Chapelle in Paris, construction had been brought to a halt when he embarked upon a (failed) invasion of France five years later. Now Edward III had both finished the chapel and exceeded his grandfather's achievements in France, another boy had been added to his large family and his daughter's betrothal had sealed a Castilian alliance. The completion of St Stephen's Chapel in more ways than one marked the fulfilment of a Plantagenet dream.

High on celebration, Edward may have been persuaded that his destiny was now set. Yet as the King jousted and danced, his nation's fortunes were being decided far away, in the Straits of Messina – that narrow stretch of water that separates the Scylla of Italy from the Charybdis of Sicily.

Much of Europe's trade with the East passed through the Straits of Messina. In the spring the ships sailed south, ready to turn eastwards to Constantinople and Cairo, to the fortified trading towns of the Black Sea and the great cities of the Levant. By late summer, the weight of traffic was heavier in the other direction. Ships' captains preferred, if possible, to make the full voyage within the extended summer months, which promised the calmer seas and clear skies that allowed navigation beyond sight of land. It was a long journey: over a thousand miles from Messina to Constantinople which, even if the winds were favourable, would take more than a month. For the larger, ocean-going, vessels, Messina was often the first port of call for some weeks. Here they would take on fresh water and replenish provisions, enough for the final leg of the journey back to Genoa and the Tuscan city-states.

In early October 1347, a number of Genoese vessels docked at Messina. The sailors were desperate: they brought news of the catastrophe that had befallen the Genoese at Caffa and of the epidemic that was raging in Constantinople. They had fled as soon as they could but several of their number had died nonetheless. Others were showing the early signs of the affliction; clearly they had contracted it from sailors already infected when they boarded at Constantinople. The disease incubated in the apparently healthy men for many weeks before the symptoms appeared, foretokens of their imminent deaths. The sick were carried onto land, where the healthy could not wait to tell of their miraculous escape. Soon, however, even those that had seemed well began to fall sick and then, not long after, so did those who had been their first contacts as they had rushed from the boat at the quay. As the Franciscan friar Michele da Piazza reported a few years later, it quickly became clear that the Genoese 'carried such a disease in their bodies that if anyone so much as spoke with one of them he was infected with the deadly illness and could not avoid death . . . The people of Messina, realising that the death racing through them was linked with the arrival of the Genoese galleys, expelled the Genoese from the city and harbour with all speed.'[8] It was to no avail. The illness soon spread through the town and caused panic. Some invoked the protection of the saints: one group attempted to bring the relics of St Agatha from further down the Sicilian coast, Catania, believing that in giving protection to that town they would bring respite to Messina. Others flocked to Catania for the same reason, hoping to escape homes now filled with the corpses of the dead. Those that made it (for many collapsed by the side of the road) found few who would put them up; the Catanians did not want to exchange their guardian relics for the dying refugees of Messina. So the Messinese dispersed, some across Sicily, others into mainland Calabria, all taking the disease with them wherever they went.

Meanwhile, delayed by autumn storms,[9] the expelled galleys arrived home at last, docking at Genoa as the Christmas festivities began.[10] Yet here again, those who at first welcomed the sailors home soon demanded their expulsion, for as soon as local people started falling ill the horrified townsmen ordered all returning ships to leave port.

Outlawed, the galleys moved west along the coast in search of a harbour where they could anchor. Meanwhile, the illness they had left behind spread rapidly in Genoa. This city was a central hub of European trade, where goods from the Orient were sent across the Continent, feeding the ever-expanding European appetite for luxuries from the East. It was only a matter of weeks, therefore, before the disease, which the Genoese still struggled to name, spread out to the other great cities that lay nearby. Gabriele de' Mussi, a notary of Piacenza, related how the epidemic unfolded with horrific inevitability: 'every city, every settlement, every place was poisoned by the contagious pestilence, and their inhabitants, both men and women, died suddenly. And when one person had contracted the illness, he poisoned his whole family even as he fell and died, so that those preparing to bury his body were seized by death in the same way. Thus death entered through the windows, and as cities and towns were depopulated their inhabitants mourned their dead neighbours.'[11]

The greatest city in the Italian north-west, the undisputed mercantile capital of Europe, was Florence – greater by far than Genoa and richer even than Venice. Over 90,000 people lived within its walls; an equal number clustered in the suburbs beyond. This urban leviathan sucked in food and drink: every year at least 4,000 oxen and calves, 60,000 sheep, 20,000 goats, 30,000 pigs and nearly 6,000,000 gallons of wine passed through its gates. Such enormous levels of consumption could only be paid for by enormous levels of wealth. The capital accumulated over several centuries of growing trade had been put to work leveraging further expansion. It had been Florentine merchant-bankers that had financed Edward III's early years of war with France, and it was a measure of the city's financial strength that it withstood Edward's default in 1345, when he reneged on loans to the Bardi and Peruzzi societies worth some £231,176. One of the Peruzzi shareholders was a merchant named Giovanni Villani. Already in his seventies by 1348, Villani watched with horror as the plague advanced from the coast towards Florence. He too had heard that the disease originated in the Orient and was aware that 'all who arrived at Genoa died . . .' The dead 'corrupted the air to such an extent that whoever came near the bodies died shortly thereafter . . . And many lands and cities were made desolate. And the plague lasted till . . .' and, with these words, his chronicle ends.[12] For by March 1348 the epidemic had reached

Florence, pulled inexorably towards the city by the very trade by which it survived, and Villani was one of its victims.

By now, the plague had been in northern Italy for three months, and to careful observers, like Gabriele de' Mussi, it was possible to discern a distinct pattern in the deaths:

> Those of both sexes who were in health, and in no fear of death, were struck by four savage blows to the flesh. First, out of the blue, a kind of chilly stiffness troubled their bodies. They felt a tingling sensation, as if they were being pricked by the points of arrows. The next stage was a fearsome attack which took the form of an extremely hard, solid boil. In some people this developed under the armpit and in others in the groin between the scrotum and the body. As it grew more solid, its burning heat caused the patients to fall into an acute and putrid fever, with severe headaches. As it intensified its extreme bitterness could have various effects. In some cases it gave rise to an intolerable stench. In others it brought vomiting of blood, or swellings near the place from which the corrupt humour arose: on the back, across the chest, near the thigh. Some people lay as if in a drunken stupor and could not be roused ... All these people were in danger of dying. Some people died on the very day illness took possession of them, others on the next day, others – the majority – between the third and fifth day.[13]

Other accounts of the symptoms – across Italy – agree with one another. Almost all conclude that the surest signs of death were what the great Florentine Giovanni Boccaccio described as 'dark blotches and bruises on [the] arms, thighs, and other parts of the body, sometimes large and few in number, at other times tiny and closely spaced'. Everywhere it was the same: a mildly uncomfortable sensation that might be mistaken for the beginnings of a cold, then the appearance of swellings in the inner thigh, armpit or throat which would soon sear with pain, sometimes a foul smell, the spread of dark blotches, fever, the vomiting and passing of blood, delirium, then death.

Sudden, painful, fatal; ravenously, yet invisibly, contagious: this terrifying disease quickly threw the people of Florence into panic. Boccaccio lived through the whole epidemic and left the most famous description of the mortality:

Many dropped dead in the open streets, both by day and by night, whilst a great many others, though dying in their own houses, drew their neighbours' attention to the fact more by the smell of their rotting corpses than by any other means. And what with these, and the others who were dying all over the city, bodies were here, there and everywhere . . . Such was the multitude of corpses (of which further consignments were arriving every day and almost by the hour at each of the churches), that there was not sufficient consecrated ground for them to be buried in . . . So when all the graves were full, huge trenches were excavated in the churchyards, into which new arrivals were placed in their hundreds, stowed tier upon tier like ships' cargo, each layer of corpses being covered over with a thin layer of soil till the trench was filled to the top.[14]

Another Florentine, Marchionne di Coppo Stefani, commented that, thus arranged, the bodies looked like a macabre lasagne: corpses piled row upon row separated only by layers of dirt.

From Genoa to Pisa, Lucca and Florence, the pestilence spread inland. Yet the diseased ships expelled on New Year's Eve were still heading their way west, docking at Marseilles before being cast out to drift westwards again. They left their dread cargo behind. From Marseilles the epidemic soon journeyed with travellers up the Rhône, to the papal city of Avignon. The pope, Clement VI, designated special cemeteries outside the city walls for the victims, whose numbers soon passed from the hundreds into the thousands. Among them was Petrarch's beloved muse, Laura; 'Death', the poet lamented, 'has put out the sun which dazed my eyes.'[15] A musician attached to the household of Cardinal Giovanni Colonna (a friend of Petrarch and another victim of plague) wrote home to Flanders to warn of the terror to come. His recommendation was simple: 'above all mix little with people – unless it be with a few who have healthy breath; but it is best to stay at home until the epidemic has passed.'[16] This was clearly a common opinion, for even the pope – having at first joined in public penitential processions – was soon quarantined in a guarded room on the advice of his doctor, Guy de Chauliac, who prescribed that large fires should be kept burning in an effort to cleanse the air of pestilence. The same logic dictated the reaction of the authorities in Milan: the city gates were shut and any household found to contain an infected person was cordoned off and the doors and windows bricked up. Inside the healthy died of starvation next to the sick and the dead. It was brutal but effective: the death rate in Milan was the lowest in northern Italy.

A cool-headed response to the epidemic was rare, however, and in many places people looked for someone to blame. In Narbonne, where the pestilence had travelled rapidly from Marseilles, beggars and travellers were quickly fingered for putting 'powdered substances' into rivers, churches, houses and foodstuffs. The men of Gerona wrote to a burgess of Narbonne, asking for advice. The reply came back stating that some of the arrested had, under torture, confessed to poisoning the town, 'admitting that they were given the potions in various places by people whose identities and names they do not know'. The aldermen and councillors of Lerida, further inland from Gerona, sought more sensible counsel. They commissioned Jacme d'Agramont, a local physician, to tell them what they could do to prevent infection by the epidemic that now threatened. His answer came in April 1348, four months after the disease arrived in the northern Mediterranean. There was much common sense amongst his waffle: it would be best, he says, to avoid contact with regions where the pestilence is aflame, although he too had clearly heard rumours of poison in Narbonne. As to causes, d'Agramont had to resort to guesswork: there were astrological and scientific causes of pestilence, but the prime reason was that it was 'sent by God because of our sins'.[17] Thus, several thousand miles from Constantinople, in the provincial town of Lerida, the same explanation for the existence of the pestilence was given as John Kantakouzenos had offered nearly a year before. Right around the Mediterranean Sea, people explained this epidemic in so similar a way that they could have been writing in concert. No wonder that the epidemic even began to be known by a common name: the Great Death.

From Narbonne this Great Death moved inland again, through Carcassonne to Toulouse. Beyond, to the north-west, was Gascony, connected to Toulouse by the River Garonne. Every twist and turn was commanded by a castle, each flying a flag – in little discernible order – of nobles partisan either to Edward III of England or Philip VI of France. It was a porous March, across which trade persisted whatever the state of the truce between the two kings. Merchants and travellers

made their way back and forth, journeying from Toulouse along the
Garonne to English Bordeaux. It was not an easy journey but it could
be done relatively quickly; at best it required less than a month.[xii] At
a time of fast-moving pestilence, Bordeaux was not far from Toulouse.

On his return to England, Sir Walter Manny – who had pleaded with
Edward to spare the wretched burghers of Calais – put his name to
a quite different petition to the king, in support of a request by his
friend Edmund Gonville for the right to found a college of twenty
scholars in the University of Cambridge. The petition was successful
and letters patent were issued in late January 1348.

Gonville was a well-born Norfolk priest who for many years had
combined his parochial duties with the stewardship of the earl of
Surrey's Norfolk estates, a post that had earned him a small fortune.[xiii]
This college was the latest in a remarkable series of endowments, each
of which had had a clear pastoral aim: thirteen years earlier in 1335
Gonville had helped to found a house of Dominican friars at Thetford in Norfolk, and before that he had established at his own home
in Rushford, just outside Thetford, a community of five priests whose
first purpose was to celebrate masses for the salvation of his soul after
his death as well as those of his family and friends. This kind of
'chantry' was becoming increasingly popular with wealthy Englishmen
in the late thirteenth and early fourteenth centuries; yet in Gonville's
new house the chantry priests were required not only to sing masses
for the dead but to minister to the local community. This concern for
the spiritual wellbeing of the people could be seen in the very first
benefaction Gonville made, to the church of St Nicholas, of
Thelnetham in Suffolk, where he had been rector in the 1320s.

Nestling in a small depression amid the flat north Suffolk landscape,
St Nicholas was not unusual, with a nave of much the same size and
proportion as churches across East Anglia. On the south side, however,
a large aisle has been added, almost as big again as the nave, thus
nearly doubling the body of the church. The aisle is simple, built by
Gonville for no grander reason than because Thelnetham church was

xii As Henry of Lancaster was to prove only eighteen months later, for which see
Ch. 12, p. 293.
xiii At the time, John de Warenne; the estates later passed to Henry, earl of Lancaster
(later duke) in 1347, although it is unclear whether Gonville served the new lord.

no longer large enough to accommodate the people of the parish. One of the windows suggests that Edmund had used the same mason who had built a similar extension in Rickinghall,[xiv] only two villages away. The church in Hinderclay, between the two, had also been enlarged. The reason these churches had been extended, at much the same time, was not due to some surge in religiosity but because, in common with much of western Europe, the population had grown significantly in the previous 150 years.

From a little over two million people when the Domesday Book was compiled in 1086, the population of England had reached perhaps six million by 1300. This rate of growth was exceptional: it resulted in part from a prolonged period of healthy harvests and an absence of epidemic disease, but was also the consequence of the rigorous imposition of feudal tenure by the Normans and their aristocratic successors. Feudalism gave the landlord an economic interest in the fertility of his tenants: not only did he derive revenue from marriages and the inheritance of land but without a thriving community living on his manors the landowner would have no one to farm his demesne and pay his dues. Lords, therefore, did all they could to promote marriage, acquiescing in the subdivision of land (which helped land-less men, who had few marriage prospects without land, to gain brides) and encouraging and coercing widows to remarry. Peasants too had good reason to marry and have a family. Children could help their villein parents fulfil labour obligations to the lord (which were fixed not by the size of family but by their landholding) and were the best insurance against old age and injury, afflictions that carried with them the fearful prospect of privation through the inability to work. So the several strong incentives for peasants to procreate amplified the effects of the benign environmental conditions that obtained through the twelfth and thirteenth centuries.

Feeding nearly three times as many mouths posed an obvious challenge. Increased demand was met, in part, by the extension of arable production into marginal land which, like the heaths of the Breck-land just to the north-west of Hinderclay, was ploughed up and sown for the first time. Moreover, a larger workforce could be used to improve yields, in digging more drains, weeding more thoroughly,

[xiv] Rickinghall Inferior.

spreading manure, removing stones, scaring birds and reaping the harvest more quickly before rains spoilt the crop. New technology helped farm the land and process its produce more effectively: improvements to the plough meant that it could cut deeper and turn the sod automatically to the side, while horses (being far quicker than oxen) began to be used to haul goods to market and fertilizer – manure and marl – around the farm. At the time of Domesday, there were about 6,000 watermills in England to grind grain; the subsequent introduction of the windmill not only allowed the number of mills to double by 1300 but aided the development of agriculture where there was no suitable river nearby. The most important technical change, however, was the spread of three-field crop rotation, enabling more of the land to be in production for longer and to be cultivated more efficiently.[xv] All of these developments point to a period of impressive agricultural improvement. Although there were shortages, even starvation in times of famine, on the whole this hugely increased population was able to feed itself.

The first consequence of the population boom was the subdivision of tenements: they became larger in number but smaller in size. Perhaps two thirds of rural households were living on tiny tenements – in some cases no more extensive than a modern allotment. Although smallholdings such as these were not sufficient to provide for a family, peasants could also offer their labour for cash, which could in turn be used to buy food at market. Landowners also benefited, as to each new tenement they could attach a new tenant, who not only paid for the privilege but owed customary service on the lord's demesne.

The abundance of labour obligations and the ready availability of cheap wage-labour from smallholders and landless wage-earners that flowed from a massively expanded population ensured the profitability of demesne farming, which in turn encouraged landlords to expand their demesnes, so that by the end of the thirteenth century they constituted about a third of arable land. As a result, the demesne was transformed from what had traditionally been a 'home farm' that provided food and fuel for the lord, his family, his servants and his

---

[xv] Indeed, in some parts of Norfolk, which through no coincidence matched those areas with the densest population, the preparation of land had reached such an advanced stage that fallowing and rotation could be dispensed with altogether.

guests into something much closer to a commercial enterprise, producing goods for market. Indeed, it was the superabundance of cheap hired labour, coupled with the attractions of commercial production, which was the reason why lords were increasingly willing to relax the old customs of feudal tenure, commuting customary works for cash – just as John Peter of Monkton Deverill had been allowed to do. With the receipts, lords (in John's case Glastonbury Abbey) hired more efficient wage-labour to cultivate the demesne – like that provided by Peter Boket, also of Monkton Deverill. In some places, the increase in villein *opera* had been so considerable that there was a surplus to the lord's requirements and so obligations were allowed to fall into abeyance.[18] Some progressive lords were making the next logical step and simply letting the land itself, turning their bondmen from providers of labour – actual or commuted – into payers of a normal cash rent.[19]

For manor managers, the key to generating profit was the correct use of labour, which was their single largest cost. Herein lay the economic justification for commuting villein obligations for a cash payment and using this cash to pay for wage-labour. Villeins were compelled to work and their labour was extracted in units of time: there was, therefore, little incentive for these bonded tenants to work with enthusiasm or to complete more than the very minimum of what they had been told to do. Conversely, wage-labourers were more often paid by their output – piecework – not by their hours. The incentive for them, therefore, was to work quickly, efficiently and effectively. Take, for example, the mowing of a meadow: villeins would scythe the grass under the supervision and direction of the hayward, filling time with as little effort as they could get away with; the wage-labourer, on the other hand, had to mow a certain amount of hay for a given price and so was motivated to do so as rapidly and professionally as he was able, if only to ensure re-employment next season. In one manor the difference in productivity has been measured: in a day a villein cut enough hay to fill a third of a cart whilst a wage-earner could manage a half. In other words, the wage-earner was fully 36 per cent more productive than the villein. In this case the demesne manager employed hired labour to fulfil about 30 per cent of his labour requirements, clearly deciding that this was the optimum balance between hard-working but expensive wage-earners and his cheaper but lackadaisical villein tenants.

Wage-labour was also essential to peasant agriculture. It was neces-sary to replace the work on the demesne that would otherwise have been done under obligation and it was essential to those few villeins who possessed more substantial landholdings.[xvi] Furthermore, in most villages, there were a few freemen who farmed and owned their land free of any labour obligations to the manorial lord; in Suffolk, as in Kent, the number of freemen was probably rather larger than elsewhere in the country. If their landholdings were extensive, and in many cases they were, these freemen would also require the services of hired labourers. Across the village economy there was a consider-able demand for wage-labour: from richer villeins, from freemen and from those lords who had commuted the labour services owed to them.

Wealthy peasants were not typical, however: the vast majority of villeins – and many freemen as well – were smallholders or owned no land at all. The expansion of the population, subdivision of hold-ings and proliferation of wage-labour meant that the majority of villagers did not have the land-capital to provide a sustainable and sufficient income. This did not mean that the peasantry became completely polarized, for there were plenty who inhabited the shifting ground between comfortable wealth and extreme hardship; it did lead, however, to an increasing distance between those who had accumu-lated relatively large landholdings – and therefore had capital wealth – and those who had not. This can be clearly seen in Rickinghall, only a couple of miles from Gonville's Thelnetham. Here was a clear divi-sion of wealth: poorer peasants married less, were more likely to migrate and relied upon employment by richer peasants and the lord's steward on the demesne. The richer peasants, however, were self-contained. They occupied most of the positions of responsibility in the village and they relied upon strong families and careful inter-marriage to maintain their land-capital. In between were a group of middling peasants who, whilst not so near the bread-line as the land-less poor, worked through their extended families and the land market to build their wealth. Many of them were scrambling to reach the safer position of the better-off peasants, who had left behind them the significant risks that went with being a smallholder. It is no surprise

xvi At a stretch, one man could farm only fifteen acres single-handedly, so a villein with a larger holding would have had to procure additional labour, both to fulfil his obligations on the demesne and to farm his own land.

that the majority of land-transfers, not to mention conflicts and disputes, are found within this group. Most villagers, however, had a relationship through an important common interest: credit. Peasants with something to spare provided credit to those in need – in both cash and in kind – to fund investments in tools, livestock and land, or simply so that they could make it through a bad year. There was, therefore, extraordinary diversity in village society, between privilege and hardship, comfort and struggle, conservatism and ambition. All this, even within the bounds of a single village like Rickinghall.

In times of crisis, these divisions were deepened and accentuated. In the first half of the fourteenth century calamities came with increasing regularity. The run of good harvests enjoyed for over a hundred years stuttered in the closing decades of the thirteenth century and then, in 1314, came to a halt. A terrible crop in that year meant that there was little seed-corn to plant for the 1315 harvest, which, like that of 1316, was blighted by appallingly wet weather. The chroniclers recalled how peasants were driven to eat dogs and cats, claiming that in some villages there were not enough people left to bury the dead. The crop yields tell the same story: on the Longbridge Deverill demesne, these years[xvii] produced 71 per cent of the average for grain yield, 51 per cent of the barley, 48 per cent of the oats and just 36 per cent of the rye. As supply of food grains fell, so the price was driven beyond the reach of many wage-earners; at the same time, the larger villeins had to cut back on hired labour to reduce costs, driving wage-earners further into penury. As a result, in some parts of the country one in ten villagers died of starvation;[xviii] at Longbridge Deverill a staggering 18 per cent of landless men died between 1316 and 1317. Those that suffered most were those that had no land to sell; small-holders were forced to part with what small property they had; many middling families were ruined; and only those who were not indebted and had sufficient land survived.[20] Indeed, the most wealthy, who had cash, were able to buy acre upon acre on the cheap. Thus the famine tended to enlarge the gap in wealth and expectations, further dividing those peasants who lived on the edge of survival and those whose accumulated assets protected them from starvation.

[xvii] 1315–1317.
[xviii] Though not in Suffolk, which was relatively unscathed.

Although the calamity of the Great Famine had a profound effect on those communities where it was felt most, it did little to alter the fundamental economic trends that were shaping English society in the early fourteenth century. So whilst famine caused considerable mortality, the levelling-off of population growth with which it co-incided had in fact begun some years before. The reasons for this were twofold. In some parts of the country, such as north-east Norfolk, all the available fertile land was being farmed and the progress being made through agricultural innovation was not sufficient to support the galloping population growth that had been witnessed a century before. More important, perhaps, was the fact that the increased use of cheap hired labour (itself a product of population expansion) removed one of the key incentives for high villein fertility, namely the desire to reduce the *per capita* labour obligations owed by a house-hold to the lord by expanding, through child-bearing, the total quantum of family labour available for that purpose. With labour obligations bought back from the lord, the relative costs and bene-fits of having more children changed. In short, the optimum family size dropped from around five to something closer to four – a reduc-tion of 20%, enough to cause population growth to flatten out. The supply of hired labour was so plentiful, however, that this did little to alter the ever-increasing use of that wage-labour on the demesne. Nor did the end of population expansion cause any widespread damage to the economy as a whole: it is true that there was a detectable downturn in some parts of the country during these decades, but the reasons are usually local and particular.[21] Likewise, the slowing of population growth did not affect to any significant degree the changing pattern of landholding that had started the previous century: although there are a few incidences of lords expanding their demesnes in these post-famine decades,[22] many more manors continued along the path of commutation and leasing. Indeed, if one generalization can be made about these first decades of the fourteenth century, it is that the slow metamorphosis of the agrarian economy increased the diversity of the rural English economy. For there were now increasingly wide variations in landholding and tenure, population densities, manorial profitability, commodity prices and wage levels. This was not evidence of stagnation or stasis; rather, in the greater heterogeneity of rural England, it is possible to see during these volatile, uncertain years the effects of irrepressible commercial forces gradually but surely overcoming the distorting restraints of feudal power.

The increasing commercialization of the relationship between peasant and lord was reflected in the growing importance of the market, through which transactions in produce, goods, land or credit, between peasants, lords and merchants, were mediated. There had always been rudimentary markets between neighbours and within villages where wage-labour, credit, land and produce were traded, and above these informal nodes of exchange there were more-sophisticated markets, with fixed locations and formal standing. For the villagers of Thelnetham and Rickinghall, a local weekly market in neighbouring Botesdale would have been the natural place for smaller transactions to take place. Perhaps a sheep or pig would change hands, a few bushels of barley or some loaves of bread. The scope of these mini-markets was small, however, for they catered mainly for the day-to-day consumption of villagers. For the bulk sale of goods, a larger centre of exchange was needed. By the middle of the thirteenth century, a network of market towns had grown up around the country, meaning that virtually everyone was within a ten-mile radius, or a day's return walk, of such a place.[xix] For Botesdale, Rickinghall and Thelnetham, this market town was Thetford.[xx] For most peasant men from this clutch of villages, a journey to Thetford would be at least a monthly event. It was here that the larger (mainly noble) producers sold their bulk surpluses, where the best prices for livestock could be had, and where tools and goods from further afield could be purchased.

It was a sign of the growing importance of market towns that rich benefactors chose increasingly to make religious foundations in these places and not in some remote monastery. Edmund Gonville's Dominican priory at Thetford, which he established in 1335, was just such a foundation. Thetford heaved on market days and it was, therefore, a perfect location for the Dominicans – who

[xix] The multiplication continued: between 1227 and 1350 the crown granted some 1,200 places in England and Wales the right to hold a market.
[xx] It is a measure of the proliferation of these markets that the next closest was Stowmarket, twelve miles to the south of the villages, which was only granted its licence from the king in 1347.

specialized in preaching – to establish a house. These 'black friars' found a ready audience among the crowds that swelled around the livestock, mounds of grains, towers of cheeses, reams of woollen cloth, piles of salted fish and proudly displayed pots and pans. Gonville's motivation in sponsoring their foundation is less obvious: so far he had concentrated on projects with which he had a direct connection. The market reveals the reason why he chose Thetford: as Rushford (where his chantry priests ministered to the local community) was four miles from Thetford, and Thelnetham (where he had extended the church) was ten miles away, Gonville knew that amongst the hundreds of villagers coming to Thetford on market day some would be from Rushford and Thelnetham. The foundation of Thetford Priory thus suited both their purposes: Gonville's concern for better pastoral oversight of his villagers, the Dominicans' for an extended reach into the western borderlands of Norfolk and Suffolk.

The Dominicans already had houses in Ipswich, Sudbury, Norwich, Yarmouth and Lynn; Thetford was a gap which, with Gonville's gift, they could now fill. It was a map that described well how Thetford fitted into a larger network of exchange, part of a web of towns linked by thousands of miles of roads that criss-crossed the country. Simple commodities were carted in bulk from the countryside to the towns and cities, feeding the urban populations that produced the goods – such as cloth and manufactured products – which went back in the opposite direction to towns like Thetford and thence the countryside around. Roads also carried goods from the coastal towns and harbours, such as salt and herring, the latter a staple of peasant and noble alike. For most villagers, white herring (salted and barrelled) and red herring (salted and smoked) were the cheapest source of protein available year-round. It was of particular importance during famine, when other important protein sources, such as eggs, were rare. Although widely available, herring came from only a few fishing ports, of which Yarmouth, due east of Norwich and connected to that city by the River Yare, was pre-eminent.

Yarmouth's position was determined by the herring, which spawned in the early summer off the coast of Scotland and by late September had arrived off the east Norfolk coast. As a result, Yarmouth became the centre of the North Sea herring industry, one of the richest towns in the country and one of its most important ports.[xxi] It was easy to see why: during October hundreds of boats with thousands of fishermen came to Yarmouth for the town's international herring fair. (Indeed, in 1339 the French estimated that if they were to attack during the fair they would find 1,000 fishing boats and 15,000 men at Yarmouth.) This flotilla was evidence of the international appetite for herring, for the boats were not just from all down the east coast but came from as far away as the Baltic and Low Countries. Thus, once collected and salted, this enormous harvest of the sea was not only sent throughout England, to Thetford and far beyond, but was also exported abroad. In return, ports like Yarmouth, London and Lynn imported those luxuries which were not available in England: furs from Muscovy, spices from the Orient, cloths from Flanders and wine from Gascony. All of these made their way inland, along roads to the towns where they were sold even to the most humble of villager. So when the villeins of nearby villages, such as those of Thelnetham, bought their month's worth of herring in the market at Thetford, and the wealthier ones among them a length of cloth or a little pepper, they were all participating in a nationwide, and European-wide, network of trade and exchange.

The Dominicans showed that this trading network reflected a pan-European society, one that was bound – however diffusely – not only by commercial ties, but also by a shared intellectual tradition and the profession of a common faith. Consider the villein from Thelnetham, stopping for a moment at the door to Edmund Gonville's new Dominican priory off the market square in Thetford. His deal done, he might venture inside the church, say a prayer, light a candle or just look around. The windows of the chancel were filled with stained glass, throwing coloured light onto an altar framed by a magnificent painted retable.[xxii] This had at its centre a moving depiction of the Crucifixion. On either side were eight saints, portrayed in vibrant greens, reds and blues on a gilded chequer-board background. There was the Italian St Peter Martyr,

---

[xxi] In 1334, by taxable wealth, Yarmouth was rated the fourth-largest provincial town in England; by this time it was probably the most important port north of the Thames.

[xxii] Now called the Thornham Retable, as it is currently displayed in Thornham Parva church in Suffolk.

with St Margaret of Antioch. St Dominic – a Castilian – was there too. It was he who only just over a century before had founded the Order of Preachers – the black friars – in Toulouse. Our villager might only have recognized one or two of these foreign saints but he will have been able to name the local martyr among them: Saint Edmund, who also provides the clue to the origin of the painting. For this retable was the product of the flourishing circle of artists who worked across East Anglia in the first half of the fourteenth century. They were a cosmopolitan group, who drew influences from far and wide. For instance, at the same time as the retable was being prepared for the new priory in Thetford, other East Anglian painters were at work at Ely, twenty miles to the west, on the decoration of a new chapel. Here was an Annunciation,[xxiii] whose Mary – with her almond-shaped eyes – showed the direct inspiration of recently completed paintings in Siena. Although the Thetford retable cannot claim so clear a provenance, its creator was working in the same tradition. Painting within the distant stylistic orbit of northern Italy, the artist worked on wood that had travelled further still. The planks were hewn from eastern European oak, felled sometime around 1322 and imported via the Baltic and an East Anglian coastal port to the artist's studio in Norwich. Now in place behind the altar in Thetford Priory, the beautiful retable made an appropriately universal display of wealth and piety for this most international of religious orders.[xxiv] More than that, it was a potent symbol of how the many constituent parts of medieval Europe – for all their apparent isolation and chaotic relationships – were bound strongly by the many things that they held in common. The villein from Thelnetham was not just a spectator in this pan-European exchange; his presence at the market in Thetford that day made him a part of it. It was for this reason, and no other, that this lone peasant in a quiet corner of England would soon be embroiled in a catastrophe that originated on the other side of the known world.

*   *   *

[xxiii] The Annunciation on the west wall of Prior Crauden's Chapel, Ely Cathedral.
[xxiv] The Dominicans were founded in Languedoc, by a Castilian, and the first English mission was launched at Bologna.

Trade carried news of the terrible pestilence before it. Ibn Khātimah, an Andalusian living in Almería, had heard from Christian merchants that the disease had started in China, from where it had spread to the Crimea and then Constantinople. At Messina word of the Great Death reached the port whilst the disease did its silent work about the town. As whispers accelerated round the Mediterranean, towns were given more notice before the epidemic itself arrived. Even so, no one could be sure that it would not just stop. Sailors coming into London, Southampton, Yarmouth and other ports around the south and east coast brought with them stories of the progress of the disease up through southern France. This was concern enough; news that it had taken hold in the papal city of Avignon, so well-known to many English travellers and clerical ambassadors, was particularly shocking. The pope, apparently, had fled.

Some paid particularly close attention to these worrying developments on the Continent, among them the bishop of Lincoln, John Gynewell, who at the time was conducting a visitation of his vast diocese.[xxv] As he moved from town to town, Newark, Grantham, Stamford, Bicester, Towcester and Leicester, messengers bringing business papers from London carried with them fresh news from abroad. By July 1348, there were suggestions that the epidemic had reached Bordeaux. Gynewell pondered the unhappy coincidence of this with the recent end of the truce with France, and indeed the incessant rain that was threatening to spoil that year's crop, and decided that the only way to avoid war, or famine, and now disease, was to pray. On 25th July, whilst staying at Newstead Priory, just north of Nottingham, he dictated a letter to a clerk to be sent throughout his diocese. He ordered first that penitential processions be made on Wednesdays and Fridays, in supplication for tranquil weather ahead of the harvest. Masses for peace were to be said and prayers for the royal family. For those who took part and who offered their confession with sincerity, the bishop promised that an indulgence of forty days would be subtracted from the supplicant's time in Purgatory. Bishop Gynewell's principal concerns were the consequences of war, which were to be greatly feared 'unless the diligent prayers of the

---

[xxv] Gynewell was appointed bishop of Lincoln and consecrated by the archbishop of Canterbury on 23rd September 1347. He had been Grosmont's steward.

faithful assuage the anger of the Saviour, who brings vengeance upon sinners in divers ways, even as it is manifest, such is the pleasure of the most High, from pestilences, stormy weather, and the deaths of men in sundry parts of the earth'.[23] It was a poor omen, in that case, that French troops, under the capable Geoffrey de Chargny, were already storming St Omer on the French border of Flanders, only twenty-five miles from the English garrison newly installed in Calais. All of a sudden, the six months of celebrations must have looked terribly premature. The French were again spoiling for a fight. Gynewell's fears were about something very much worse. He did not have to wait long to have them confirmed.

3

Pestilence Arrives

July–December 1348

Deth cam dryuyng aftur[i]
William Langland, *Piers Plowman*[1]

The Shipman is one of the more faintly drawn characters in Geoffrey Chaucer's *Canterbury Tales.* Certainly he made his presence felt: he was bearded and strong, and his torso was browned from standing at the helm under the sun. His crew was drawn 'from every land' and he imposed discipline on them with his fist; it was perhaps the only language that they could all understand.[2] Other than that, his fellow pilgrims had to rely on inference to get the measure of his shadowy figure. He was from the West Country, but beyond that, no one could be sure: 'For all I know', the narrator explains, 'he was from Dartmouth', no doubt because the post was a famous haunt of pirates and smugglers.[3] Not for nothing did this mariner know every creek and haven between the Baltic and the Bay of Biscay, for his trade was often illicit. Even when shipping wine legally from Bordeaux, it would not trouble him to draw off a good measure from the barrels whilst his client-merchant slept elsewhere on the boat, unaware. How fitting that his boat was called the *Magdalene*, a controversial patron in an age when ships were named after more conventional saints. Yet the Shipman's eccentricities did not make him unusual; indeed, he was unmistakeably an archetype. He was a lonely figure but he was free, neither bound by the ties of land nor fastened by its precepts and laws. Crowded together on their wooden island, the Shipman and his sailors

[i] Death came driving after.

were creatures of their own floating domain. It is a timeless picture
and a believable one for it.

The shipmen of the middle of the fourteenth century sailed ships
that were designed, above all, to be versatile. They had to carry every
kind of cargo, from wheat and spices to wine and soldiers, across
stormy oceans into the tightest coastal harbours and up narrow inland
rivers. Boats were, therefore, only large enough to transport their
merchandise safely – typically 80 feet long and 20 feet across the beam,
with fore- and after-castles and one mast in between. Oars would be
used to move the vessel down the river to the sea, where a sail would
be unfurled to harness the power of the winds. What these boats
possessed in versatility they lacked, however, in navigability. A primitive
rig and sail system made it difficult to tack, and even if the wind was
in the right direction the cloud-covered northern skies made stellar
navigation unreliable. As a result, on long voyages across open seas –
such as that between Gascony and the south coast of England – a
ship's master might well, through adverse winds or an unhelpful night
sky, arrive some distance from where he wanted to be. There was
usually a port nearby, however – one of a whole string that had grown
up in response to the unpredictability of navigation on the open seas.
Having put his ship in to rest, taken on fresh water and replenished
provisions, the master would make for his intended destination, joining
the considerable coastal traffic of ships, fishing boats and barges, sailing
past the little coves and remote beaches that lay between larger harbours.
This was a pervious coastline, as the Shipman's littoral knowledge
attested well.

Sometime in late May 1348, two ships made their way out of the
English port of Bordeaux and began the journey home. One at least
was bound for Bristol; most likely both carried (as did the Shipman)
a cargo of wine. Up the western coast of France, the ships rounded
the Breton arm that reaches out into the Atlantic sea. Rather than
attempt to cross the English Channel at its widest part, they made for
the Channel Islands off the western edge of the Norman Cotentin,
before sailing north for England and thereby cutting the open-sea
crossing in half. The journey so far will have taken about three weeks;
it would be another couple of days before land appeared on the
horizon. The ships' masters will have been pleased to see the familiar
promontory of Portland Bill extending out into the Channel, forming

a natural breakwater, behind which they could escape into the haven of Weymouth Bay and the narrow mouth of the River Wey. Squeezed between the dock on one side and the Bay on the other was Melcombe Regis, the northern part of modern-day Weymouth. Melcombe Regis was well-situated: almost midway between disreputable Dartmouth and Southampton, the largest port on the south coast, the town had a prosperous hinterland, full of noble manors and great estates. As a consequence, the town enjoyed local pre-eminence in the import of wine and export of grain, and was a popular departure point for English Gascony. Melcombe was by now a little *entrepôt*, attracting shipmen from across northern Europe and sometimes beyond, bringing all the usual disputes between locals and foreigners. (Indeed, in 1347 the town elders had been ordered to welcome Venetian ships in an amicable manner.) Such was the town's importance that Edward III impressed almost as many ships from Melcombe Regis during the Siege of Calais as he called on from the far larger ports of Bristol and London.

The two ships, having completed the three-week voyage from Gascony, docked in Melcombe Regis in early June 1348. One of them was just pausing before making for Bristol but in the meantime both crews disembarked. Amongst them were some Gascon sailors who had become sick during the Channel crossing and had to be carried ashore. They were soon inspected and their bodies found to be covered in dark blotches and large ulcers in the groin and under the arms. No one was sure from what disease the sailors were suffering, not least because they had been completely healthy on leaving Bordeaux three weeks before. Within days of their arrival at Melcombe, the Gascon sailors had died. It did not stop there: as soon as they had been buried, other crew-members started to cough up blood and show similar symptoms; as the days and weeks passed more sailors died, until a greater part of the crew had been taken. As yet, the epidemic had not spread to local residents, so the fate of the Gascon sailors was kept quiet for fear of scaring people from bringing their goods to the town. Within the month, however, a few inhabitants of Melcombe were showing the first signs of the mystery illness. The course of the disease was precisely as it had been for the hapless Gascons – the rash and ulcers appeared, the patients fell into a fever and after three days had died. It was Monday, 23rd June 1348, Midsummer Eve, and the Great Death had claimed its first English victims.

As the pestilence quietly established itself on the Dorset coast, elsewhere in England merchants and sailors were stepping onto piers not with news of an English epidemic but with more accounts of the terrifying progress of pestilence through the Continent. It was almost certainly via the trading community of York that Archbishop Zouche heard that the disease was fast approaching. Pacing the rounds of his castle at Cawood, Zouche – who was a reflective, if not scholarly, man – looked back on the successes of the last few years, of the king's victories at Crécy and Calais, and of his own at Neville's Cross. It seemed that Edward and England's glory could grow no greater (indeed, Edward had even been offered the German Imperial Crown, an offer he wisely rejected). Zouche pondered all of this, and then considered the reports of the advancing plague. How could God, so favourable to the English in war, threaten to punish them so terribly in peace? On 28th July, Zouche wrote to his official, nine miles away in York, with an answer:

Since the life of man on earth is a war, no wonder if those fighting amidst the miseries of this world are unsettled by the mutability of events: now favourable, now contrary. For Almighty God sometimes allows those he loves to be troubled while their strength is perfected in weakness by an outpouring of spiritual grace. There can be no one who does not know, since it is now public knowledge, how great a mortality, pestilence and infection of the air are now threatening various parts of the world, especially England; and this is surely caused by the sins of men who, while enjoying good times, forget that such things are the gifts of the most high giver. Thus, since the inevitable human fate, pitiless death, which spares no one, now threatens us, unless the holy clemency of the Saviour is shown to his people from on high, the only hope is to hurry back to him alone, whose mercy outweighs justice and who, most generous in forgiving, rejoices heartily in the conversion of sinners; humbly urging him with orisons and prayers that he, the kind the merciful Almighty God, should turn his anger and remove the pestilence and drive away the infection from the people whom he redeemed with his precious blood.[4]

The prelate went on to prescribe processions and masses, just as Bishop Gynewell had done three days before in his diocese of Lincoln. Many days travel from the south coast, neither bishop nor his audience knew yet what horrors were unfolding in Melcombe Regis.

From Buckinghamshire to Northumberland, the bishops' instructions were read from lecterns in parish churches. Meanwhile, death was making its way round the Cornish peninsula, up the Severn estuary and into the mouth of the River Avon. Whether it was the Bristol ship that had first landed at Melcombe, piloted home by what remained of the crew, or another ship from infected France, is not known. The chroniclers are agreed, however, that by the middle of August the pestilence had arrived in Bristol.[5] The city lay within the diocese of Bath and Wells, whose bishop – the much-loved and ever-conscientious Ralph Shrewsbury – was spending the summer months in his manor house of Evercreech in Somerset, about twenty-three miles away. It seems that he too had heard of the imminent arrival of pestilence, just as Gynewell and Zouche had before him. On 17th August he sent instructions throughout his whole diocese, commanding prayers, processions and the encouragement of contrition in the whole population. That this bishop thought the epidemic had still to leave 'a neighbouring kingdom' – presumably France – suggests that it had indeed only just arrived in Bristol and that the outbreak in Melcombe had not spread beyond the town. It is doubtful that Shrewsbury had seen either of the other episcopal letters despatched so far; nonetheless, his mandate echoes the standard explanations they give for the threatened catastrophe. This was an act of God, he claimed, who was angry at the sins of men, an anger that could only be assuaged by prayers for mercy and expressions of genuine atonement. Only then, the bishop concluded, will God 'grant peace between Christian countries and send healthy air'.[6]

Entreaties for peace were of little consequence to the humiliated French, who were busily cutting off the supply lines to English Calais and diverting the streams that supplied it with water. Perhaps due to the plague, they were unable to follow these small acts of sabotage with the kind of full-blown attack that was needed to retake the town. Edward, too, was diverted from a return to campaigning, preparations for which had begun in earnest after rain had drowned out the final tournaments of the post-Calais celebrations. Dreadful news had just arrived from Gascony: Princess Joan, who had been despatched to marry Pedro of Castile but a matter of weeks before, had, on 1st July, been struck down by the pestilence.[7] Her chaperone, Sir Robert Bourchier – Edward's first lay chancellor and an esteemed diplomat – had also died. The Great Death had travelled up the Garonne from Toulouse to Bordeaux, where it had not only infected sailors about to make the journey to England (the very same sailors who landed at Melcombe Regis) but had also claimed the life of young Joan, who was staying in the castle of Lormont nearby. By this wicked coincidence the princess had become one of the first English victims of the pestilence. Edward was devastated. Before he could work out how to unwind the intricate diplomatic arrangements that had propelled his daughter to Castile, he was to be consumed anew with grief: his infant son William, conceived on his return from Calais and born only a couple of months before, had also died (not, however, from plague). The baby was accorded a full royal funeral on 5th September – a sombre conclusion to nine months of rejoicing.

The bishops had explained the pestilence as God's punishment for belligerent Man; pestilence had now inflicted an early blow on England's principal warmonger. Although the coincidence cannot have been missed by acute observers, Edward was not inclined to moral prevarication. Besides, he was distracted both by events in France and by the need to deal with a further death: that of his one-time antagonist John Stratford, the archbishop of Canterbury, who died at his manor of Mayfield on 23rd August. Edward had only recently asked Stratford to arrange for prayers to be said throughout the Canterbury province to beseech God for protection from the pestilence. (As with little Prince William, however, it was not plague that carried the archbishop away: he had been suffering from an unrelated illness since June.) Edward, in whose side Stratford had been a particularly painful thorn, was keen to ensure that the archbishopric did not fall into unreliable hands again: he knew he had to act quickly in order to secure a favourable replacement. However, within a week of Stratford's death, the obstinate monks of Canterbury confounded the king by electing a new archbishop themselves, rashly asserting their rights without seeking the customary guidance of the monarch.[ii] Their choice, Thomas Bradwardine – a brilliant theologian and mathematician – was no enemy of the king. On the contrary, he was a royal chaplain

---

[ii] On Saturday, 30th August 1348.

and had accompanied Edward on the Crécy campaign, where, upon hearing the news of the victory at Neville's Cross, the scholar had preached to the king and assembled nobility on the text 'Now thanks be unto God, which always causeth us to triumph in Christ'.[8] The sermon was delivered in English – an unusual but for that all the more pointed reference as to precisely *which* nation had triumphed in Christ. Nonetheless, Bradwardine was perhaps too mercurial for the moment. Edward wanted power concentrated in the hands of those whom he absolutely trusted, and who would wield it as he bid them while he was abroad. So, over the heads of the Canterbury chapter, he lobbied the pope to appoint his chancellor, John Ufford, to the see, a request that was granted.[iii] In the end, seeking the pope's approval proved unnecessary: even before Clement VI's letter had arrived in England, the monks had been bullied into a new election and Ufford was their inevitable choice.[iv] It was a measure of Edward's intent to renew the war in France that he moved so decisively to reinforce his regent administration.

Meanwhile, the prior of Canterbury, Robert Hathbrande, who exercised spiritual authority during the vacancy of the archiepiscopal throne, sent out the letter that had been requested of Stratford before his death. Stung by his treatment at the hands of the king, Hathbrande launched into a critique of the war that was more overt even than Gynewell and Shrewsbury had dared to propound. Bradwardine had professed God's preferment for the English king; now Hathbrande observed that 'those whom [God] loves He censures and chastises'. Leaving no one in any doubt as to the cause of the impending disaster, he pointed to the 'growing pride and corruption of the English, and their numberless sins', amongst them the wars 'which are exhausting and devouring the wealth of the kingdom', leaving it on many occasions 'desolate and afflicted'. War was, Hathbrande suggested, both the agent of God's cleansing anger and its cause; its own devastating effects were now to be compounded by 'the pestilences and wretched mortalities of men which have flared up in other regions'.[9] Sufficiently carefully worded to avoid censure, Hathbrande's message was nonetheless perfectly clear.

[iii] By a bull issued on 24th September 1348.
[iv] On Sunday, 28th September 1348.

Edward did not concur, despite the grievous loss he had already suffered at the hands of the plague. In a letter sent to Alfonso XI of Castile concerning the death of Princess Joan, Edward gave a remarkable show of royal grief, without the slightest suggestion that he felt in any way culpable:

> We are sure that your magnificence knows how, after much complicated negotiation about the intended marriage of the renowned Infante Pedro, your eldest son, and our most beloved daughter Joan, which was designed to nurture peace and create an indissoluble union between our royal houses, we sent our said daughter to Bordeaux, en route for your territories in Spain. But see (with what intense bitterness of heart we have to tell you this) destructive Death (who seizes young and old alike, sparing no one, and reducing rich and poor to the same level) has lamentably snatched from both of us our dearest daughter (whom we loved best of all, as her virtues demanded). No human being could be surprised if we were inwardly desolated by the sting of this bitter grief, for we are human too. But we, who have placed our trust in God and our life between his hands, where he has held it closely through many dangers – we give thanks to him that one of our own family, free of all stain, whom we have loved with pure love, has been sent ahead to heaven to reign among the choirs of virgins, where she can gladly intercede for our offences before God himself.[10]

Amongst all his pitiable expressions of sadness, Edward gives no indication that he saw his daughter's death as part of a divinely ordained punishment. Indeed, he seems to have held that precisely the opposite was true – had he not been preserved 'though many dangers'? Edward's letter gives the unavoidable impression that his vaunted 'trust in God' was a self-fulfilling piety.

The pestilence had been steadily incubating through the summer months in Melcombe Regis. Fewer visitors than normal came during August, for, in between the downpours that had persisted since late June, most people were in the fields frantically gathering in the harvest. It was inevitable, however, that the plague would soon break the bounds of the town and make its way into the countryside beyond. The deaths of priests, which were recorded in the diocesan registers, give an indication of how the disease spread. At the beginning of September, the parish priest of West Chickerell – a village just a couple of miles north-west of Melcombe – fell ill and died. It is just possible that the disease had already claimed the life of a priest on the Isle of Portland, but this death at West Chickerell was the first to give sure evidence of the creeping epidemic.[11] Perhaps the rector became infected on a trip into Melcombe; maybe it passed to him as he gave confession to a dying parishioner. We shall never know.

Whatever the cause, the over-riding priority for the diocesan authorities in Salisbury was to get a replacement rector into the parish as soon as possible. The ecclesiastical bureaucracy worked rapidly to that end. Having consulted the patron of the church (who could be a local noble, the bishop, an abbot or even the king), a candidate would be proposed, briefly examined to ensure he was qualified to take on the parish, and then instituted as the new rector. From the point of death to the institution of a new priest, the process would typically take about twenty days.[12] Where problems arose in finding a suitable candidate, the appointment could take far longer, but canon law stipulated that in no event should a parish be without a priest for more than six months. Twenty days was the norm, however, at least under normal conditions. Accordingly, at West Chickerell, where the rector was dead by early September, his replacement had been instituted, if not yet installed, by the end of the month. He was not to stay there long.

Melcombe Regis and West Chickerell sit on a triangular beach hemmed in by an arc of hills. On this plain, almost contained by the downs and the sea, the pestilence established itself through July and August. It was only a matter of time before the disease pushed out along the principal roads that led from the town, a journey hastened by the first movement of wagons carrying the August harvest. To the east, on the way to Wareham, the priests of Warmwell and Wool (about seven and fourteen miles from Melcombe respectively) had both died by the end of September. The next-nearest town of Dorchester, eight miles to the north, was also affected that month. Once it had taken hold in this local market, the disease quickly fanned out into the Dorset countryside around, its progress marked by the loss of priests in the parishes nearby

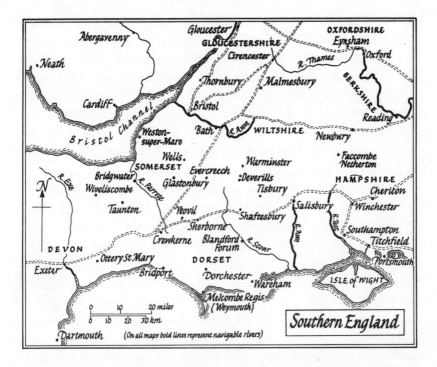

during October: Langton Long Blandford (on the way to Salisbury) to the north-east, Cerne Abbas (on the road to Sherbourne) to the north, and Toller Percorum and Kingston Russell (respectively on the way to Crewkerne and Bridport) to the west. At Abbotsbury, on the coast west of Melcombe, Abbot Walter de Saunford was probably the first head of a religious house to be killed by the pestilence. The Benedictine abbey of Sherborne soon lost its prior and the hospital of St John the Baptist in Shaftesbury its warden, William de Godeford.

Much of Dorset had succumbed to pestilence by mid-autumn but further progress overland was still comparatively slow, creeping through the countryside at no more than a few hundred metres per day. The disease had moved from Constantinople to Messina in the same time that it had taken to spread from Melcombe Regis to Blandford Forum. In part this was because Dorset was relatively remote: other than Melcombe it possessed no great trading hubs and had no town or city with the pull of Bristol, Norwich or Coventry. Dorset was also, therefore, avoidable; no doubt people steered clear of the county once news got around that the plague had taken hold.

The people of Dorset, however, were not immobile and the disease moved with them. Slow across land, it travelled more rapidly along the coast. Thirty-eight miles west of Melcombe, at Ottery St Mary in Devon, many of the canons of the collegiate church had perished by early autumn. This was some distance along the coast from the abbey at Abbotsbury and far from any village yet infected by land. It is almost certain, therefore, that the epidemic came here by water, probably with the little fishing boats that worked off the long beaches that ran west from Melcombe. On the other side of the town, however, were high cliffs, where Chaldon Down and the Purbeck Hills met the sea. Here the villages of East Lulworth, Tyneham and Worth Matravers all lost their priests in quick succession during the autumn. This was a secluded corner of a quiet county, yet it still had trading links with the rest of the country – the Purbeck Hills were quarried for marble, most recently sending stone for the west front of Exeter Cathedral; the majority will have been shipped by sea and this may explain why the disease seems to have come inland from the coast. There may be another explanation, however: these villages sat atop the coves and caves of the Purbeck cliffs, the sort of coastline with which the Shipman would have been particularly well-acquainted. Perhaps it was an illicit night-time errand on the shoreline below that brought the pestilence in from the west.

It was most probably fishermen or smugglers who introduced the pestilence further east along the south coast, at the point where the mouth of the little River Meon forms a tiny haven off Southampton Water. The first village inland was Titchfield, lying two miles up the river just before the abbey that was the lord of the village, haven and surrounding lands. At the manorial court held on Friday, 31st October 1348, eight tenants were reported to be dead. As there had been only five deaths (out of about 150 tenants in all) through the whole of 1347, it was immediately clear that an epidemic of some sort was present. Among the dead was John Swein, a relatively affluent villager who held a house and about fifteen acres at Titchfield Common on the west side of the manor.[v] In order that John's wife Isabella should take on the holding, she would have had to appear at the next manorial

---

[v] The inheritance tax (called a heriot) payable to his lord, the abbot, was a mare worth 3s, i.e. £0.15.

court held in the village, which under normal circumstances might have been in some weeks' or months' time. But such was the impact of the disease that the abbey was forced to call another court just a week later, on 7th November. Isabella Swein was among those due to appear to claim their holdings, but the court was informed on the day that she was sick. Although she was given until the next court to claim the land, the fact that she could not make the short journey on this occasion suggests she was unlikely to last until then. At the same court it was reported that a further twenty-five tenants had died in the previous seven days; in a little over a fortnight, Titchfield had lost 22 per cent of its tenants and (it must be assumed) a similar proportion of wives, children and free households. So great a number of deaths could only point to the presence of pestilence. The Titchfield court must have been a miserable, wretched scene that early November day.

In this little corner of Hampshire the disease spread even more slowly than in Dorset: other than a couple of deaths recorded in the hamlets adjoining Titchfield, there was no apparent increase in mortality in any of the neighbouring villages also owned by Titchfield Abbey. Nearly half a century later the chronicler Henry Knighton would claim that the pestilence entered the country via Southampton, only ten miles north of where Titchfield Haven meets the Solent. Given Southampton's pre-eminence among the ports of the southern coast, we should expect there to be good evidence to reinforce Knighton's claim, yet there is none: Southampton was to remain untouched for some time yet. The little village of Titchfield, then, was the Great Death's first foothold in Hampshire. It was to remain an isolated island of epidemic for some months to come.[13]

Like a slow-moving fire, the contagion which had just set a small corner of Hampshire alight was steadily burning its way through Dorset. Already it had claimed the lives of thousands. Yet the epidemic moved so slowly that people would have been forgiven for thinking there was still a chance that it could be contained, if only by prayer. On 24th October, just as the first victims started to die in Titchfield, Bishop Edington wrote a letter from London to be distributed throughout his diocese of Winchester, making the now-familiar order that processions and intercessionary masses be held. He spoke with horror about what he had heard of the advance of the disease:

We report with anguish the serious news which has come to our ears: that this cruel plague has now begun a similarly savage attack on the coastal areas of England. We are struck by terror lest (may God avert it!) this brutal disease should rage in any part of our city and diocese.[14]

Edington will have known that Bristol was one of the 'coastal areas' so far afflicted, as the pestilence had been present there at least since the middle of August, brought in by an infected boat from Melcombe Regis or perhaps even directly from abroad. Bristol was an ancient, large and wealthy place, whose port communicated not only with English Gascony but with the many harbours of English Ireland as well. As a regional mercantile hub, Bristol enjoyed a similar role in the West of England to the one played by London in the East. It reached out into central England through a direct road to Oxford and into the Midlands via Gloucester and Worcester. The road to London, which the modern A4 follows all the way to the capital, was probably the single most-travelled route in the country; no doubt it was along this road that news came to London of Bristol's distress. Yet little has been recorded of what happened once the Great Death took hold. Here narrow streets were packed in on either side of a loop in the Avon, bounded by St Mary's Redcliffe to the south and the sheriff's great castle in the north, and the lanes running from the dockside were jammed with merchandise and commodities just brought in or being made ready for shipping. It is not difficult to imagine how pestilence made its way swiftly through the hubbub. Henry Knighton later claimed that 'almost the whole population of the town perished, snatched away, as it were, by sudden death, for there were few who kept their beds for more than two or three days.'[15] It does not appear that this was exaggeration after the event, for the monk of Malmesbury (a contemporary, whose monastery was only twenty-two miles to the east) stated that 'very few were left alive.'[16]

On the outskirts of Bristol, the hospital of St Katherine in Bedminster, which had been founded to care for the needs of the sick, infirm and needy traveller, lost its master – most likely infected by some such traveller carrying the disease. Keynsham Abbey, a little further out on the road to Bath, lost its abbot, Nicholas de Taunton, while the monks soon stopped serving the doles they traditionally handed out to the poor, probably because so many brothers had died that there were not enough left to serve them. It was not only the poor who suffered, however: fifteen of the city elders died during the months of the Great Death, more than a third of their number. Given that these were precisely the people who could most easily flee the panic, it is probable that the proportion of Bristol's overall population that perished was far higher. It is not hard to imagine what immediate effect such mortality had on this bustling town. Edington had heard how 'cities, towns, castles and villages, . . . which rang with the abundance of joy . . . have now been suddenly and woefully stripped of their inhabitants by this most savage pestilence' and that 'as a result no one dares to enter these places, but instead flees far from them, as if from the caves of wild animals . . . and they become instead places of horror and desolate wasteland.'[17] There is every reason to suppose that Bristol was reduced to the same pitiful state.

The Great Death soon burst from Bristol's walls. Just as it had done in Dorset, the disease followed the coast and the roads out into the countryside around. The route north through the Vale of Berkeley to Gloucester was the principal means of getting goods between Bristol and the Midlands; about twelve miles out of Bristol on this road, the merchant-traveller would have passed the small borough of Thornbury, which sits between the fields that lie before the broad River Severn.[18] Much land had been reclaimed here behind a sea wall, which separated agriculture from marsh and the Oldbury Sands – work that had nearly doubled the acreage of land under cultivation since the time of the Domesday Book, a clear sign of the growth in the population of this part of England. It was a substantial manor, with several constituent hamlets,[19] all run by a considerable manorial administration – a survey of 1322 described a manor hall, kitchen, dairy, two barns, and a cowshed. Instead of an open fire with a vent in the rood, the lord's chamber had a chimney – still very unusual in the middle of the fourteenth century. The steward, the bailiff and 'Augustine the clerk' all had separate chambers of their own, each sized according to their status. Yet despite the extent of its operation, its amenities and its pleasant aspect, Thornbury received only irregular visits from its lord, Sir Ralph Stafford. The manor was thus left to the lord's officials and his tenants, about 230 of whom were spread across the various hamlets and sub-manors. Rents and feudal dues were fairly low, and this, together with the retention of so much woodland and marsh, showed that although the population had grown, it was still comfortably within the carrying capacity of the land. As elsewhere, some of the people who lived in Thornbury had to deal with severe hardship, and disasters were not unknown: the villagers feared that the river might break through the sea wall, just as it had done fourteen years before in 1334 when it had killed livestock and flooded crops. Yet it seems that Thornbury was by and large a comparatively prosperous place and the tenants were correspondingly quiescent.

Then the Great Death came to Thornbury, rupturing its regular, peaceful, estuarine existence. All was well at the court held on 10th August, when rumours of the disease had just arrived from Bristol. Perhaps Thornbury men stopped going there for business and avoided travellers making their way up the Gloucester road, but it would have been to no avail. For in late August a little boat made its way up the creek to Oldbury Mill, bringing with it the deadly pestilence they had been trying so hard to avoid.[20] As whispers got round that someone was showing symptoms of the disease, panicked villagers skirted round the house of the infected victim. For many, however, it was too late – they had already been infected, and had carried the sickness home, to their children, wives and husbands, completely unawares. We can only imagine the fear with which people went about their daily lives, as friends, neighbours and relatives fell ill without warning or apparent reason. If a session of the manorial court took place in September, it was not recorded; perhaps Augustine the clerk was an early casualty. On 20th October, however, the court records resumed. The villagers reported that twelve villein men and two villein women had died, all from Kington, Morton and Oldbury – the cluster of hamlets that straddled the creek. Although the epidemic had yet to show its full force, this was already seven or so more deaths than could be expected in a normal year. The villagers had every reason to be terrified. As a precaution, they decided to elect three reeves and three beadles, instead of the usual single nominee for each post. Thomas Thurstan, John Marsh and Richard Fortheye were duly selected as reeves and Richard Mason, Walter Sanford and Robert Andrew as beadles.

The worst fears of the Thornbury villagers were to be confirmed in the month that followed. When the surviving tenants met again, on 24th November, they heard officially what they already knew: that the pestilence had now spread to the hamlets on either side of the

Bristol–Gloucester road. Whether they had been infected from Thornbury or from passers-by mattered little to those who were now left to try to survive in the aftermath. After each death had been reported, the bailiff would ask if there was a relative to 'enter' the land. This was the official moment of family conveyance. In an average court, with few deaths, there would have been just one or two who needed to make their claim. Not on this November morning, however: death after death was announced. Yet, for all their grief, the tenants were not stunned; they responded, as people would come to do across England, with stoical – ruthless even – pragmatism. One poor villager, John Gibbs, was reported dead; his widow Alice said that she would take on his cottage and four acres of land. Another poor villein, John Fish, said he would take on the house and six acres of Isabel Lynch, who had also died, paying just 6d.[vi] for the land. Thus, although the weekly toll of death was continuing to rise, these people were taking the opportunity to enter land. They were simply betting on their survival – a good bet, given that the investment was cheap and it would matter little if they did not make it.

With so many husbands and wives perishing in the plague, some saw the opportunity for an expedient marriage. Bartholomew Thatcher, who held a house and four acres, died sometime in October or November, leaving his widow Matilda all alone. Barely had his body been carried from his bed to the grave than a certain Thomas Wilcox pledged his troth to Matilda, widowed for still less than a month. The death of Bartholomew and marriage of Matilda were announced at the November court, Wilcox taking on the Thatcher holding by right of his marriage. If this had not set tongues wagging, the manoeuvrings of Robert in the Hale certainly would. Robert had a very substantial holding on the eve of the Great Death – at least eighty acres built up by judicious acquisition over the previous two decades. (Already, this was more than twenty times the size of the holdings just taken on by John Gibbs and Thomas Wilcox.) Yet in this November court Robert stepped forward to say that he was marrying Amice, widow of Robert Theyn, thereby adding another sixty acres, a house and more besides. For this he paid 73s. 4d.[vii] – more

[vi] £0.03.
[vii] £3.67.

than a hundred times the entry fee paid by John Fish. John, Robert and all the others who benefited in this way were taking advantage of the mortality to get hold of land and set themselves up for the future.

Others, however, were keen just to defend their inheritance. Old Edward Willes had been ill for so many years that it will have surprised no one that he had at last died. The death of his son Robert in the same month suggested that – in the end – it was the plague that carried him away. Edward had been a beadle, and his significant position within the manor was indicated by the substantial holding that he left. It was this tenancy that now became the cause of an unpleasant tussle between his younger daughter, Agnes, and his grandson (through Robert) – Walter Pill. The court heard the pleas of each and weighed up the merits of the different claims, before announcing that Walter was to inherit; Agnes was left with nothing. For Agnes, this will have been a considerable loss, coming on top of the sorrows that she – like everyone else – was undoubtedly suffering. Many others, however, left the court in a much-improved position: newly engaged, richer or the proud holder of new land. It had been the longest court session that anyone could remember and, at its end, the complex web of relationships within the village had been recast, reflecting the losses the community had endured and the opportunities its members had already sought to exploit.

With profound grief came immense confusion. All of a sudden, wives who had lost husbands were left to tend their holdings alone. Newly orphaned children were passed from one family to the next, as overburdened relatives took on the duty of their care. Infants were now the unexpected responsibility of grandfathers, who had long forgotten what little they had ever known about caring for a small child. But all of the survivors, from the destitute and dispossessed to the winners of the November court, were at least alive. Continued survival had its own imperative: however profound the grief or great the bewilderment, the daily need for bread and water remained the immediate concern of most of Thornbury's peasant villagers. As we have seen, the security with which peasants could face the future was determined in large part by the size of their landholding. There should be nothing surprising or unseemly, therefore, about the rush for marriages and the arguments over bequests. It is true that for a few villeins such as Robert de la Hale this was an opportunity to enlarge an already impressive landholding. For most, however, the results of the court would determine whether they could expect to survive the Great Death – if they were to survive it – with a secure expectation of food and a basic income. If not, they may well be condemned to a new poverty, one which would in all likelihood bring a slow death from hunger, even if they had escaped the quick kill of the pestilence. This was a stoicism borne of necessity.

There was a corporate interest in survival too, which was why the tenants prepared for the worst by electing treble the number of estate officials than usual. They were wise to do so: of the six officials selected in that special October court, three had already died. It was a rate of mortality consistent with the deaths of tenants across the manor. By the court held on 15th December, with pestilence still raging strong, ninety-four of Thornbury's tenants – 40 per cent of the manor's tenantry – were dead. There is every reason to believe that this figure will have been repeated amongst the freemen, their families and the kin of the villeins too. It was an almost incredible death toll.

Just as Thornbury had been infected by some little boat going from inlet to inlet along the Severn estuary, so in the same way the disease travelled south along the southern shore of the Bristol Channel. By the end of November, it had moved west through Somerset from Portishead, Clevedon and Weston-super-Mare to the inlets headed by Bridgwater and Barnstaple in north Devon. Infected almost all at once, these little harbours then spread their deadly import inland. Just as it crept out from Bristol, going north, to Thornbury and beyond, the epidemic also edged south, towards the area of infection already established in Dorset, which had by now spread west into Devon almost as far as Exeter and east to the border of Hampshire. A thin sliver of uninfected ground separated these two 'fronts', in the middle of which was the bishop of Bath and Well's manor of Evercreech.[viii] It was from here that Ralph Shrewsbury had sent his letter commanding prayers in mid-August, unaware at the time that the pestilence had already reached England. By the end of the following month, however, the scale of the epidemic was all too apparent. He made the short

---

[viii] Just eight miles east of Glastonbury and almost midway between the abbey and the Deverill villages just over the county border in Wiltshire.

journey to his cathedral city of Wells (separated from Bristol only by the Mendips) then moved on to his other diocesan seat at Bath,[ix] staying there until the end of October. Then suddenly he disappeared. In a normal year, Bishop Ralph would spend the autumn touring his diocese, but he appears instead to have left Bath at the beginning of November and made straight for his most distant and remote manor house, at Wiveliscombe, tucked beyond Taunton on the edge of Exmoor. It was fortunate that he had done so, for on 19th November he had to approve the institution of a new rector to the church at Evercreech, the former priest having died a few weeks before. The pestilence had thus moved from Bristol into the middle of Somerset almost as soon as he had left it; indeed this may even have been the reason for his hasty exit from Bath.

The patron of Evercreech was the hospital of St John the Baptist in Wells, founded by one of Bishop Ralph's predecessors. There were soon troubles here too. The prior died some time in 1348, most probably another victim of the epidemic: the disease had killed other brothers and soon there were no more than two remaining to care for the sick. As the number of brethren had fallen below the quorum required to elect a new prior, Bishop Ralph was forced to impose a nominee. Evercreech and Wells formed the centre of a diseased crescent, separated from Longbridge and Monkton Deverill, which lay to the east, by only a little over ten miles of ground and the screen of Selwood Forest. Hardington, to the north-west of the Deverills, lost its priest around Christmas. Mells, another Glastonbury property, was fast losing tenants.[21] Then there was Castle Cary, where the incumbent died about a fortnight after his colleague at neighbouring Evercreech. Further south in Yeovil, a new rector – Hugh de Rissingdone – was appointed on 18th December; his predecessor could equally easily have been a victim of the Dorset epidemic stretching north or the Bristol infection stretching south. In any event, it seems that it was at this point that the two fronts of the epidemic met, separating uninfected Devon and Cornwall from the rest of as yet healthy England. It was here too that the encirclement of Longbridge and Monkton was completed. Like a noose drawn tight, so the disease closed round the terrified villagers, who – had not the plague already arrived by

[ix] To his manor of Claverton.

Christmas – cannot have been in any doubt as to what awaited them in the New Year.[22]

The atmosphere at Edward's court could not have been more different, where Christmas was celebrated with merry abandon. The royal family were the guests of the new archbishop of Canterbury, John Ufford, at the archiepiscopal palace at Otford in Kent. The lavishness of the great feast matched that of the previous year's extravaganza. Edward's entourage was dressed in tunics of green and red, threaded with gold, their faces covered by masks with painted male and female faces, crowned with lions' and elephants' heads, bats' wings or the heads of 'wodewoses' – wildmen. Into this bizarre mêlée the king himself rode, horse and rider wearing a matching ensemble all spangled with silver. The king bore a shield emblazoned with one of his several enigmatic mottoes: 'Hay hay the wythe swan, by goddess soule I am the man.'[x]

Edward evidently felt that he deserved his fun and games, for he too had had his share of travails that autumn. Hard on the bitter news of Princess Joan's death, with which the long-negotiated Castilian alliance had also deceased, Edward had received word that another key ally, the oligarch confederation of Flanders, had collapsed. Louis de Mâle, count of Flanders and exile in the French court, had launched a successful raid into the Low Countries and by the middle of September controlled most of the principal towns. This was a serious blow for Edward, although not as great as it could have been: had it happened a year earlier, the Flemish upheaval would have denied Edward his only safe point of entry onto the Continent. Now, at least, he had a firm base of his own – Calais. But here too the French had been causing problems, instigated in the main by the redoubtable captain, Geoffrey de Chargny. Forced to stall for time, Edward had arranged a temporary truce with the Count of Eu,[xi] one of the king's French hostages, before the earl of Lancaster was despatched to Calais with William Bateman, the bishop of Norwich, to treat more formally with the French. There they sat protected, swapping points

[x] 'Hay, hay the white swan, by God's soul I am the man.' The 'white swan' has been reputed to be the Countess of Salisbury, whom Jean Le Bel accused Edward of raping in 1342. The motto would later be appropriated by the dukes of Lancaster.
[xi] The Constable of France. The truce was signed in London at the agreement of Philip VI and Edward III on 13th September 1348.

of difference with their French counterparts, who were ensconced just down the coast in the castle of Boulogne. At the same time, English diplomats opened negotiations with the new Flemish regime, aiming to bring the Low Countries into alliance with England again. Back across the Channel, Edward made great show of preparing to do battle: on 8th October he sent out orders for a muster of troops at Sandwich in twenty days' time, a proclamation that was read aloud throughout London within twenty-four hours. Two weeks later the king announced that he would sail from Sandwich in person and instructions were sent out to the bishops to order prayers for a successful campaign. On 29th October the warrior king led his throng of troops through the prosperous streets of Sandwich, between the tall timber-framed merchant houses, onto the waiting vessels, and set sail. So while the diplomats spoke softly, Edward wielded a big stick. The ploy worked: the French agreed terms on 13th November, promising to pursue a permanent peace in March the following year. Not a month later, on 4th December, Edward's ambassadors then delivered their *coup de grâce*: a meeting in Dunkirk with Louis de Mâle, now fully in control of his county of Flanders, at which a secret treaty of peace and possible alliance was signed by both men. Lancaster and Bateman had pulled a diplomatic triumph from the set-backs of late summer. Edward returned to England and had paused in London only to ratify the treaty, which he signed within the walls of the Tower. Then, on 10th December he had made straight for Otford, eager for the festivities to begin.

It was precisely the peace 'between Christian countries' for which Ralph Shrewsbury had ordered prayers back in August. By the same mandate the bishop had also prayed that God send 'healthy air' and 'turn away his people from this pestilence',[23] reminding his congregation of God's mercy on the people of Nineveh, who had been spared because – quoting the prophet Jonah – they had 'turned from their evil way'.[24] Unlike Nineveh, however, England's fate was already sealed. Shrewsbury seems to have anticipated as much. For the passage he quoted from Jonah follows immediately the account of how the men of Nineveh had been led in repentance by their king, who had covered himself with a sackcloth and sat in ashes, declaring a fast throughout his city in an appeal to God's mercy. But the king of Nineveh was conspicuous by his absence from the bishop's letter. The implication was clear: far from seeking to assuage God's anger in the hope that plague might be averted, Edward had indulged in tournaments. Had the terrified inhabitants of the Deverills and of Gloucester known of the frivolities of the king's Christmas celebrations, they too may have noted a similar contrast.

4

Colonial Ireland

October 1348–May 1349

Ich am of Irlaunde,
And of the holy londe
Of Irlande.

Gode sire, pray ich thee,
For of sainte charite,
Come and daunce wit me
In Irlaunde.

Anonymous[1]

The monastery of St Mullins, which for more than 700 years had watched over a bend in the River Barrow, had never seen such crowds. Hordes of pilgrims had come to this ancient place, each wading thigh-deep upstream in the quick-flowing waters of the little tributary that led down from the monastery to the river. They were all making their way to the tiny stone hut that sat atop the opening of the brook. On reaching the submerged threshold, each would enter through the low doorway that framed the stream. Inside the dank room, the pilgrim faced a stone wall, pierced at head-height with a hole about the width of a span. Water gushed from this hole into a small pool in the floor. One at a time, the pilgrims put their hands into the water, splashed their faces, crossed themselves, perhaps even kissed the well-head itself. Their sanctifying ablutions complete, they moved towards the exit, urged on by the impatient devotees behind. Emerging into the daylight the pilgrim could look down on the stream-full of people, snaking its way up to the well. It was a mixed crowd: mighty and humble, holy and penitent. Trudging up the stream was all part of this watery rite, so nothing was to be gained from jumping the queue. Most were peasants and labourers who had walked in from the surrounding manors, but others amongst them had come from further afield: priests and monks, the occasional noble and perhaps even a bishop. Some mouthed prayers alone in their approach, others further back chatted: there was little English mixed amongst their soft Gaelic tones.

It was the same every day through September and October 1348: hundreds, sometimes thousands, seeking protection from the plague that was already well-established in nearby ports.[2] Those unfortunate enough to see someone struck down with the disease reported how the victim 'died of boils, abscesses and pustules which erupted on the legs and in the armpits'.[3] It was natural, therefore, that people sought the protection of St Mullin,[i] who was cured of skin ulcers when he walked against the current up to the well he had built to supply his monastery. Others with similar ailments had since been restored to health. The pilgrims hoped that these holy waters might act as a prophylactic against this unknown disease, which manifested itself on the skin of its victims too. The chronicler who records all this makes it quite plain that the pilgrims were there because of 'their fear of plague';[4] by implication there were none who were as yet showing any signs of the disease. Yet in the midst of the queues and crowds of penitents there were some who were already infected, even though they seemed perfectly well. Unwittingly, these votaries of St Mullin were spreading pestilence all around; their fellow pilgrims were not to know that the feared contagion was already moving among them.

The Great Death travelled to Ireland through commerce. The island was very much on the periphery of European trading networks, but its commercial links were nonetheless strong and well-established. The Vikings had founded trading stations long before the Anglo-Norman entry into Ireland in 1169: they had built Dublin and Wexford on the east coast, Waterford and Cork on the south and Limerick in the west. Whilst the Vikings had not attempted to conquer Ireland's forbidding interior, for their Norman cousins this was the principal object of their invasion. The pioneering barons carved out huge patrimonies from

---

[i] Anglicized from St Moling.

their newly won territory, dividing them into manors just as in their home estates in England and Wales. Whilst agriculture was not new to Ireland, the creation of a manorial economy brought a huge increase in production, delivering a quantity of produce far greater than the domestic market could possibly consume. The colonists established new ports for their possessions, the better to sell their surpluses overseas: to the old Norse settlements were added Carrickfergus on the eastern coast of Ulster, Dundalk and Drogheda north of Dublin, New Ross and Youghal on either side of Waterford, and Galway in western Connacht, to the north of Limerick. Except for Carrickfergus and Dundalk, all of these towns (Norse and English) sat at the mouths of rivers – the Boyne, Liffey, Slaney, Barrow, Nore, Suir, Blackwater, Lee and Shannon – each bringing the fruits of inland manors to the coast for export abroad.

Trade was principally with England. Most goods were sent to Bristol but Chester had strong links too, as it gave better access to Coventry and the cluster of Midlands towns that surrounded it. By the end of the thirteenth century, vast quantities of grain were carried across the Irish Sea. However, increasing disorder during the first decades of the fourteenth century reduced the shipment of grain, to the point where Ireland was no longer a net exporter of agricultural produce. Other than timber and fish, the bulk of exports now consisted of products of the (far older) pastoral economy: hides, coarse wool and the hardy Irish mantles that were so famous at the time. Nonetheless, there were still merchants, government officials, nobles and senior clerics in Ireland, all of whom retained an appetite for the kind of luxuries that could only be imported from overseas: cloth from Flanders, spices from the Orient, and wine from Bordeaux. Ireland also lacked the more workaday things that the colony required, so iron was brought from Galicia and salt transported from the Bay of Bourgneuf in Brittany. Much of this import trade came via London or Bristol but the largest Irish ports – New Ross, Dublin and Waterford – enjoyed direct trading links with the Continent. Indeed, Dublin and Waterford maintained European connections that dated back to their occupation by mercantile Vikings more than three centuries before.

The extent of these trading connections is revealed in a court action of 1319. In that year Thomas Mustard, a merchant of Bristol, sent his agent Walter atte Strode of Waterford to Bordeaux by boat, carrying wool worth £100. He was instructed to exchange the wool for wine and to purchase additional stock for cash. Unfortunately, Walter died in Bordeaux before he had completed Thomas's business; Thomas, therefore, had to sue for the return of his goods and went to Bordeaux to prosecute his case. He soon found a merchant from Waterford who had seen Walter selling the wool and who was able to vouch for the fact that Walter was acting on Thomas's behalf. Thomas also called on the evidence of one of Walter's acquaintances, who also hailed from Waterford. He stated that it was well-known that Walter was working for Thomas; he himself had discussed how business was going with Walter on a number of occasions. This little court case demonstrates how, at one moment in 1319, there were at least three merchants from Waterford in Bordeaux, all of whom knew each other. One of them was trading via Bristol, engaged in a three-way exchange that extended over 1,500 miles. There was nothing unusual in what these men were doing: their activities were so normal as to enjoy the regulation of civil law. It is a remarkable statement about the degree to which the Anglo-Irish colony was integrated into the networks of international trade, a commercial milieu in which these Waterford merchants mixed freely and with ease.

Thomas Mustard's original intention may well have been to ship his consignment of wine to Dublin, as the administrative capital of Ireland was also its greatest consumer of claret. Dublin was Ireland's largest city and yet, by English and Continental standards, it was relatively small. Its walled area enclosed only forty-four acres – roughly a fifth of a square kilometre. Indeed, this space was too small even for Dublin's modest population. Many Dubliners lived outside the walls along the roads that ran out from the city centre. At most the city and these suburbs had an extended population of 25,000, certainly no more than modern-day Drogheda or Dundalk. They were more tightly packed, however. Beggars and hucksters, labourers and traders, clerics, nobles and merchants: the whole array of urban life thronged the streets, beneath a gabled skyline pierced by the towers and spires of the many stone churches – Christ Church Cathedral rising chief amongst them. To the casual eye it was a typical, if rather down-at-heel, medium-sized English town but to the keen ear a clear difference was detectable: for here West Country and Welsh accents mixed with spoken Gaelic, betraying the unusual jumble that was Dublin's population and the unusual nature of this city.

Dublin had suffered from the decline in the Irish grain trade, a situation made worse by the silting of the Liffey in its final approach toward the sea, forcing larger boats to dock elsewhere. The downturn was palpable: at the turn of the century well over a thousand tuns of wine had been imported by Dubliners every year, most of it destined for distribution within the colony. By the 1340s, however, little more than a tenth of that quantity was being brought in.[5] Nonetheless, there was still demand for wine within the city and so a few large ships continued to make the journey from Gascony, up the eastern Irish seaboard and round Dalkey Island into Dublin Bay. The bay was embraced by two promontories: Dalkey Head and Howth Head. Ships with deeper draughts, now unable to proceed into Dublin itself, had to drop anchor by one of these headlands and unload their cargoes into riverine barges for transport into the city. There was nothing remotely unusual, therefore, about the ship that moored in Dublin Bay some time in July 1348. Like Thomas Mustard's intended shipment, it had probably sailed direct from Bordeaux.[6] Before anything could be unloaded, however, the crew lowered several sick seamen into a tender, and they were then ferried to land to die. So it was here, in a little

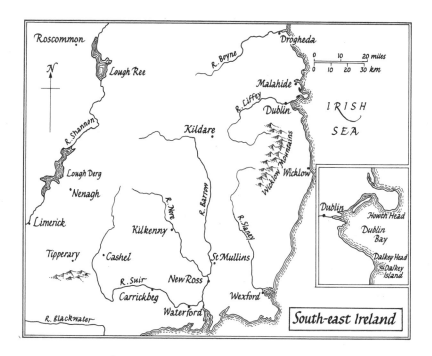

fishing village overlooking Dublin Bay, that the pestilence claimed its first victim on Irish soil.[7]

Very soon the small communities on both sides of the bay had been struck with plague. At Dalkey, almost as soon as news had gone round that pestilence had arrived, the little Celtic church of St Begnet started receiving the victims. The speed with which people died would have been as shocking as the number. Death was always present, unpredictable and capricious, yet – accidents aside – was more often lingering, not least because illnesses which today require only simple medication were then the cause of gradual debilitation and a drawn-out demise. Such a slow end was not altogether unwelcome, however: the unforeseen and hasty death was greatly feared, as the expectation of salvation depended to an important degree on the manner in which the Christian exited this life for the next. Preparation was all, therefore, and planning often began, just as now, long before the end threatened.

If a will were required and none had been written up, then it could be dictated to the priest, who was probably the only literate person in the village. The medieval will was concerned with both spiritual and material bequests: the testator would first bequeath their soul to God, requesting the intercession of the Virgin Mary and maybe a favourite saint; a place of burial would be chosen, and prayers sought from those left behind. Only then, after the soul and body had been legally disposed of, would a statement be made as to the distribution of worldly goods. Whilst the testator was able to make preparations for their absence from this world, as death neared, they placed themselves in the hands of the church, whose duty it was to prepare the dying for their journey to the next. First the priest would encourage his parishioner to meditate on a Crucifix, hung on the wall of his room within sight of the deathbed. For the faithful believer, the contemplation of Christ's Passion, preceding as it did the joy of His Resurrection, would have been a moment of great comfort. A contemporary mystic, Brother Peter of Farne, described the meditation on the Crucifixion like this:

> Thus do mothers in their tender love for their little ones. When they see them afar off, and would have them run quickly back, they straightway stretch wide their arms and bow their head, and the children, taught by nature and eager for kisses, run and leap into their mother's embrace.[8]

When death was close, the priest would hear a final confession and make a final absolution. The performance of penance, upon which full absolution depended, was expected in Purgatory. Then, taking a phial of holy oil, the priest anointed the forehead of the dying penitent. It was a ritual cleansing, recalling the gift of myrrh at Christ's Nativity and His embalming after death. Just as the oil of chrism, applied at baptism, proclaimed life but was a reminder of death, this deliberately symmetrical ritual announced death with the promise of eternal life. Finally, the priest would administer the *viaticum*, bread transubstantiated as the Body of Christ in the Mass now given as – literally – 'one for the road'. It was the last of the three sacraments given to the dying, the reception of which was the earnest wish of every Christian. The church proclaimed its power to open the gates of Heaven to the baptized faithful: the ritual of confession, extreme unction and last communion was the fulfilment of that promise. The pestilence generated such horror in large part because it so often robbed men and women of this sanctified death. The priest of Dalkey must have been frantic with visiting the dying: too lengthy a final confession with one person may well deprive another of their Last Rites. Worse still, even for those whom a priest could be found, their ability to make confession, receive anointment and take the *viaticum* was often horrifically impaired, as so often they 'died in a frenzy, brought on by an affliction of the head or vomiting blood'.[9]

When pestilence had taken its victim (anointed or not) the deceased was sown up in a shroud – a ritual clothing that was appropriately undertaken by a woman. Thus the dying had been cared for by family or neighbours, ministered to by a priest and prepared for interment. These final contacts were well-meaning, indeed essential; they were also almost certainly fatal. John Clyn, a Franciscan friar of Kilkenny, explained how 'the pestilence was so contagious that those who touched the dead or the sick were immediately infected themselves and died, so that penitent and confessor were carried together to the grave'. So the disease was passed on: to surviving sailors, to the bargemen who conveyed the ship's goods to Dublin, to those who had tended the first victims of the disease. They in turn took the pestilence with them, to their families and the communities around. Thus, from person to person, it was not long before the plague had taken hold in Drogheda and – not far at all from Dalkey and Howth – in Dublin.[10]

There were the same flu-like fevers, the pustules and the boils. Many went home to die, closed their doors to neighbours, even to their family. Those who wished for company were frequently disappointed: as Friar Clyn related, 'because of their fear and horror, men could hardly bring themselves to perform the pious and charitable acts of visiting the sick and burying the dead'. It was a hellish scene. Clyn noted that 'since the beginning of the world it has been unheard of for so many people to die of pestilence, famine or other infirmity in such a short time.' It is no wonder that he considered 'that the whole world is encompassed by evil'.[11] How could it have seemed otherwise, when the grief-stricken were all of a sudden torn as to whether they should go through with even the smallest dignities for their recently dead?

In this way the Great Death made its rapid entry into Ireland. In all probability, the disease attacked several Irish ports, almost simultaneously. To these it came, if not directly from Bordeaux, then from Bristol or by coastal transport and fishing fleets that went out from Drogheda and the two towns of Dublin Bay. New Ross – and by implication Waterford too – were infected early enough to encourage the mass pilgrimage to St Mullins. By late autumn 1348, the pestilence had got firm footholds in the east and south-east of the island. Where there was as yet no infection, rumour preceded contagion. In truth, no exaggeration of the disease was possible, so those who had only heard of what was threatened had little less to fear than those who had seen the symptoms for themselves. Spurred on by witness or mere rumour, they flocked to St Mullins to seek protection from the horrors of the plague. There too they mixed, prayed and fretted together. Unseen, the phantom thread of pestilence wove its way between them. They went out from St Mullins in the belief that they were now in the safekeeping of the saint. They had in fact exposed themselves to infection. Tragically unaware, the pilgrims took the pestilence back with them to the scattered villages and towns of Leinster whence they had come.

In October 1999 the banks of the River Ward at Windmill Lands, Swords, between Malahide and Dublin, were eroded by particularly heavy flooding, leaving what appeared to be human bones protruding from the ground. Excavation revealed five bodies – three women, a pre-term foetus and a newborn baby – all dumped together, hastily and apparently without ritual. For all the time that had passed, it was still a pathetic sight. The covering of midden material contained coins and pottery fragments indicating that the bodies were deposited – at the latest – in the early fourteenth century. This could not be a plague-pit then, as it predated the Great Death's arrival in Ireland. Nor is it likely that these were the victims of famine: no matter how poor, they would have been buried in consecrated ground. This grave pit was, in all likelihood, evidence of the mayhem that was rife in much of colonial Ireland throughout the fourteenth century.

Swords was a typical Anglo-Irish manor, of the model imported by English lords to eastern Ireland in the early thirteenth century. It was owned by the archbishop of Dublin (who held nearly a quarter of all the land in County Dublin), was cultivated in large part by unfree Gaelic Irish villeins (called 'betaghs'), and produced staple cereal grains in a three-field rotation. There will have been a large surplus from the considerable portion of the manor that was farmed directly as demesne – a surplus sold, no doubt, in the market at Dublin. The bodies in the river bank give the lie to this picture of manorial stability, however. Although Swords possessed all the apparatus of the English manor, it was a world away from Thornbury or the Deverills. Swords sat in an Anglo-Irish pocket of eastern Ireland, one that had once extended into the centre of the island but which now comprised little more than a vulnerable exclave, with Dublin at its centre. Although Dublin was the administrative centre of the Anglo-Irish colony, it had become virtually besieged by the Gaelic Irish. They came from all sides but attacked principally from the Wicklow Mountains in the south. From there they descended to plunder at will; as soon as the colonists had brought a force together to repulse them, they fled back to the mountains' craggy sanctuary. As a result, the villages that lay around Dublin were being deserted: Dalkey failed to render any burgage rents in 1326 because of the deprivations caused by the Gaelic Irish, while at Boly Minor (hard by the archbishop of Dublin's palace at St Sepulchre) the betaghs did not dare to stay in their houses at night for fear of attack. The year before at Tallaght, another of the archbishop's manors, it was reported that the tenants were leaving owing to Irish attacks; much of the land in his more distant manors of Clondalkin, Rathcoole and Ballymore Eustace was in the hands of the Gaelic Irish, whilst the estate around Castlekevin, in the middle of Wicklow, had long been deserted by its Anglo-Irish settlers. So serious were the attacks in the immediate vicinity of the city that in 1319 and 1334 the mayor and commonalty requested a reduction in the taxes they owed to the crown, on account of the repeated burning of the suburbs by the Irish.

The never-ending violence around Dublin begat constant troubles for its inhabitants. The supply of food from surrounding manors was disrupted; manorial incomes declined; rents inside the city were depressed. In short, Gaelic Irish attacks had succeeded in crippling Dublin's economy – as was so clearly evinced by the poor fortunes of the once vibrant wine trade. Worse still, Gaelic incursions and attacks meant that Dublin had become cut off from that (larger) part of the colony that lay to the south and south-west. In 1340 the justiciar (the king's vicegerent in Ireland) complained that merchants could no longer make the overland journey to Kilkenny for fear of being set upon.[ii] The situation deteriorated to such an extent that in 1345 the Exchequer and Common Bench were removed by royal mandate from Dublin, as the city had become utterly isolated from much of the portion of Ireland it was meant to control. Deprived of its administrative purpose, its trading life withered, and so much land around the city reduced to abandoned waste, Dublin's colonial *raison d'être* had, by 1348, been battered away.

Dublin and its manors were not alone in suffering from the Gaelic Irish menace. All over Ireland, the colonial lordships were being riven one from another. The Anglo-Irish colony, laid down so swiftly in the latter part of the twelfth century and consolidated so surely in the thirteenth had, by the middle of the fourteenth century, been reduced by the resurgent Gaelic Irish to four settler enclaves. There was Dublin and Drogheda, with the troubled hinterland of Meath and Kildare, to the north of which lay Ulster, only the very eastern portion of which was in Anglo-Irish possession (and this more closely resembled a marcher outpost than a successful colony). On the west coast was the remnant of colonial Limerick, and in south Leinster there were the fertile estates of Kilkenny between the Barrow and the Suir, reaching

[ii] Named as Ossory, the ancient kingdom of south-west Leinster which had Kilkenny at its centre.

north from New Ross and Waterford into Tipperary. This latter part was the largest of all four enclaves, and by far the richest. Unsurprisingly, the manors here presented juicy targets for the Gaelic Irish neighbours, the strongest of whom were the MacMurrough hereditary kings of Leinster.[iii] Anthony de Lucy, one of the few justiciars to attempt to get a grip on the deepening crisis, had tried to bring the MacMurroughs under control, proffering the carrot of payments whilst wielding the stick of excommunication and fines. The landowners also tried a similar ploy, buying off the Irish to gain a modicum of peace: Lady Elizabeth de Burgh's[iv] steward on her manor of Lisronagh, for instance, paid for the 'protection' of Richard Tobin rather than fighting him off. In the long run, however, none of these were sustainable strategies. No matter what threats the Anglo-Irish made, the native Irish still coveted what they did not control, whilst collusion in Gaelic Irish protection rackets served only to encourage the very behaviour that the colonists wished to prevent. The native Irish, whom the colonists had once sought to overrun and completely suppress, were now insurgent; for the first time in centuries Anglo-Ireland was receding.

The behaviour of the colonists did as much damage to the colony as did the wounding Gaelic Irish attacks. Some of the more fractious Anglo-Irish nobles displayed the same flexible loyalties and unpredictability as could their Irish opponents. A prime culprit was Maurice fitz Thomas FitzGerald, the 1st earl of Desmond, who during the 1330s and 1340s allied his private army with that of the Gaelic Irish strongman of Thomond, Brian O'Brien,[v] terrorising settlers from Limerick across to Waterford. For all his bluster about becoming the king of Ireland, the earl of Desmond was no more than an old-fashioned marcher baron, of the kind that had caused such trouble to Edward III's father and grandfather in Wales: jealous of his rights as an independent lord, he resented any interference from the officials of the colonial administration. Wary of stirring up a situation in Ireland whilst preoccupied

---

[iii] Anglicized from Mac Murchadha.

[iv] Lady Elizabeth de Burgh (1332–63), daughter and sole heir of William de Burgh, 3rd earl of Ulster. She is not to be confused with Lady Elizabeth de Clare (1295–1360), who owned extensive lands in England and Wales and was sometimes known by the same name.

[v] Anglicized from Brian Ó Briain.

with France, Edward III did almost nothing – a brutal piece of *Realpolitik*, the subtleties of which the English settlers were unlikely to appreciate. Desmond's actions were particularly disruptive, yet even the most loyal Anglo-Irish nobles found it hard to focus all their energies on their native enemy. Fulk de la Freigne, a warrior knight in the service of the earl of Ormond, had served on the justiciar's privy council and participated in the siege of Calais. He was one of the Tobin clan's most successful adversaries, expelling them from Tipperary in 1344, and during July and August 1348 – just as the pestilence was creeping along the east coast – he recaptured Nenagh, a feat that – according to Friar Clyn – 'everyone had thought impossible'.[12] But just a decade before, de la Freigne had been languishing with his son Oliver in Kilkenny Castle, having been imprisoned by the royal seneschal after a family feud threatened to spread anarchy throughout Kilkenny. Thus, even this stalwart of the settler nobility could not boast an unblemished record of service in support of the colony.

Anglo-Irish sparring exacerbated the effects of Gaelic Irish raids, making lawlessness endemic and hastening the depopulation of out-lying manors. On the extensive de Burgh estates in Tipperary and Meath, the tenants were deserting their holdings through the 1340s, giving up their land just as the tenants of the archbishop of Dublin had done twenty years before. Lady Elizabeth's steward eventually had to lease much of her estate, as did the earl of Kildare. The widespread withdrawal from direct farming reflected an increasing reluctance on the part of English landlords to spend time in Ireland, or at the very least maintain a staff on their Irish estates, leaving a vacuum in local power that the Gaelic Irish were more than happy to fill. Absenteeism became neglect, exposing colonial land to recovery by the Gaelic Irish. Thus, as at Grean (Co. Limerick) in 1331, much demesne and betagh lands rendered little or nothing because they had been overrun by the Irish. In many places, it only took the threat of Irish incursions to make colonial agriculture impossible, as the earl of Ormond had found earlier in the century: he lost his land in Tipperary for good, because 'no one dared to lease them'.

As the dramatic fall in exports out of the colony's coastal ports bore testimony, declining agriculture entailed a decline in trade. Inevitably, all of this soon fed through to the cash revenues generated by the crown, which experienced a substantial drop in the first half of the fourteenth century, both from its own lands in the colony and from the receipts of customs and taxes levied on the colonists.[13] For the first time in a century, the colony found itself barely able to cover its own costs. It was a far cry from the lordship of Edward I, when Ireland had been a rich and stable source of both supplies and revenue. Ultimately, the fault for the pitiable state of the colony lay at the crown's feet. For while feudalism could be an effective tool of colonization, devolving as it did police and judicial powers to a small cohort of barons who shared an interest with the crown in keeping the peace, to be effective the colonization had to be complete. Indeed, this was the most important lesson that the first Norman king of England, William the Conqueror, had taught. Subsequent Anglo-Normans had failed to follow his example in Ireland and as resistance to their presence increased, the distractions of the other frontiers in Wales, Scotland and France drew them away. The results of such negligence revealed themselves in good time; for what had once been a prized and profitable possession became, both for the crown and for landlords, an embarrassing encumbrance.

Ireland could never be abandoned by the English, however: not only would an exit have been an insufferable blow to the prestige of the crown, but it was still felt that this island that had once returned such a bounty must still be capable of doing so again. Indeed, it was the financial pressure of funding the war in France that eventually forced Edward to think anew on the problems that afflicted his lordship of Ireland (a sure demonstration of the interrelationship of the crown's several fragile frontiers). In 1341 Edward III demanded that the colony make the same returns that his father had enjoyed. The king decreed, moreover, that all crown officials should hold either lands or benefices in England, as it was thought this would make their loyalty to the crown much more certain. The reaction in the colony was predictable, and that distance which permitted the king to act with such magisterial insouciance also afforded the colonists the ability to be more than a little blunt in their reply. The opportunity came at the parliament at Kilkenny in October that year. To the primary charge that all king's officials should retain connections with England, the colonists angrily rejoined that it was precisely because of their English interests that so many ministers were absent from their posts in Ireland. The king's English ministers, they protested, treated their positions as sinecures. The colonists railed against the king's justiciars: they knew nothing of warfare, a necessity in a land of war. On that point, the Anglo-Irish had specific recommendations: life would be far easier, they suggested, if the king maintained his castles and kept them properly garrisoned. The anger of the colonists was hardly synthetic: the king had questioned their loyalty and had singularly failed to understand their predicament – a great part of which, they insinuated, was the direct result of the policies of the crown. Edward saw that there was nothing to profit from an attempt to counter the settlers' arguments, so he made a decorous withdrawal.

The following year, 1342, the citizens of Cork pleaded for relief from their rents, as none could be collected owing to the raids by the Irish. Predictably, the earl of Desmond was behind the trouble (this time he was in league with the MacCarthys[vi]) and was once again entertaining notions of becoming High King of Ireland. Yet although the new justiciar, Ralph d'Ufford, moved against Desmond in 1344 and made him an outlaw the following year, there was no concerted campaign to bring the earl to heel, nor any attempt to remove his powerbase. In Ireland, everything seemed to be turned on its head. The English settlers of Cork, who were amongst those who had made representations at Kilkenny, received no royal protection – despite their suffering – from men like the earl of Desmond, who behaved like the worst of Gaelic Irish brigands and yet escaped punishment because of their Anglo-Norman pedigree. In the end, Edward ignored them both. Cork – bourgeois, law-abiding and tax-paying; the earl of Desmond – aristocratic, anarchic and destructive: the Anglo-Irish, of whatever ilk, were once again to be left to themselves. It was a dangerous policy, not least because it added a degree of cultural separation to the geographical divide already enforced by the Irish Sea. As a consequence, the Anglo-Irish colonists – whether they had pulled hard away from mother England or had been rudely pushed – all now felt a common sense of divorce. For when in 1341 the Kilkenny parliament claimed that 'the land of Ireland stands on the point of being lost from the hands of the king of England', the Anglo-Irish were not just referring to the efforts of the Gaelic Irish kings. 'At no previous time', they went on 'had there been such a remarkable and overt division between

[vi] Anglicized from Mac Carthaigh.

the English born in England and the English born in Ireland.' The colony was less than 150 years old and yet already, between native Ireland and Anglo-Norman England, a new nation was being forged in the fires of adversity.

On Palm Sunday, 1348,[vii] three months before the arrival of plague in Dublin Bay, a rumour whipped round Toulon that the Jews were responsible for the pestilence that was spreading through the city. The vengeful mob made its way to the Jewish quarter, sacked it, and murdered forty Jews in their homes. There were similar (but unconnected) incidents in Barcelona and other Catalan towns. By July, the victimization of Jews had taken on a more organized form: in Dauphiné they were accused of poisoning the wells and fountains, thereby causing the spread of the pestilence among Christians. The charge had been levelled before. In 1321 Jews across France were accused of poisoning wells, in league with lepers. There were show trials, massacres and burnings; those lepers that survived were shut in colonies whilst the Jews that escaped murder were expelled. As a result, the Jewish community in France was much depleted by 1348, which perversely limited the persecution they suffered during the plague. Tragically, this was not to be the case elsewhere. Where they had not been expelled, Jews were still excluded from most livelihoods, except money-lending. Usury had long been condemned by the church but the Jews were expressly exempted from this prohibition. Although this gave Jewish communities an important role in the expanding European economy, it defined and further reinforced their moral separation from the rest of society. There was thus official sanction for the prejudices and petty jealousies that were directed at the Jews, who also attracted the inevitable resentment of failed or aggrieved debtors. Like the leper, the Jew had become a scorned outsider; unlike lepers, the Jews were now a necessity, as they could not be removed without losing the credit they provided. The Jews found themselves, therefore, in an invidious position: they were hated but needed, and were thus suspected of somehow having a 'hold' over people, fears that easily transmogrified into a ready belief in the myths that for centuries had adhered to Jews across Europe: the blood libel (the ritual killing and cannibalism of children), deicide

[vii] Sunday, 13th April 1348.

(the heretical accusation that only the Jews had murdered Christ), and well-poisoning. All of this made Jewish communities particularly vulnerable in times of general civil disquiet. Suspicions found a public voice as anti-semitic legends were regurgitated, leading to attacks on Jewish communities. This violence was frequently a proxy for wider protest, not least because those that depended on the usury of the Jews – the 'ruling' classes of merchants and nobility – were themselves often deeply unpopular. It was for this reason that the city authorities of Cologne wrote to the burghers of Strasbourg in January 1349, warning that a massacre of the Jews arising from the 'rage the common people feel against the Jews' might well precipitate a 'popular revolt'.[14]

For these city burghers the threat of a pogrom was a matter of public order; for the pope it was a source of great moral concern. Clement VI, who was unusually sympathetic to this afflicted community, was so exercised at the mounting accounts of persecution of Jews that he reissued the ancient bull *Sicut Judæis*, which brought the Jews 'under the shield' of the papacy's protection. The mandate, formulated first by Gregory the Great in 598 in defence of Jewish worship, was frequently repeated and expanded by medieval pontiffs. Clement's form of the bull prohibited Christians from committing any act of violence or theft against a Jew, under pain of excommunication. This was the gravest sanction that the church could impose on the faithful, as it caused the sacraments to be withdrawn and the exclusion of the excommunicate from church. In a time of mass mortality, the threat that the Last Rites and a Christian burial might be denied was indeed a serious one. First issued on 5th July 1348, the bull was sent out again in September and October, and was sterner on each occasion. The plague was a punishment sent by God, the pope claimed, inflicted on Christians for their sins. Clement scotched the idea that the Jews had anything to do with the epidemic, pointing to the fact that not only were Jews dying of plague but that the pestilence was also present in England, from where the Jews had been absent since their expulsion by Edward I in 1290. The true criminals, the pontiff averred, were avaricious Christians, who falsely accused the Jews merely in order to get hold of their wealth.

There was much truth in this final allegation, which was why the pope's 'shield' ultimately had little effect.[15] For sure, there were many who genuinely believed the charges of well-poisoning. It is easy to see how credulous citizens – hearing commixed whispers of mortal pestilence and Jewish malevolence – might well be whipped up into a paroxysm of retribution. However, all too often the accusations thrown at the Jews were merely an excuse for people to seize the property of Jewish families with impunity or rid themselves of their debts to Jewish lenders. For many, no doubt, the two motives – fear and greed – existed side by side. For similar reasons, city councils and law officers everywhere turned a blind eye to the bloodshed, fearing the consequences if they were to intervene but conscious of what they might gain from confiscated Jewish property. Their collusion further fanned the flames of persecution: as Clement VI protested, 'while such behaviour goes unopposed it looks as though their error is approved'.[16] Thus, as the plague moved steadily though Savoy, Switzerland and Germany, the butchery of the Jews swept before it. The persecution assumed a life of its own, quite beyond the control of any civil authority or indeed the injunctions of a well-meaning pope. This was now an epidemic in its own right, one which accompanied the first rumours that the plague was about to arrive. Just as the bodily signs of the pestilence had their inevitable, fatal, conclusion, so too did the symptoms of this man-made terror – rumour, suspicion, denunciations, forced confessions – all lead inexorably to the torture-wheel, sword and stake. Thus, by St Valentine's Day, 1349, the Jews of Strasbourg were burning before the complicit eyes of the burghers, despite the strong warnings the town had received from Avignon and Cologne; the number of Jews was so great that it took six days to complete the massacre. The persecution of Jews across Europe had become a holocaust.

The Anglo-Irish port of Dundalk, just below Ulster's eastern bulge, was a natural place for Richard FitzRalph, the new archbishop of Armagh, to deliver his first sermon, on 24th April 1348. Not only was the town midway between the two principal cities of the archdiocese – Drogheda and Armagh – but it was also where the archbishop had been born, nearly fifty years before. FitzRalph had left Dundalk for Oxford in or just before 1315, the year in which the town had been devastated by a Scots invading force. The local boy had since done good: having gone to Oxford in his mid-teens, he had gained a doctorate in theology, studied for a year at Paris and been appointed chancellor of Oxford, all by the age of thirty-two. In 1334 he went to Avignon, where he played an important role in some of the developing theological controversies of the day, leaving to take up the position of dean of Lichfield Cathedral in 1335. Appointed to the archbishopric of Armagh by pope Clement in 1346, FitzRalph did not go to Ireland until he had completed a self-imposed apprenticeship in pastoral work, under the careful tutelage of his patron, John Grandison, the bishop of Exeter. It was nearly two years, therefore, before the new archbishop addressed his expectant flock for the first time, in Dundalk.

FitzRalph's opening words (which he must have considered many times in the months before his arrival) were appropriately dramatic. His sermon would be on the Lord's Prayer, he explained: just as he had now returned to his own people, he would preach on the very first prayer that Jesus had taught the people of *his* own blood, the Jews. It was a striking (if incongruous) statement: not only was the new archbishop identifying himself with the Anglo-Irish community, but he was by implication recognizing their tribulations. There was also a silent paradox in this comparison: much of the early growth of Anglo-Irish ports had been built on Jewish capital, a source of funds extinguished for ever after the Jews were expelled from England and its possessions fifty-eight years before. The outcast Jews may have been a distant memory now but the congregation will have quickly grasped to what end FitzRalph associated the forgotten Anglo-Irish of Dundalk with the despised and rejected Jews.

The Gaelic Irish of Ulster, who dominated FitzRalph's archdiocese, were equally enthusiastic in their reception of the new archbishop. As the successor of St Patrick, the archbishop of Armagh was treated with extraordinary respect in Ireland and especially in Ulster, a reverence that one later traveller would claim verged on that usually reserved for a pope. This had afforded archbishops of Armagh past – whether they were Irish or English – the power of peacemaker between the native Irish and Anglo-Irish, a position of which both prelate and king were eager to make best use. Thus it was probably by mutual agreement that Edward, on 12th August 1348, gave FitzRalph full powers to make peace with the Gaelic Irish chieftains who opposed the king and fought his subjects. By the time the order reached Ireland, however, pestilence had swamped much of the east coast and was starting its deathly spread through the rest of the island.

Friar Clyn states, with great certainty, that between August and Christmas 1348, 14,000 people died in Dublin alone – over half the population of the city and its suburbs – and that Drogheda was nearly emptied of its inhabitants. Almost the entire body of Franciscan friars in Drogheda and Dublin died before Christmas,[17] by which time the pestilence had spread around the coast, to New Ross, Cork and Youghal. In Cork it was said three years later that 'the greater part of the citizens of Cork and other faithful men of the king dwelling there all went the way of all flesh.'[18] Just as a later chronicler would claim that coastal communities were particularly hard hit,[19] Richard FitzRalph himself commented the following year that the plague had been most severe among those who lived near the sea, especially fishermen and sailors. From the coastal ports the disease quickly travelled up the arterial rivers inland. Clyn heard the news of the mass pilgrimage at St Mullins; some of those that told it probably brought the disease back with them, so Kilkenny, up the Nore from New Ross, was also infected by Christmas. Eight of the Dominican brothers died there between Christmas, 1348, and 6th March 1349 (the middle of Lent); if so, here too the majority of the brothers were taken away.[20] These scant details of religious deaths are more than a dry accounting of the pestilence: they give an idea of the stupendous mortality, not just across towns and cities but within a single house, in this case one inhabited by friars. As Clyn explained, 'it was very rare for just one person to die in a house, usually husband, wife, children and servants went the same way, the way of death.'[21]

There is no record of Richard FitzRalph having busied himself during the period of the epidemic; his survival suggests that he kept a safe distance from the towns which were the principal places of infection.[viii] Then, on 25th March 1349, the feast of the Annunciation of the Virgin Mary, the archbishop broke cover. The pestilence was now on the wane on the eastern coast and this traditional start to the year – Lady Day – presented an appropriate moment for the archbishop to comment on the catastrophe. It was announced that he was to preach a sermon, in the Carmelite church of Drogheda. His congregation was much reduced – perhaps less than half the number

[viii] Presumably he went to the archiepiscopal manor of Dromiskin, between Dundalk and Drogheda, as it was the more remote of the two manors to which he could have withdrawn.

now sat before him than had been there when he had last preached in Drogheda but a year before.[ix] Everyone present will have lost members of their family and numerous friends and acquaintances; many will have expected their miseries to have been understood, indeed explained, in the sermon the archbishop was about to give. They were to be disappointed, however: for instead of a consolatory message of hope, FitzRalph launched into a vigorous denunciation of the errors of the Anglo-Irish community, grappling his subject with a passion that betrayed his great frustration at the many months of pastoral inactivity that had been forced on him by the raging plague. The archbishop identified two key problems, both of which had become abundantly clear to him during the past, extraordinary year. He had been struck by the 'great wickedness of men' in the colony, a capacity for sin that was exacerbated by the general ignorance of the Anglo-Irish, who lived a long way from any source of education and learning. These twin faults of wickedness and ignorance did as much to threaten society as the 'inundation of pestilence' that the colony was experiencing. FitzRalph drew attention to the never-ending conflict between English and Irish in Ireland, which he condemned as not only wrong in its own right but also an abrogation of conscience. Finally, FitzRalph challenged the 'law of the March', which excused heinous acts perpetrated on the enemy community. The colonists had long exculpated themselves for their robbery and murder, on the pretext that they were acting in defence of the king's rights; FitzRalph showed them the fallacy in their arguments – that whilst their actions might not offend the king, they violated God's law, which was not suspended for the ease of the colonists. The archbishop's strictures may have seemed obvious enough to mainland Englishmen but for a frontier community such as this they made for uncomfortable listening. Although the Anglo-Irish believed themselves to be camped near the frontier of civilization, FitzRalph showed them that any notion of a 'moral frontier' was in fact a sham, as there was nothing to distinguish the actions of Gaelic and Anglo-Irish, both of whom had descended into a barbarous orgy of plunder and bloodshed.[22]

It was an unapologetic denunciation of the colonial enterprise. Put next to the archbishop's sympathetic introduction to the colony nearly

[ix] 4th May 1348.

a year earlier, it was a complete *bouleversement*. The terrible year of 1348–9 had clearly given the archbishop a rude awakening to the realities of his old homeland. On the face of it, the plague seems to have played little part in the archbishop's analysis of the errors of his countrymen: it is mentioned in the sermon once and then only for context. It would be a mistake, however, to think that this meant that it played no role in FitzRalph's thinking. All disease, to a greater or lesser extent, was believed to be a divine punishment, the humble forbearance of which was an earthly substitution for the far greater pains of purgatory. It is easy to see why, therefore, pestilence was universally understood to be a more general punishment for man's sins. This, at least, is the reason for the almost unquestioning repetition of the fact by the chroniclers and clerics. It was a view that had firm roots in the prevailing theology of the church, which is precisely why Clement VI's exhortation to spare the Jews and Richard FitzRalph's condemnation of the Anglo-Irish employed similar arguments.[x] For both archbishop and pope, violence against the outsider was a transgression of divine law, a breach in which the civil power wickedly colluded. In punishing the sins of men, pestilence further exposed the extent of their wrongdoing. Plague was the divine backdrop, against which the shape of human sin was all the more sharply defined.

Soon after Richard FitzRalph had admonished Drogheda, the archbishop set out for Dublin, ostensibly to investigate allegations that the archbishop of Dublin, Alexander Bicknor, had sheltered heretics. The journey had another purpose, however. There had been a long-running dispute between the metropolitans of Armagh and Dublin as to which prelate could claim the primacy of all Ireland. The fact that the Dublin archbishop was traditionally the supporter of the Anglo-Irish colonists, a cause that FitzRalph had only just profoundly questioned, gave an additional piquancy to the anticipated engagement. Showing a complete lack of guile and sensitivity, the Armagh archbishop entered Dublin preceded by his primatial cross; a few days later he had his rights to the primacy of Ireland read out in the presence of the principal Anglo-Irish dignitaries, including Walter de Bermingham, the justiciar, and John FitzRichard, the prior of the

[x] As did also, albeit by sleight of hand, the bishops' condemnation of Edward's war with France.

Knights Hospitallers of Kilmainham – a major Dublin landowner. Not surprisingly, they refused his demand that they recognize him: the magnates would take no lessons from this cosmopolitan smart alec. They had already heard about the Drogheda sermon; quite why they would wish to accept the archbishop's claims was beyond them. So he was told, in no uncertain terms, to leave. FitzRalph returned to Drogheda in a fury and, believing that the great men of Dublin had been paid off by Archbishop Bicknor, excommunicated the lot of them. Armagh was to have its way, however. Within days FitzRalph received news that the prior of Kilmainham was on the point of death; most probably he had been struck down by pestilence. As the sentence of excommunication was still hanging over him, the prior feared he would die without the benefit of a final confession, extreme unction, the *viaticum* or even burial in consecrated ground. The threat was certainly a powerful one, for the prior recanted his opposition to FitzRalph's primatial status and begged for absolution. FitzRalph duly absolved him but it was too late: before the message could be returned, the prior had died. The supporters of Bicknor clearly saw this as a divine judgement on their obstinacy and hastily made their way to Drogheda to pledge themselves to the archbishop of Armagh's cause. Thus was FitzRalph victorious, not, in truth, through his own diplomatic efforts, which had been execrable, but rather through the agency of the plague.

Alexander Bicknor did not have to suffer his humiliation long. The prelate was in his eighties and had been ill for some time, so his death on 14th July 1349 – whilst inevitably linked by others to pestilence – was more likely simply a result of old age, for the epidemic had long burnt out in Dublin. It was still working its way towards the frontiers of the colony, however, leaving those brave communities further debilitated and all the more vulnerable to attack. The Gaelic Irish, who were yet to receive the disease, seem to have made full use of their advantage; certainly no one outside Drogheda – English or Irish – took notice, or even heard the archbishop of Armagh's rousing call for an end to bloodshed. Indeed, on 17th June the violence claimed a prominent victim: the inveterate warrior Fulk de la Freigne. Friar Clyn, who gives us this report, alleged that he had died as a result of trusting too much in the treacherous promises of the native Irish. It was the last of Clyn's entries in his chronicle. The plague may well have receded from Dublin and Drogheda but Kilkenny, on the rim of what remained of Anglo-Ireland, was still aflame. Perhaps the ageing friar fled to the more remote Franciscan house at Carrickbeg, of which he was guardian.[xi] If he had tried to escape, it was in vain. The next line on the parchment roll is in another hand. It says simply: 'Here it seems the author died.'[23] Friar Clyn had known that he was 'waiting among the dead until death comes'; now he had joined them – probably another victim of the epidemic he had taken such care to record, lest 'anyone survives' to read what calamities had befallen him and the people of Anglo-Ireland.[24]

[xi] The house had been founded in 1336 by the earl of Ormond and could maintain twelve friars. As Fulk de la Freigne is reported to have died on 17th June 1349, Clyn may well have perished shortly after this date. Indeed, this may give us a date for the presence of the plague around Carrickbeg, indicating the relatively slow movement of the epidemic through Ireland.

5

London Succumbs

October 1348–May 1349

*Among the noble cities of the world that Fame celebrates, the City of
London of the Kingdom of the English, is the one seat that pours out
its fame more widely, sends to farther lands its wealth and trade, lifts
its head higher than the rest.*

William FitzStephen, c.1173[1]

Pulteney's Inn, the house of the great merchant and financier Sir John
Pulteney, was well-known to be among the most magnificent houses
in London. Not only was this mansion exceptionally large (occupying,
with its garden, an entire block of precious London ground) but it
was also exquisitely furnished. In the great hall fine silverware was
displayed on large oak tables, the walls were hung with tapestries
decorated with the legend of Tristan and Isolde, surrounded by
griffins and wreaths of white roses on a red and green background.
The chambers upstairs were no less beautiful: there were hangings
and bedcovers patterned with fleur-de-lys, eagles, lions, popinjays and
apple blossoms, all in gold, blue, pink, green, violet, and red. It was
a most powerful statement of Sir John's success, evidence of a fortune
gained not by inheritance but through a lifetime of industry and the
prodigious accumulation of wealth.

On Monday, 4th August 1348, John Goldbeter, a successful merchant
from York, knocked on the main entrance door of Pulteney's Inn.
Admitted by a servant, he was ushered through the house to the
garden, where Pulteney himself stood in the sunshine, flanked by his
two other guests, Walter Chiriton and his business partner Thomas
Swanland. It was a pleasant place in which to do business, and a

welcome opportunity to enjoy the sun in what had been a summer drenched by incessant rain.

The reason for the meeting was this. The year before, in 1347, Chiriton and Swanland had secured the right to farm the customs at English ports on goods being exported to the Continent. It was an arrangement into which the crown had been forced by extraordinary financial pressures: the Normandy campaign that had ended with the battle of Crécy had been expensive and the protracted siege of Calais threatened to be exorbitantly so. The king was unable to meet the repayment schedule of existing loans, mostly made out to foreign lenders, but a consortium of financiers, led by Chiriton and Swanland and backed by both Pulteney and Goldbeter, offered him a way out of his predicament. The deal was complicated: Chiriton would give the crown an agreed sum of money in instalments over a set period of time, the payments being weighted towards the short term; he would also take on the debt owed to foreign creditors. In return, Chiriton's company would have the right to collect the customs, the receipts of which could be set against the advances made to the king. The theory was that the crown would gain by ridding itself of some of its borrowings and would benefit from bringing forward the customs revenue; for the merchants the incentive was to farm the customs more efficiently than the government had managed and thereby make a profit. Inevitably, things had not turned out as planned: the receipts from the customs had been worse than expected, a situation not helped by the partial embargo on the export of wool imposed during the first half of the year; furthermore, those foreign debts devolved from the king were still falling due and yet the company was not generating the cash required to meet them. In short, the company needed to be baled out, and they wanted Goldbeter to do it. Chiriton and Swanland knew, however, that Goldbeter would take some persuading. He had already extended a short-term loan of over £2,000 to the company in April that year, nearly half of which was still outstanding. So, although like Pulteney he had an interest in seeing that the company remain solvent, he could also decide to refuse the risk and cut his losses. Worried that he may take the latter course, which would hasten the ruin of the company, Chiriton and Swanland had turned to Pulteney to give credibility to their request.

This, then, was why these four merchant grandees now strolled in

Pulteney's garden: they were thrashing out the terms of a deal. The ploy worked, but Goldbeter attached precise conditions to his agreement: he would lend the company another thousand pounds but only in return for some extraordinarily elaborate guarantees – Pulteney may have been able to charm Goldbeter into advancing the cash but he could not prevent the wily Yorkshireman from covering his back. It was not a time to take unprotected risks, for there were few people in London who did not know that the rumoured pestilence was now very close and likely to strike at any moment.

The metropolis that lay before John Goldbeter, as he arrived from York for his meeting with Chiriton and Pulteney, was many times more impressive than the city William FitzStephen had described 200 years earlier. London now spread all the way from the grim fortress of the Tower in the east to the twin landmarks of Westminster Hall and Westminster Abbey in the west. The skyline in between was serrated by a hundred spires, the tallest and most magnificent of which belonged to St Paul's Cathedral. The centre of the city was still crammed

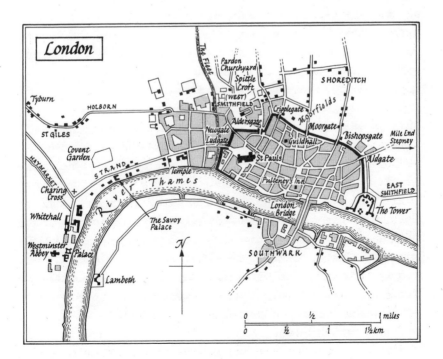

between the river on one side and its Roman walled enclosure on the other three: this much FitzStephen would have recognized. But London had long since burst from these bounds, spilling into suburbs that ran out from each of the city gates. The largest of these lay to the west. Here were the legal schools and lodgings of the Temple and the many great houses that abutted the Strand – the wide road that ran parallel with the river, connecting London with the royal capital of Westminster. This suburb was divided from the city by the Fleet River, which had for a long time doubled as an open sewer, into which the butchers of Smithfield upstream threw the entrails of slaughtered animals. From the point where the Fleet met the Thames by the great convent of Blackfriars, along the water's edge all the way to the Tower of London, lay the tightly packed docks and warehouses of the Steelyard, Billingsgate, Wine Wharf, Haywharf and Timberhithe. Their line was unbroken, except by the inhabited bridge – London Bridge – which crossed the Thames to Southwark, where brothels, bear rings and cockpits sat hard against the priory of St Mary Overy and the Bishop of Winchester's Inn.

Since FitzStephen's time, London had doubled in size – now almost 100,000 people lived in or around the old city walls. Although half the size of Paris, London housed a higher proportion of the national population, perhaps one in every sixty. The city was a prodigious consumer, devouring over 1,000,000 bushels of grain a year, which required the cultivation of some 250,000 acres of land. The stoves of London's homes and furnaces of its workshops worked their way through the equivalent of a large wood each year, a quantity increasingly supplemented by coal shipped from Newcastle and the north-east, fuelling the forges, tanneries, dyehouses and the near 200 other trades practised off the city's narrow and crowded streets. Pepperers and grocers, fishmongers and cordwainers, leather-workers, goldsmiths, pewterers – almost every business that existed save farming, quarrying and mining took place within the city's boundaries. But London's primary business – then, as now – was trade. From hides to cloth, iron to alabaster, gold to spices, almost every single kind of tradable commodity and finished product passed through London's docks, wharves, and merchant warehouses.

Rising above the boats squeezed along the embankment between the Steelyard and Haywharf was Coldharbour, another of the properties owned by Sir John Pulteney. It was the most impressive of the river-side mansions, as befitted a man who had made more – and spent more – than any other trader within the city. Pulteney, who came from a minor Leicestershire landowning family, arrived in London in his late teens to be apprenticed as a draper. By 1316, when he was in his mid-twenties, he had established himself as a citizen; not more than eleven years later he became a member of the Drapers' Guild and was elected an alderman (the councillors who represented and ran London's twenty-six wards) in the Coleman Street ward, in the north of the city. Pulteney also began providing services to the crown: in 1327 he was granted the right to collect customs, on which he took a percentage, along the whole length of the Thames from the city to the sea. Between 1331 and 1338 he was mayor of London no fewer than four times and became a major lender to the king, for which service he was rewarded with a knighthood and the gift of lands from Northamptonshire to Kent. In this latter county, at Penshurst near Tonbridge, he had built a country retreat, whose deliberately anachronistic style betrayed his pretension to nobility.

By 1348, Pulteney had passed sixty and was able to enjoy the almost unparalleled wealth which he had amassed. However, as was to be expected of a self-made man, he continued to work as well as perform the duties proper to a city father, using the mansion of Coldharbour as his office. The five-minute walk between Pulteney's Inn, just off Candlewick Street,[i] down the hill to Thames Street and across the road to the land-side entrance of Coldharbour was a journey that Sir John must have undertaken many times, taking him through all the enormous variety of medieval London. Immediately outside the magnificence of Pulteney's Inn were the cramped and dim streets that twisted and turned across the city. From the mansion's perfumed splendour, the rank smell was almost overpowering: the giant manufactory that was London created a great ferment, brewed up by tanneries, ale-houses, soapmakers and vinegar makers, coal and wood fires, dung heaps, slaughterhouses, fishmongers and salters, rubbish tips, cesspits, and sewers. The noxious brew stewed in the confined streets of central London, of which St Lawrence Lane – where Pulteney's Inn had its entrance – was just one of many. Stepping out of the magnificence

---

[i] Candlewick Street is now Cannon Street.

of the Inn into the grime of St Lawrence Lane, Sir John turned his back on the small stone-built church that gave the street its name and walked between the two facing rows of timber-framed terraces, whose upper storeys jutted so far out that a person upstairs on the second floor could shake hands with someone leaning out of a window on the opposite side of the street. Down the middle of St Lawrence Lane ran an open sewer into which refuse and ordure were swept in anticipation of enough rain to wash it down the hill, from which it would eventually reach the Thames. 'Rakers' were appointed in each ward to keep such channels clear and regular enactments were required by the city authorities to ensure that this open sewerage system continued to function. In another ward the citizens had recently been censured for 'casting out of ordure and urine' whilst to the west, in Foster Lane, fourteen households were indicted for throwing 'ordure and urine' from their windows, 'the which annoys all the people of the ward'.[2]

At the bottom of St Lawrence Lane, Sir John crossed Thames Street, busy then as it is today. The streets teemed with carriers and carts moving goods to and from the wharves which separated Thames Street from the river, whilst merchants picked their way between the traffic, crossing and recrossing between counting rooms, guild buildings and warehouses. Once he had negotiated this hubbub, Sir John could slip down Haywharf Lane, pressing his back to the wall to allow the passage of handcarts piled high with freshly unloaded produce, before arriving at the entrance to Coldharbour which lay at the bottom near the quay. Once inside, he could at last enjoy the view: a spectacular panorama of the River Thames, heaving with ships and boats of every conceivable size – from small ferries taking no more than a couple of passengers, through barges carrying grain up and down the Thames, to the largest of ocean-going vessels which plied the trade routes with the Baltic and Mediterranean. The river provided an attractive prospect, so long as the wind carried its fumes to the south: with the Fleet in the west, the Shoreditch in the east, and the Walbrook, which ran through the centre of the city to the quayside, all pouring their filth into the Thames, the stink was such that Edward III was forced to complain twice to the mayor and aldermen about the threat posed by the river to Londoners' health. Despite the king's protests, the condition of the water supplies did not improve. Industry in London, especially tanning, dying and brewing, required large quantities of water, yet the few conduits that brought a fresh supply from the spring up at Tyburn, by present-day Marble Arch, had long been insufficient. So Londoners used and drank water not only from the Thames but also from the many wells that stood in the lanes and yards around the city, despite their pollution by the hundreds of seeping cesspits that leaked effluent into the ground. These privies were a constant source of friction between neighbours. In 1348 an angry citizen, Ralph de Cauntebrigg, complained to the mayor and aldermen that the wall of his neighbour's latrine was 'not sufficiently thick, so that the sewage . . . penetrates and defiles his whole premises'.[3] The neighbour concerned, William Bragweyn, was ordered to build a new stone wall around his tenement to prevent a reoccurrence.

As Pulteney would readily have recognized, these problems were not symptoms of decay but the signs of a thriving city outgrown and overstretched by a burgeoning population. What allowed some semblance of civilized life to continue was the significant degree to which London's civic government could exercise control over Londoner's daily lives. Since William the Conqueror reaffirmed the city's ancient rights by charter, London had enjoyed considerable independence and effective self-government. Managed by the aldermen, headed by a mayor selected from among their number, London held privileges in nearly all the matters of government that elsewhere were the preserve of the crown. This was no democracy, however: the mayor and aldermen, who together formed the city's council, represented the interests of an elite – the citizens – who had inherited or been granted the freedom of the city. As most of these citizens were involved in either trade or craft of some sort, the council had become a merchant oligarchy which, as in other English cities, worked for the maintenance of their urban privileges and the increase of its wealth. The power and wealth of London, however, meant that this city's patriciate more closely resembled those that controlled the trading cities of the Mediterranean than the petty town councils of provincial England.

Although enshrined in ancient charters, London's freedoms were nonetheless bestowed at the pleasure of the crown. However, as Chiriton's dealings indicated, the relationship between the city and the king was more equal than the grant of liberties might at first suggest. Increasingly, English monarchs had come to depend on

London merchants, not just for the collection and payment of customs revenues but also for the loans that made possible their foreign campaigns. Edward III learnt to manage this association to his great advantage. Between 1337 and 1349 his total borrowings exceeded £120,000, an extraordinary sum, much of which came from a small handful of merchants whose combined wealth was well in excess of the Exchequer's resources. As royal government came more and more to rely upon London's vast wealth to sustain its ever-expanding requirements, it was inevitably pulled within the compass of the city. Traditionally, some offices of state had had no permanent home but travelled with the monarch. However, during the reign of Edward III, royal administration, as well as the courts, coalesced around Westminster. The proximity of royal government and the mercantile centre of England served to confirm London's pre-eminence within the realm, giving its citizens a degree of influence that few other commoners enjoyed. It had been the mayor and aldermen who had organized the revels in the Guildhall on Edward's return from Calais in 1347. They made sure to put on a good show: such festivities had never been seen before. It was a last moment of mutual self-congratulation and pride before the miseries visited on the city by plague.

Londoners knew of the pestilence long before it had secured its first foothold on the Dorset coast. Merchantmen setting alongside the jetties that sprang out all around Coldharbour brought news of the horrors that they had left behind in the Mediterranean. No doubt some Londoners received these first rumours with some scepticism; even Boccaccio, who saw the pestilence in Florence with his own eyes, said that he 'would scarcely dare to believe it, let alone commit to paper', even if he had heard it from a person whom he could trust.[4] Even those who were disposed to accept the news would not have been unduly worried: Florence and Genoa were a long way away, so people carried on as if there were no serious threat. This complaisancy can only have lasted a few months, however, since by early summer the plague had reached Bordeaux. It was from there that the vintners who plied between Gascony and London had brought the news that the king's daughter had died in the outbreak. Then word came that it had reached English soil: Bristol, somewhere on the south coast, Ireland even – no one was quite sure. Yet wherever it was, the contagion was

still some way off, distant enough to cause serious worry but not immediate panic. Writing on behalf of the king on 28th September,
demanding prayers, the prior of Christchurch, Canterbury, was still
under the impression that the disease was so far only in 'other regions'.[5]
Conversely, the chronicler Geoffrey le Baker, writing in Oxfordshire,
claimed that the first cases of the pestilence in London occurred
'around Michaelmas' – the very next day.[6] Although le Baker's dating
is a little early, in one sense he was entirely right: plague-infected
people probably did arrive in London around this time, although these
were unwitting carriers, whose symptoms were yet to appear. Nearly
a month later, on 24th October, William Edington wrote to his diocese
commanding confessions, penitent acts and the now standard routine
of processions, stating that he still believed the epidemic to be confined
to 'coastal areas';[7] he cannot have heard that the plague was already
present in his Winchester diocese, around Titchfield on the Solent.
He would certainly have known had the pestilence broken out in
London, for he was writing to Hampshire from his palace in Southwark,
on the south bank of the Thames. Nonetheless, he may well have
been ignorant of plague's presence, for behind closed doors, hidden
from prying eyes, people were probably already dying – those very
first men to bring pestilence to the capital. Where they came from
is uncertain. Bristol, which had been infected for two months, was
120 miles away, yet it is still just possible that the disease had made the
journey to London direct from the West Country, perhaps carried by
an apparently healthy trader or official. It is more likely, however, that
pestilence arrived first on London's quayside, with the same sailors who
brought the very latest news from the Continent. Virgil claimed that
there was no swifter ill than rumour, yet pestilence clung to rumour's
tail, arriving – silently – with the whispers that warned of its approach.[8]

Orders for acts of public devotion and repentance – masses, sermons
and processions – had been issued in London at the end of September.[9]
Civic pageantry in London revolved around a calendar of processions:
on the patron saints' days of guilds and companies, at midsummer
and at Corpus Christi. The greatest of them all, the day of the mayor's
appointment, was imminent – 28th October. Yet for the incoming
mayor, the fishmonger John Lovekin, it was to be a far more solemn
affair than was usual. Already guilds, fraternities, sometimes entire
wards, were walking ceremonial routes, from one church to the next,

led by priests holding crosses and candles. Psalms and hymns were sung and a litany of prayer repeated; sermons were preached at both the beginning and end. Detailed reports of these liturgies are scant, but three centuries later a tanner of Barcelona, Miquel Parets, would write of processions that will not have been all that different. There were, he said, 'so many processions of clergy and monks and nuns carrying so many crosses and so many rogations that there was not a single church nor monastery which did not carry out processions both inside and outside their buildings'.[10] Similar lines of penitents would have snaked over London in the autumn months of 1348: people from all over the city, from every trade and of every status, joining together in a united plea for deliverance from the coming plague.

These processions were much grander than those at St Mullins; they would spread the disease about all the same. The first infected men had arrived around the beginning of September. They had chatted by the dockside, done business, negotiated over a meal in the tavern. Some had bought trinkets, others sold their wares. Many had drunk in the ale-houses, a few consorted with whores, most had gone to Mass and all of them had slept in the inns. As they were embraced by the city, they passed the disease on. So it spread from person to person, moving invisibly between them as they talked, kissed, argued, slept together, or even just brushed up against each other in the scrum of the street. One incubator infected another, they another and soon one had become thousands, all ready to break out into infection. The time when one person could infect another was only a portion of the period of infection, but it is likely that this stage started before the symptoms appeared: indeed, there can be no other way that the epidemic spread as it did. The result was an explosion – from nothing, then a rumour of a couple of cases, to mass mortality, all in the space of a couple of weeks. Robert of Avesbury, a chronicler working for the archbishop of Canterbury at Lambeth Palace, reported that the epidemic started in London around 1st November, just a week after Edington's letter was sent. London Bridge, which connected Southwark and the city, soon filled with an impromptu procession – a terrified crush of Londoners, forcing their way through the narrow lane that divided the houses on London Bridge, desperate to flee what had been rumoured, then feared but had now, finally, arrived.

Many of those that could, fled. Bishop Edington, who could see the mayhem on London Bridge from the windows of his palace, made for his manor house at Esher.[ii] Sir John Pulteney, however, decided to stay – at least for the meantime. On 20th October he attended the funeral of his fellow former mayor, Sir John Hammond, an alderman for thirteen years whose death (which was unconnected with the plague) was of particular loss to the Guild of Grocers, in which he had been a leading light. Most guilds had a rule that as many members as were able should attend the funeral of a fellow guildsman; in Hammond's case, all but four of the whole company of grocers turned up. As was the custom, those grocers who could not come were obliged to pay a donation to charity by way of a fine. However, when the chaplain of the guild was struck down by the plague a month and a half later, only ten grocers out of the entire guild turned up for his wake.[iii] They had not died; it was too early in the course of the epidemic for there to have been that degree of mortality. More likely many members had simply taken flight, preferring to pay a fine rather than risk contracting pestilence. Unsurprisingly, the Guild soon suspended the levy of fines for non-attendance at funerals: it was unreasonable to penalize people for avoiding such an obvious risk. Pulteney himself was aware of the danger. On 14th November he made out his will, naming his executors as none other than Sir William de Clinton, earl of Huntingdon, and the bishop of London, Ralph Stratford, the nephew of the lately deceased archbishop of Canterbury. In the event of his death these two important men were charged with administering Pulteney's enormous estate, the vast bulk of which he had built up himself in his extraordinary life. Having updated his will, Pulteney may well have left for Penshurst, in the comparative seclusion of the Kentish Weald. Most did not have this choice. They had nowhere to flee and instead had to face the pestilence as it spread and killed amongst them.

Sure signs that plague had taken grip of the city came in the very first days of the New Year. For in the first week of January the wardens of the glovers' trade came before the mayor's council to request that

[ii] Edington wrote again to the diocese on 17th November 1348, from Esher. He then joined the king on his mock-expedition abroad, sometime between the signing of the treaty with Louis de Mâle on 4th December and the king's return to London before going to the Tower on 10th December. Edington's register states that he returned on 12th December.

[iii] 2nd December 1348.

they be granted new ordinances. They wanted prohibitions on outsiders selling their wares – in this instance gloves – within the bounds of the city; in this they were in line with most other London trades. Yet the wardens also requested that the mayor impose some rather more novel regulations: restrictions on master glovemakers enticing away the servants of their fellow masters, and byelaws preventing glovers' serving-men charging more for their work than they had done two or three years previously. This was an odd petition, which in its provisions on servants was quite unlike anything that had been put before the mayor's council before. The reason, simply put, was pestilence: tales of the disease had been swirling round London for months and the one thing that everyone knew from what had been relayed from Italy was that to touch a diseased person was to risk certain death. With pestilence now in Londoners' midst, there had been a run on gloves. Master glovemakers had desperately sought to meet this extraordinary demand, and on finding that they had insufficient labour, had sought to lure away their competitors' workers. These men, suddenly conscious of their new-found worth in this specialized trade, raised their rates. Meanwhile, every other fly-by-night operator in London had set themselves up in glovemaking, enticing away the workers of legitimate tradesmen to staff their new shops. This kind of commercial anarchy was anathema to the city fathers, who had prospered through tightly regulated and restricted trades. The mayor and his council had no hesitation in acting on the glovemakers' petition, granting them on 6th January the ordinances they had claimed they required.

This was the city fathers' first bureaucratic response to the pestilence. Thus far, they had acted almost as if in denial of what they knew was about to happen. Unsure of what precaution they needed to take, the government of the city, comprising the mayor and his council, did all they could to keep to their time-honoured routine, spending the anxious months of early autumn 1348 not in preparation for the coming epidemic but in supervising the day-to-day business of local administration. (In the last week of September, for example, as episcopal letters made their way around the kingdom imploring congregations to pray for salvation, the council found time to hear a dispute between the wardens of London Bridge and the rector of St Margaret Moses concerning the course of a gutter.) In October the council had attended to the raising of troops in preparation for the end of the most recent truce with France,[iv] and, as custom dictated, the Court of Husting (where the wills of wealthy Londoners were granted probate) had returned from its summer recess on the first Monday after the Feast of St Luke.[v] Like other London institutions, this court carried on with a sense of almost studied normality. In November 1348 only three testaments were brought before the court, marking those few natural deaths that had occurred during the previous, plague-free, month.[vi] The court did not sit in December; this would be its final respite before the full onslaught of pestilence was felt. In January 1349 eighteen wills were enrolled, five more than the court had proved in the previous six months. This in itself was sure confirmation that the plague had begun to have an effect before Christmas. During February and March the court proved eighty-three wills, nearly four times the number of wills enrolled through the whole of 1348 and a figure reached now in only two months. Then, in April, because of Easter, the court did not sit and the record stops. Many Londoners must by now have wondered whether it would ever meet again.

Yet wondering helped no one: those who still survived were occupied enough dealing with the effects of the unceasing mortality. The deaths of friends and family meant that there was much to be done: even in times such as these the first duty of the living was to act upon the final wishes of the dead. In mid-February, for instance, the fish merchant William Greyland was charged with executing the terms of a particularly elaborate will, made out by a friend, which involved complicated property transfers witnessed by none other than Pulteney and requiring confirmation in Chancery at Westminster Hall. Within two months, however, the pestilence was claiming members of his own family: his sister Joanna, his daughter Katherine, and then his niece's husband, who only weeks before had seen William in the Court of Husting – both of them attending as executors to the recently dead.[vii] Then, at the end of April, William's friend Henry Cross died

---

[iv] On 25th October.

[v] 18th October 1348.

[vi] Last wills and testaments, already signed and witnessed, were brought before the court to be proved as soon after the testator's death as the executors could manage. There was a court, on average, every three to four weeks, so the number of wills enrolled in one month more or less reflected the number of citizens who had died (and had written a will) in the month before.

[vii] On 23rd March.

and he was called on to supervise the execution of another will. By serendipity Greyland had survived thus far but this latest obligation may well have brought his luck to an end; perhaps he caught the disease from his dying friend. For on Monday, 4th May, William went to the Guildhall to sit once again in the Court of Husting, this time to see Henry Cross's will put through probate. In the Guildhall he appeared a healthy man; unbeknownst to him and to everyone else in the packed room, he was in fact infected. By the following week, he was feeling ill and feverous; a couple of days later the tell-tale spots had appeared and then the swellings under his armpits and in his groin. On Friday, 15th May, he made out his own last will and testament, and very shortly after, he was dead. The pathetic final months of William's life had still not found a conclusion, for he was forced to ask his own executor, his brother Simon, 'to administer the goods of Thomas Francis and Henry Cross, not yet administered by the testator'.

Underneath a giant slab in the south-east corner of the cloister of Westminster Abbey lies the body of Simon Bircheston, abbot from 1344 to 1349. With him are the remains of twenty-seven of his monks, about half the total number of conventuals in the house. The stone is one of the few memorials to the victims of the Great Death that remain. All of those who lie there were carried off by plague in early May 1349, leaving only half the monks to tend the sick in the Abbey's hospital. Abbot Bircheston, who died in a retreat house on the abbey's manor of Hampstead, was not greatly missed. He had previously assaulted a royal stonemason, and a monk who survived the plague bitterly recounted that 'he left Westminster greatly burdened with debt, the result of his own extravagance and the fraudulent depredations of his household and kinsmen.'[11] Simon Langham, an exceptional monk and one of the survivors, was made abbot in Bircheston's place. Immediately he set about dealing with the abbey's many problems, and thus pestilence became Westminster Abbey's salvation. The hospital of St James, not far the from the abbey, was not so lucky. There the master, all the sisters and all but one of the brothers were killed, leaving only Walter de Weston, who became master – despite his manifest unsuitability – by default. Elsewhere, the dean of St Martin-le-Grand was another probable victim, as were the master and many brethren of St Thomas's Hospital in Southwark. Within the walls of London itself, the greatest of the city's religious houses – Greyfriars – lost about a hundred brothers. At the time London's clergy accounted for one in every twenty of the city's inhabitants. As a sample, these figures alone give an idea of the huge number of deaths in the capital.[12]

The penitentiary processions instigated when pestilence still only threatened the capital most likely ceased as the plague took hold. Certainly people still felt the need for prayer but public gatherings soon became associated with contagion. As the death toll mounted, far grimmer processions made their way across the city: rakers, leaving their daily routine cleaning the gutters to act as makeshift pall-bearers, were now conveying the dead to the grave. From the moment the morning bell of St Thomas Acon marked the lifting of the curfew, bier after bier would pass out of the city gates towards the two cemeteries which waited to receive the dead. The first of these, Holy Trinity Churchyard, lay beyond Tower Hill to the east of the city wall and had been established within weeks of the plague's arrival in 1348. The benefactor was an otherwise anonymous clerk named John Corey, yet it was likely that he was acting as an agent for the king, not least because the following year Edward banned the digging of another cemetery nearby, most probably to protect the revenues of his own burial ground. (Corey had the cemetery consecrated by the bishop of London, Ralph Stratford, as Holy Trinity Churchyard; after the Dissolution the land provided a victualling yard for the Royal Navy and premises for the Royal Mint.) Thousands of bodies of those who died in the Great Pestilence have lain underneath ever since. Even now we cannot be sure how many, but in 1881 a large repository of bones was discovered during building works and recent excavations have revealed parts of several mass graves. Some of the skeletons had disarticulated limbs, not as a result of a hurried interment but because they had putrefied before burial, either through fear or unavoidable neglect – or simply because there was no one left to arrange their interment. However, no matter how they arrived at East Smithfield, the bodies of those who were buried there were treated with solemnity and respect. Corpses were placed with care next to each other, neatly resting shoulder to shoulder some distance below the surface. In the end not all the land bought was needed: it may well have been that the opening of a new, far larger, cemetery on the other side of the city rendered Holy Trinity Churchyard obsolete.

Bishop Ralph was also involved in the creation of this new cemetery, which was just north of Smithfield. A four-acre strip of ground called Pardon Churchyard was purchased by the bishop in late 1348 for the express purpose of burying the bodies of plague victims. Within a matter of months it proved to be insufficient, so the bishop turned to Sir Walter Manny to fund an extension. Manny approached the master of St Bartholomew's Hospital nearby and asked them if he could purchase the land they owned adjacent to Pardon Churchyard. It was a measure of the urgency of his request that they agreed that he would rent the land until he could provide an alternative site in exchange. So he took possession of Spittle Croft, constituting a further thirteen acres to the south of the existing burial ground. The two were amalgamated and enclosed by a wall. On 25th March, the feast of the Annunciation of the Virgin Mary, the bishop went to the new cemetery with Manny to consecrate the new ground, giving a sermon on the word 'Hail!', it being the feast day of the angel Gabriel's revelation to Mary that she was carrying God's child. Manny clearly took this to heart, for he founded a chapel on the site, dedicated to the Annunciation. The knight's prestige and the bishop's imprimatur soon attracted further benefactions to the chapel, with merchants falling over each other to make contributions, perhaps in the hope that they would be associated with the great warrior himself. Remarkably, in sight of the mounting bodies, the prelate and the knight still found cause for some hope. Perhaps they clung fast to the angel's words to Mary: 'Fear not.' This extraordinary faith was indeed the only hope that Londoners still had.

The great sixteenth-century antiquarian John Stow reported that in this cemetery, which is still partly visible, there stood a cross, which carried the following inscription:

> A great plague raging in the year of our Lord 1349, this churchyard was consecrated; wherein, and within the bounds of the present monastery, were buried more than 50,000 bodies of the dead, besides many others from thence to the present time, whose souls God have mercy upon. Amen.[13]

This figure may well not be entirely accurate, but surely the precise number is immaterial.[14] For it is certain that between St John's Street and Goswell Street in Clerkenwell lie tens of thousands of people, the greater part of that half of London's population that did not survive the Great Death. Smithfield must have been a hellish sight. The quantity of corpses cannot possibly have been accommodated with the polite spacing enjoyed by the bodies in John Corey's graveyard. This was no mass grave but a burial pit: rather than laying the bodies in rows, they were stacked on top of each other starting from one end of the giant hole, so as to make sure that the rakers need not tread over the decaying remains when interring the next cartload. All day the rakers came, with bodies piled high on their carts. According to Robert of Avesbury, 'more than two hundred corpses were buried almost every day in the new burial ground next to Smithfield, and this was in addition to the bodies buried in other churchyards in the city', of which there were about a hundred.[15] Only nightfall brought respite. It is enough to imagine the sorrowful stillness that came over the city as St Martin-le-Grand rang the curfew at nine o'clock. The last pall-bearers had returned through the great gates of London and one by one – Cripplegate, Ludgate, Aldgate, Newgate – they closed for the night.

Contrary to what many Londoners must have feared, the city did not collapse. The Court of Husting resumed its business on 1st May 1349. They proved in this one sitting a remarkable eighty-three wills, the same number enrolled in those two unprecedented months before Easter. A further thirty-seven testaments were brought before them in May, confirming a pattern of mortality that corresponds with Robert of Avesbury's assertion that the deaths in the city peaked during eleven grim weeks between 2nd February and 12th April (from February 1349 to January 1350 a total of 341 wills were brought before the aldermen sitting on the Court of Husting). After May there was a dramatic decline in the number of wills being granted probate but the rate does not return to trend until November; most of these later instances were most likely delayed grants of probate, reflecting a death earlier in the year.[16] These records are inherently imbalanced: they deal only with that very small minority who were passing on substantial estates, not with the journeyman and the cook, or the inn-keeper and the huckster, or indeed the imprisoned and the destitute. Nonetheless, the wills of the wealthy explain much about the proportionate effect the pestilence had on London's wider population. The fifteen-fold increase in wills enrolled at the Court indicates that, given an (optimistic) average life expectancy of forty, over a third of those who were in a position to make out a will fell victim to the disease in 1349; and these were the people most able to flee, to hide away, and therefore to survive. Given the considerable anecdotal evidence and what is known about cities elsewhere, we may suppose with some certainty that the number of Londoners who died was far greater than a third of the city's population: it was more likely a half, possibly even more.[17]

London endured this extraordinary mortality in part because Mayor Lovekin and the aldermen insisted that city life should continue, as far as was practicable, as if the plague were not there. The Letter Book of the Guildhall provides a crude guide to the extent to which this was achieved. A variety of actions are recorded in 1349: the confirmation of property deeds (five cases), the enrolment of royal writs (eight), guardianship hearings (thirteen), guild appointments and trading standards enquiries (ten) and Guildhall appointments (five). Nowhere is there any evidence of an operation to deal with the bodies which the churchyards had no room to receive, nor of any measures to care for the sick and the destitute: these were things traditionally (and more competently) organized by others. It was hard enough to ensure that the rudiments of city administration continued through the panic and disruption caused by the epidemic. Indeed, because the city's rakers (now much reduced in number) had been diverted from street-cleaning to carting bodies to Smithfield, stinking sewage had begun to foul London's streets, so much so that the king was forced to order the mayor to have the streets and lanes cleared of 'human faeces and other filth', the accumulation of which was causing the air to be infected and 'poisoned to the danger of men passing, especially in the mortality by the contagious sickness which arises daily'.[18]

As the great seventeenth-century historian of this period Sir Joshua Barnes observed, the pestilence was 'contrary to humane Precaution'. Even had they been able to fulfil the King's unhelpful command, the mayor and his officials must have known that there was in fact nothing they could do to halt the raging epidemic.[19] Barnes was well placed to know, for he had seen London suffer a bout of plague second only to the Great Death, followed swiftly by a catastrophic fire. Then, as in the aftermath of the first pestilence, London had rapidly recovered because of the same inextinguishable commercial instincts of its citizens, instincts that were shared by the mayor and his aldermen, whose common interest it was to create an environment where trade and enterprise could flourish. Thus, during the terrible months of epidemic disease and mass mortality that afflicted the city from late 1348 to mid-1349, Lovekin, his officials and councillors did all that they were supposed to do, which was maintain the unglamorous but necessary administration of those civil matters that lay within their direct jurisdiction: the guardianship of wealthy orphans, civic appointments, the supervision of what trade continued, the certification of property deeds, and keeping the peace. The difference this year was the extraordinary volume of business: the exceptional number of guardianship cases heard because of the high mortality; the property deeds confirmed on newly inherited landholdings; the replacements for deceased officers of the Guildhall and guild fraternities. The problems were not in themselves unusual; the quantity, however, was unprecedented. It was to John Lovekin's credit, and the credit of his administration, and indeed the credit of the city as a whole, that London kept on going.

Nonetheless, London was not the place it had been when John Goldbeter came to Pulteney's Inn, on that hot August day the previous year. Then the streets had bustled with traders, carts, carriers and merchandise; now the traffic was mostly wagons piled high with the dead. Everywhere there was evidence of death: empty shops and houses; the orphaned child led by the uncle, grandmother or sibling; the grim procession of funerals and constant tolling of bells; the smell of death and the sight of it. This was no place to do business, even for those that were brave enough to attempt it. It surprised no one, therefore, that on 15th March the king's serjeants seized the lands and assets of Walter Chiriton and his partners. Finally their obligations to their creditors and to the crown had overwhelmed them, the plague making a precarious situation untenable. In the administrative confusion of the plague year, it is unclear whether John Goldbeter managed to retrieve the £1,000 that he had reluctantly lent them less than seven months earlier; subsequent litigation suggested that he did.

Pulteney too had sunk money into Chiriton's company, so the news that it had collapsed, whilst not unexpected, must have been a considerable irritation. He did not allow the loss to distract him, however, as he had much to attend to besides. On the very day Manny and Bishop Stratford consecrated the cemetery at Smithfield, a chaplain in his chantry chapel of Corpus Christi in the church of St Lawrence Candlewick Street, just near Pulteney's Inn, died. Four days later Pulteney wrote to Bishop Edington from Poplar, asking him to appoint a replacement.[viii] Pulteney stipulated that he 'should be of good disposition, able to read and sing well and take charge as soon as convenient'.[20] It was a business-like communication, which nonetheless betrayed Pulteney's acknowledgment that such were the times that this minor appointment might have to wait. No doubt Edington did indeed find it 'convenient' to keep Pulteney's request in the pending pile. It meant that Pulteney most probably never met the chosen successor. For whether as a result of his premature return to London from Kent or because of a belated infection caught elsewhere, Sir John contracted the plague in May. After a couple of weeks he was suddenly and hopelessly struck down, and was dead by the beginning of June. His funeral was attended by the mayor, the recorder, the sheriffs, the common pleader of the city, and the master of the chapel of Corpus Christi – all of them in dutiful attendance despite the still-present risk of infection. For this act of memorial was as much an affirmation of London's ambition, one in which a provincial son could join the ranks of the great city fathers. In the extended peal of bells, the richness of vestments and dignity of the mourners, the ceremony said much about what London had been – a great European city that in turns was fostered and built by an aristocracy of merchants, artisans and tradesmen, many of them self-made. It remained to be seen whether London, ravaged by plague, would be able to sustain such glory.

[viii] The bishop had the right of appointment to this post.

6

Winter Crawl

January–April 1349

After Crystenmasse com þe crabbed Lentoun

Sir Gawain and the Green Knight[1]

As soon as the people of Gloucester heard that the pestilence had arrived in Bristol, they shut the gates to those travelling up from the south, 'believing that the breath of those who had lived among the dying would be infectious'.[2] It was a wise precaution. Through the final months of 1348, the Great Death had marched from Melcombe Regis through Dorset, meeting another front of pestilence coming down from Bristol through Somerset. The coasts of Devon were infected and the western portion of Wiltshire – in which the little Deverill villages sat – was braced for infection. The epidemic crept up the road from Bristol towards Gloucester and took hold of the countryside in between, including the borough and manor of Thornbury, on the southern bank of the Severn. Gloucester, however, remained untouched, despite sitting astride the busy road that led from Bristol into the west Midlands. Conversely, London – on the other side of the country – had taken no precautions whatsoever and was in the grip of the disease by the beginning of November. As the king's extravagant Christmas celebrations got under way, his kingdom was being attacked from two fronts: the west, where the epidemic now reached from the Severn estuary to the Devon and Dorset coast; and the east, in London. Moreover, Dublin and Drogheda, the easternmost part of the English colony in Ireland, had been suffering for over four months, and English Gascony had been ravaged since before the middle of the year. If the king had pondered what the New Year held, he cannot have arrived at a very pretty prognosis.

Edward, like everyone else, was well aware of how the pestilence might be caught, and so on his return from treating in Flanders he stayed in diseased London only as long as he absolutely had to – and then only within the walls of the Tower. He had then made quickly for the comparative safety of the archbishop of Canterbury's palace in Kent. The security was only partial, however, for the epidemic was already showing an ability to surprise: there was the isolated outbreak in Titchfield on the banks of the Solent and there may have been other outbreaks too – in Farnham in south-west Surrey, Codicote in Hertfordshire, and as far away as Crowland in the southern fens of Lincolnshire. All of these places were separate from the main locations of the epidemic but were not themselves out of the way. Farnham was on the main road from south-west England to London; Codicote was sandwiched between Watling Street and Ermine Street, two residual Roman routes from London to the north; and Crowland Abbey was amongst England's greatest wool farms, with active trading links of its own with London and the Continent. A merchant coming from Melcombe Regis could have stopped off in Farnham for the night; a Codicote farmer might have made the round trip to infected London, where one of Crowland Abbey's officials may well have gone to sell a consignment of wool. So, although the epidemic had assumed a couple of broad fronts – in the West of England and in London – it was also capable of establishing itself in forward positions elsewhere.

This pattern was quickly understood for what it was: a reflection of the simple fact that the pestilence was being spread by people. The epidemic started in ports because they were the main points of entry from the Continent; from these landing points, fishermen and coastal shippers spread the disease quickly along the shoreline. Inland, the majority of frequent journeys were very local, and the constant to-ing and fro-ing spread the epidemic town by town, village by village, house by house. Before the epidemic had gained a large carrier population, the speed with which it spread was fairly slow, especially out of little Melcombe into the Dorset countryside around. Gradually, however, as more and more were infected, the rate at which it covered ground increased, particularly once Bristol had been struck: Somerset and south Gloucestershire quickly shared in that town's horrors. Then, however, the cold months of winter came, slowing everything – the epidemic included – to a crawl. There was little reason to go to market and as far as it was possible people stuck to the warmth of their homes. By contrast, the business of urban life was less affected by the seasons, as trade, government and justice continued through the winter months, involving much direct exchange between the urban hubs of the realm. As a consequence, the epidemic leapt from one town to another, leaving miles of disease-free countryside untouched. For it took only one visit from infected travellers for the disease to become established, and once inside a town, with people living close by and on top of one another, pestilence quickly spread within families, amongst friends and between neighbours. It was for precisely this reason that the men of Gloucester refused entry to the fleeing citizens of Bristol. Yet although contemporaries understood how the pestilence moved, they were not to know at what length the disease incubated itself. So the precaution of the burghers of Gloucester was to no effect: for pestilence had already sneaked in, and was invisibly making its way around.

After his murder in Berkeley Castle in 1327, the body of Edward's hapless father, Edward II, had been taken to the Benedictine abbey in Gloucester, where the abbot was obliged to receive the skewered corpse and make provision for its burial. On reaching his majority in 1330, Edward III immediately moved to give his father a suitable tomb and began to develop a plan for the improvement of the choir of the abbey in which he was buried. This was not mere filial duty: it was important for the young king that the royal body was treated with dignity, and to do otherwise might give tacit approval to regicide – something he could never be seen to condone. On the other hand, the king's foreign commitments dictated that what was essentially a glorified mausoleum should not cost too much. So he commissioned Thomas of Canterbury, his master mason, to do his best with the existing structure.

Thomas was certainly equal to the task. He had recently been working on the chapel of St Stephen at Westminster, begun by Edward I in response to the great Sainte-Chapelle in Paris, the *nonpareil* of the French Gothic achievement. The English attempt, by comparison, had been a failure. It took fifty-six years to complete, and both brief and architect had changed several times during the course of the project. The chapel was, therefore, a muddle – a cuboid topped by a pitched roof and finished at the corners with ungainly turrets, with three rows of windows perforating the sides, unrelated in size and unconnected with each other. Thomas had brought some degree of order to this imbalanced building by applying the same moulding used in the window mullions to the walls in between, forming panels on the stone walls. The effect was to apply tracery to the entire side of the building, not just the window apertures, thereby bringing coherence to the façade. It was decorative rather than structural, but a success nonetheless, giving aesthetic purpose to what had been an ungainly mess.

The project at Gloucester was just as sensitive. The abbey of St Peter was an ancient foundation which had been refounded by the Norman royal family and had retained strong royal links ever since. The east end of the abbey church, finished around 1100, was built in heavy Norman Romanesque. The fact that some side chapels had been beautified in the early fourteenth century made the prospect of the total demolition and complete rebuilding of this massive edifice even more unattractive. So Thomas devised a plan. Work would start in the south transept, where there had been some damage from a recent fire: this space would afford him the opportunity to test his new idea. In spring 1331, he took down the roof and removed the clerestory which formed the upper range of the walls. Then, grafting on new vaults to the existing piers, he created a new – Gothic – roof. This much had been achieved elsewhere before. However, the result had always been unsatisfactory, as it produced an all-too-obvious mixture of styles: round-arched Romanesque topped with a pointed Gothic ceiling. To avoid this, Thomas took the blind tracery he had developed at St Stephen's and tooled it onto the flat Norman walls: a Gothic appliqué on a Romanesque surface. At high level he was able to squeeze in some new clerestory windows; awkward, just as they had been at St Stephen's, but they unified the whole by using his new panelling effect. Finally there remained the aisle arches at ground level. These were still round-headed heavy Romanesque affairs which could not be removed without jeopardizing the structure. Thomas's solution was driven by the exigencies of that inheritance and yet it would become the defining component of late-medieval English Gothic. He saw that were he simply to insert a pointed arch inside the Norman curve, it would produce an unsatisfactory and ill-proportioned apex, requiring much unsightly and tricky stone infilling. Instead, his new arch, which was of slightly more complicated geometry, could be better accommodated within the existing Romanesque curve. Given the limitations of the site, it was the ideal way to gothicize a Romanesque façade. Only the keen eye would see what was actually going on: this was a Gothic sketch on a Romanesque palimpsest.

The techniques used by Thomas of Canterbury in Westminster and Gloucester were so successful, and so flexible, that other masons quickly took note, one of them being a young mason from Norwich, William Ramsey. Ramsey had grown up surrounded by masons: his brother, father and uncles had been connected with the construction of the cloisters at Norwich Cathedral and, indeed, with St Stephen's Chapel at Westminster. Families often specialized in a craft, with fathers and uncles apprenticing sons and nephews in the family trade. Ramsey's early progression, however, shows a precocious ability. He was born at the turn of the fourteenth century, was apprenticed in his early teens as a mason and by 1323 was mentioned as a mason working on a passage linking St Stephen's Chapel with the Painted Chamber in the palace at Westminster. In 1326, William was back in Norwich, his home town, working on the south walk of the cathedral cloister. By now he was called 'master', meaning that he had long since achieved his apprenticeship as a stone mason and had worked as a journeyman – the standard degree of competency in any craft. As a master mason, Ramsey was qualified to design buildings alone and supervise their construction, overseeing gangs of masons, carpenters, glaziers, plasterers and painters. The nearest modern-day equivalent is the architect, although it should be remembered that the master mason had worked his way up through the manual craft itself. It is an important distinction. The master mason not only had a good understanding of geometry and an ability to draw, design moulds and even model; crucially, because master masons had learned their skills 'on the job', they also possessed a physical 'feel' for how buildings stood up, giving them a structural intuition that enabled them to perform the kind of architectural gymnastics that remain so breathtaking today. Unfortunately, there were few opportunities for master masons in the early fourteenth century to demonstrate their bravery and inventiveness, as large building projects were few and far between. The nave of York Minster – a huge structure in the French style, recently terminated with an extravagantly flamboyant west window – was one such;[i] St Stephen's in London was another. Beyond rare opportunities such as these, master masons such as Ramsey had to compete for less grandiose improvements, of which the new cloisters at Norwich Cathedral were a good example. These commissions posed challenges of their own: fashionably elaborate stonework (like that at York) was too expensive and often difficult to integrate into the existing fabric of a building. An innovative response was called for: a fresh architectural palette, one that could be used successfully within the many existing buildings whose improvements were now the mainstay of master masons' business.

The answer came in 1332, when Ramsey was instructed to build a cloister and chapter house for St Paul's Cathedral – a commission prompted by Sir John Pulteney, who was at the time serving one of his periods as mayor. It was by far the most significant new project of the time, giving Ramsey an unrivalled opportunity to apply his original architectural thinking. Constrained by space, William placed the chapter house within the square cloister garth. This was a difficult trick to pull off – a cloister should be light and engender a sense of peace, but this was hard to achieve if a large stone edifice had to be placed right in the middle. Ramsey's solution was doubly novel: first he used the stone itself to create a feeling of lightness. The lower part of the cloister was built in Purbeck marble but the upper was in Caen limestone; limestone alone was used for the octagonal chapter house. He then employed the device which had been used so successfully in Westminster and took the window mullions right up to the curved sides of the arch, giving a sense of upward thrust to the façades. Square panelling and blind tracery were again used on the flat stone surfaces, articulating the whole and giving a tight unity to the mass of the chapter house. Put together, the two tones of stone in the cloister gave a light, floating feel to the arcades, whereas the careful and coherent surface articulation of the chapter house endowed the building with a unified vertical presence. Far from being an overbearing mass of

---

[i] By Ivo Raughton, c.1330. The nave was begun in 1291 and was coming to its conclusion by the mid-1340s.

stonework, the central chapter house formed a powerful focal point. It was a *tour de force*, which not only guaranteed William Ramsey a continued stream of work but was soon copied by other – less able – masons elsewhere. At St Paul's, William Ramsey had succeeded in creating a new architectural language, one that eschewed the rich sculptural curves seen in York for a more ordered, versatile, rectilinear style.

When Thomas of Canterbury died in 1336, Ramsey was made his successor as king's master mason south of the River Trent and became, therefore, responsible for the ongoing work at Gloucester. As soon as the French expedition of 1346–7 was over, Edward and the abbot agreed that the next stage of the improvements could begin.[3] They decided to tackle the choir, the very place where Edward II was entombed, which had become a place of pilgrimage. Although this new popularity was unexpected, the abbey was not going to interfere, for the income derived from visitors funded in part the improvements to the fabric that they wished to make. Ramsey worked up the plans for the next phase of building. The highest part of the structure was removed. Then, suddenly, the news of the pestilence arrived.[4] The city closed its gates, the pilgrims ceased to come and supplies of stone could no longer be assured. The abbey was left with an uncovered choir and no immediate prospect of a new roof being built. All the abbot could do was wait for the plague to pass.

Medieval Gloucester sat on the east bank of a great bend in the river Severn, which formed one side of the town's defensive boundary, the remainder being provided by a high wall. Even though they closed the gates, the townsmen could not stop the flow of traffic on the river. Gloucester was on a crossroads – it was the lowest bridging point over the Severn, carrying the road from London into Herefordshire and then on into Wales. Traffic from the south came by the road from Bristol, proceeding on to the Midlands, and by river on the flat-bottomed barges that could cross the shallow water. It must have been from one of these that the pestilence got inside the town, no doubt from one of the little fishing settlements that supplied fish to Gloucester's market. It might even have come from Oldbury in Thornbury manor, which was infected at least by October 1348. So the disease established itself by early winter 1348, and by the New Year the town was infected. (Maybe the townsmen's precautions, in delaying the entry of the pestilence, did indeed have an effect. At the abbey, it is probable that about a quarter of the monks perished; however, at Llanthony Priory[ii] just outside the city walls, nineteen of the thirty canons were killed – a death rate approaching two thirds of their community.) The pestilence had shown itself to be irresistible. As the Malmesbury monk commented only a few years later, the plague 'travelled northwards [from Bristol], leaving not a city, a town, a village, or even, except rarely, a house, without killing most or all of the people there'.[5]

Irresistible but not inescapable. The Great Death had made considerable progress in the countryside to the south of Bristol, forcing the bishop of Bath and Wells, Ralph Shrewsbury, to move from one place to the next in a desperate effort to avoid the disease. Eventually he had taken refuge, in his manor house at Wiveliscombe, on the edge of Exmoor. This was a sensible precaution: Wiveliscombe was as remote a place as could be found in Somerset, but it was still close enough to allow the continued administration of the diocese. There was much to do. Just before Christmas he had ordered the institution of a new rector at Yeovil,[6] yet in the course of little over a month, he had to institute another two clerics to the same parish: the people of Yeovil had no fewer than four priests between December 1348 and January 1349. Indeed, villages all over north and east Somerset were losing their priests – at least fifty parishes by the end of 1348 and another fifty within the first two months of 1349. Around Bath alone, the parishes of Bathampton, Weston, Twerton, Batheaston and Freshford all lost their priests in January; the new incumbent in Batheaston was already dead by February and in Bathampton there were to be three further institutions. The records of parish appointments not only give a crude indication of the terrible mortality suffered in those places; by implication, many parishes were now lacking – at least for a few crucial weeks – someone capable of giving the Last Rites. Realizing the gravity of the situation, Bishop Ralph sent an ordinance throughout his diocese on 10th January 1349, in which he set out the challenge he and his flock faced: not only were priests dying and leaving their

---

[ii] 'Canons' here being monks following the Augustinian, rather than Benedictine, rule. The house was properly called Llanthony Secunda.

parishes destitute, but it was becoming increasingly difficult to find replacements who were willing to visit the sick for fear of contagion or infection. Shrewsbury's anger at the failings of his clergy, unwilling (he claimed) to risk their lives for the 'salvation of souls', was palpable. So to ensure that everyone who died had been able to make a final confession, he instructed that if a priest could not be found, then the dying could make their confession to a layman; if a man could not be found, then a woman would suffice. In this moment of crisis, when priestly mediation was needed most, the bishop effectively delegated sacramental powers to the laity: Shrewsbury had been forced to concede the complete incapacity of the church in the face of this overwhelming catastrophe.

The procession of priests making their way to Wiveliscombe will no doubt have helped to draw the epidemic into west Somerset, only a couple of miles from the Devon border. The disease had already independently infected the harbours of the north Devon coast and so now the county was threatened from three points – the north shoreline, west Somerset, and the Great Death's first locus in south Dorset. The Cistercian monastery at Newenham on the Dorset–Devon border had lost nearly all its monks,[7] whilst the collegiate church of Ottery St Mary, a little further into Devon, had also been struck hard. The foundation at Ottery had been established by John Grandison, the bishop of Exeter, whose diocese took in Devon and Cornwall. It was a striking version of Grandison's other great building project – Exeter Cathedral – in miniature, where work was currently underway on the west front, overseen by the mason William Joy.[iii] The stone for this project was being shipped from the Purbeck Hills, where the pestilence had struck early on. Perhaps the plague came with a boatload of marble, perhaps with the fishermen, perhaps from a visiting priest from nearby Ottery: whatever the source, Exeter was infected just before Christmas 1348. At the hospital of Clyst Gabriel, just outside the city, the first of the aged and infirm priests who were patients there died on New Year's Day. Guy de Okehampton had been a resident for over twenty years (the longest in the community) but was the first to perish; eight more patients died by the end of March, the last of whom – Richard Molyns – was more than sixty years old. There

---

[iii] The work was probably begun by Thomas Witney and taken on by William Joy.

were then no more deaths for nearly a year, so we may assume that in Exeter the epidemic had burnt itself out by the middle of spring. In three months, however, it had killed well over half the parish priests in the city, a rate of mortality that cannot have been far different from that suffered by the general populace.[8] One of the victims was almost certainly William Joy, which was enough to disrupt the building on the west front of the Cathedral. So far only one tier of niches had been completed on the west front screen and only some of these had been filled with the statues for which they had been designed. Now, with the architect dead and most probably some of the sculptors too, Bishop Grandison's great project stalled when not even halfway to completion.[iv] Yet with half of his parishes losing priests through 1349 and the need to institute a legion of new candidates (264 in that year alone) there was business enough for this well-regarded prelate without worrying about the building work on his beloved cathedral.

The band of disease that now stretched from the Severn to the south Dorset coast expanded slowly across the countryside through the cold winter months, west through Somerset and Devon and east into Wiltshire.[v] Men had little need to travel and everyone stayed at home to conserve heat and their energies as best they could. Yet although the pace of the epidemic's spread was slowed by winter stasis, its potency was undiminished. At Tisbury, for instance, just over the border from infected Dorset in west Wiltshire, the tenants started falling ill late in 1348. In January, at the first manorial court of the new year, seventy-five of the tenants were found to have died, a figure which suggests that already several hundred in this village had perished. Two villages either side of Tisbury give some idea of the proportion of the village population that this might have been. Seventeen miles due east in the manor of Downton, the death rate was 66 per cent of the tenantry; eleven miles due west in the village of Gillingham, 190 of the 300 tenants died during the winter of 1348–9.[9] It is likely

---

[iv] Although it is likely that basic maintenance work continued nonetheless, and offerings from the public at the cathedral altars was unaffected.

[v] The infection may have spread into Wiltshire before 1348 was out: the master of De Vaux College in Salisbury, Baldwin de Mohun, died in November or December and the prior of Ivychurch a couple of the miles to the south-east died in the first few months of 1349.

that in Tisbury, therefore, more than half the village had died before January was at an end.

Tisbury was only a couple of hours' walk from Monkton Deverill, the southernmost village in the little chain of Deverill settlements hidden in a fold in the West Wiltshire Downs. The pestilence may well have made it to the Deverills by the end of 1348, and certainly had the villages within its grip by the first weeks of the New Year. Agnes Panel, who had lost her husband nearly nine years before and had managed his considerable holding on her own since, was soon dead. John Cutel, the reeve, who will have been present at the manorial courts when the first deaths were announced, also died. For nearly twenty years he had derived much benefit from his position within the village; it may well be that it was his office that brought him into early contact with the disease. Not everyone was unlucky, however: John Peter, the *pater familias* of the large and comparatively well-off Peter family, saw the year out, as did his wife Agnes, although it is possible that his two sons, Robert and Stephen, did not make it. Peter Boket, the landless wage-earner and brewer, was a survivor, as were just over half his fellow landless labourers in the Deverill villages. These men were certainly fortunate, as on other Glastonbury Abbey manors well over half the landless died. What can account for the fact that fewer landless men perished in Monkton Deverill, where Peter Boket lived? It is not clear, for this epidemic worked in mysterious ways, but perhaps the sheer isolation of the village, out of the way of travellers and traders, saved it from the worst the disease could do.

Meanwhile, the small outbreak of disease in Titchfield, on the east bank of the Solent in Hampshire, continued to simmer – by March two thirds of the tenants had died.[vi] The surrounding towns and villages seemed impervious to the epidemic, however; perhaps word had got out and everyone avoided contact with people from Titchfield. Yet it could only be a matter of time before the disease spread out. Whether Southampton, sitting at the head of the Solent, caught the infection from Titchfield to the south, or from Dorset or Wiltshire to the west, or independently from infected ships coming into its port, it is impossible to know. Indeed, it is surprising that Southampton, which was

---

[vi] It is possible that the disease also entered Hampshire from the west over Christmas: the rector of Fordingbridge, just south of Downton but across the county border, died in December 1348.

the most important port on the south coast of England, stayed free of infection so long: its resilience may have had something to do with the predominance of its trade with northern (as opposed to southern) France. Eventually, however, the epidemic arrived, finding the town already in a bad way. A vicious attack by the French a year into the war had left Southampton dilapidated and impoverished. God's House, a hospital for the poor and once fairly wealthy, had to be remitted local tolls and taxes in 1347 because of its depressed condition, never having recovered from being set alight by the invaders nine years earlier. In the same year the endowment of the town's leper hospital was given to the local priory of Augustinian canons, which was suffering considerable hardship as a result of its sacking by the French. The arrival of plague – marked tellingly by the increase in merchant wills that began in early 1349 – only heaped despair on Southampton's indigence.

Winchester, the ancient capital of Wessex, was twelve miles up the River Itchen from Southampton. It too was in a state of slow decline: after the royal Treasury and Exchequer moved to London in the 1170s, Winchester could boast little of importance other than the annual St Giles's Fair, held on a hill just outside the city – one of several English fairs which enjoyed international repute.[vii] The purpose-built shops and market squares found more and more in English market towns made these fairs increasingly irrelevant. Some of the very oldest inhabitants of Winchester could probably remember the exciting fortnight of the fair – when traders would come from all over the country and abroad to buy and sell all manner of goods, from grains in bulk to the finest manufactured goods from the Continent. Yet those days were now gone: where once mercers from Flanders and merchants from Italy choked the old narrow streets of the city, now the fair was lucky to draw people from more than one county away. The impact of this had been felt in the town: shops had gone and two of the city's fifty-four churches had been closed for want of parishioners. Although about 10,000 people still lived in Winchester,[viii] unlike almost every other town in England the

[vii] The others being in Northampton, Stamford, St Ives, Boston and Lynn.
[viii] The population today is about 40,000; pre-Great Death Winchester was thus about a quarter of the size the city is now.

population had not grown since pre-Conquest times. The city had become a provincial backwater.

Nevertheless, Winchester remained an important local market and the centre of administration for the vast estates of its bishop, scattered from Surrey to Oxfordshire, Berkshire, Hampshire and Somerset. It may well have been one of the bishop's officials returning from the West Country that brought the disease in; it could equally have come from Southampton or Titchfield in the south or direct from London itself. Indeed, there would have been a terrible irony if the pestilence had been introduced by the messenger who bore William Edington's letter from his palace in Southwark. Bishop William sent his instructions ordering prophylactic processions and prayers on 24th October, believing as he did that the pestilence was still confined to coastal regions. He clearly suspected that many deaths were imminent: before he left for the Continent with the king, he devolved his powers of absolution reserved to the bishop (those sins considered so wicked that only the bishop could absolve them) to local representatives, helpfully reminding them that 'sickness and premature death often come from sin; and that by the healing of souls this kind of sickness is known to cease'.[10] Yet no amount of repentance would stop the advance of the pestilence, which took hold in Winchester within a month of Edington's mandate, well before Christmas 1348. It was not long before the graveyards were full and Bishop William, noting the 'present and increasing mortality', had hastily to consecrate an extension to the cathedral cemetery.[11] Unfortunately, the chosen site had for a long time been used by the townsmen as a market place and its annexation as a burial ground irritated them greatly. In the middle of January a mob attacked a monk of the cathedral priory, Ralph Staunton, who was in the middle of burying one of the many dead. The unfortunate brother was beaten, prevented from completing the burial, and the body carried away and dumped on the town tip. Edington was outraged: he condemned the attack, arranged a notice of censure by the king and instructed the clergy to preach on the importance of burial in consecrated ground for the eventual resurrection of the dead. It seems that the bishop's admonitions had little effect, however, for the protests continued; within a month the townsmen had torn down the perimeter fence and started building market stalls in the cemetery, in an attempt to prevent further burials. Not only was this an act of sacrilege but during construction the half-decomposed cadavers of the recently interred plague victims were dug up and flung outside the burial ground. When the monks remonstrated with them, the contumacious townsmen threatened to burn their cathedral down.

In truth, while the encroachment into the market was an irritation, the root of the townsmen's anger most probably lay with the fees levied by the priory for burying the dead. As an occasional charge, these payments were manageable; but when half a family had died, the costs of burial were especially burdensome to those who remained. Since both bishop and priory insisted that the dead be buried within their own sanctified ground, the fees were unavoidable; indeed, it was hard not to feel that the priory was exploiting its privileges in order to make a heartless return on the widespread mortality – a grievance with which the extension of the cemetery would become inextricably bound. The charges will have appeared all the more oppressive given that the people of Winchester could see that they were effectively contributing to the rebuilding of the cathedral choir, which was at that time wrapped in scaffolding. But William Joy was the mason here too and his death, with that of so many of his workmen, soon brought this long-running project to a halt; the window tracery was to remain uncompleted for many years. The priory's poor relations with Bishop Edington did not help matters. On the death of the prior in early March 1349, the monks elected a replacement contravening all their own laws of due process, and so Edington made them repeat the exercise (although, in the event, they ended up with the same result). Despite such mortality and misery, William Edington remained a stickler for the rules. It was a glimmer of normality amid the horror of epidemic disease, as was the townsmen's willingness to assert themselves in defiance of episcopal and royal power. For if the pestilence did not dull the bishop's sense of impropriety, nor did it diminish the townsmen's feeling of grievance. At the very least, these disputes demonstrated that everyone believed there would be a future worth fighting about.

Although the city of Norwich was also an ancient town, its fortunes were wholly different from those of Winchester: the sale of cheap worsted cloth and a pre-eminence as a market in its rich East Anglian hinterland had brought sustained growth over the last couple of hundred years. With 25,000 people by 1340, it had two and a half times the population of ailing Winchester and a quarter the number living in London. The citizens' civic aspirations were correspondingly ambitious. Norwich's wealthiest citizen, Richard Spynk, not only personally paid for the completion of the city walls but purchased a memoranda book in which the acts of the community were to be noted. In this there is the first mention of an elected body of twenty-four citizens, six from each of the four wards (or 'leets') that made up the city. This was municipal government in the making, forged in part by the citizens' desire to take control of their own affairs. For here too there had been ructions between the townsmen and the cathedral authorities and in 1344 the city successfully petitioned the king to be given police jurisdiction over the cathedral enclosure. This was granted and by way of thanks the burghers of Norwich sent twenty-four herring pies to the king every year, the recipe for which was recorded in Spynk's book. The pies were extravagantly spiced – ginger, cinnamon, cloves, pepper, galingale and the exotically named 'grains of Paradise'.[12] A certain Hugh de Curson was deputed to deliver these choice pies to the king, containing the first fresh herrings of the year. It is safe to assume that these fish would have come from Yarmouth during the great autumn herring fair and the spices brought from London. Once the pies had been made up, Hugh de Curson would have to travel to the king's court and back, probably via the capital, to deliver the city's gift of thanks.

In all probability Hugh had nothing to do with the transmission of plague to Norwich, but the ingredients of his pies – and their destination – provide good tangential evidence of the connections that spread the pestilence around, precisely those links which ensured that Norwich contracted the disease so early. With plague ravaging London, the threat extended not only to those places very near, such as the villages that surrounded the city, but also much further away, where the frequency of administrative journeys and vibrancy of trade made the transmission of the disease all the more likely. So Wandsworth, only six miles south-west of London, caught the plague from the city at about the same time as Canterbury, over fifty miles to the south-east. Similarly, in January 1349 nine tenements in the village of Stepney, less than a mile from the city's eastern wall, were reported to be vacant owing to the deaths of their tenants, just as word got round the citizens of Norwich – a hundred miles away to the north-east – that the pestilence had broken out in their city.[13] Sadly, entries into Richard Spynk's book of memoranda cease in 1349, most probably as a result of the pestilence. It is one of the reasons why so little is known about the effects of the disease in this important city, although a sure indication is given by the fate of the Friars of Our Lady, every one of which perished.[ix]

Bristol, London, Southampton, Winchester and then Norwich: pestilence made the jump between the larger cities of southern England with depressing inevitability. Canterbury, however, was not a large town; its early infection had more to do with its proximity to the ports of Kent and the capital. Moreover, this ancient place was the metropolitan seat of the Primate of All England, and its high concentration of ancient religious institutions ensured that the citizens' experience of the pestilence was recorded in somewhat finer detail than was the case in far larger Norwich. The Canterbury chronicler, Simon Birchington, wrote that barely 'a third of mankind were left alive' – a claim borne out by the taxation returns covering the years of the Great Death, in which two thirds of the taxable population disappeared from the record.[14] Whereas the prior of Winchester Cathedral Priory perished, the prior of Christchurch Canterbury survived, as did almost all his brothers. In part because they benefited from their own water supply, the monks had been able to barricade themselves into the priory, denying themselves all contact with outsiders and thereby preventing the ingress of the disease.[15] Of seventy-five monks in the priory, only four died during the months of plague; it was surely not without coincidence that every monk who stayed within the priory bounds survived. Thus the priory monks of Canterbury succeeded where the citizens of Gloucester had failed, proving that it was indeed possible, by maintaining strict isolation, to keep the pestilence at bay.

William Ramsey had come far since his apprenticeship in Norwich. He was now a wealthy, respected man, and an elected alderman of the city of London. His was a remarkable tale of advancement through

---

[ix] 'De Domina', or Friars of St Mary – a lesser order of friars which had arrived in the city in the late thirteenth century and had a house just next to the church of St Julian, now off King's Street.

talent and hard work, together with the assiduous courting of men of influence. He probably got his break at St Paul's as a result of the patronage of Sir John Pulteney; it is not hard see why the great mercer liked the young architect so much. Both Pulteney and Ramsey were ambitious and gifted sons of the provinces who had made it in the capital and become men of national importance in their respective fields. Both provide evidence that for the very able at least, some degree of social mobility was possible in mid-fourteenth-century England.

In Ramsey's case, this advancement had not been uncontested. When, in 1331, he arranged the engagement of his daughter Agnes to Robert Hubert – the heir to a large property portfolio – Robert's guardian, John Spray, refused to allow the union, not wishing to permit his ward to involve himself with the daughter of a mere mason. So, on a November night, William – with his wife Christina, father and brother – stole into Spray's house, where they abducted the fourteen-year-old fiancé. Spray lodged a complaint in the courts but young Robert protested that he wished to remain with Ramsey. Perhaps he really was in love. John Spray could not, however, have complained at the subsequent progress of his ward's father-in-law: Ramsey was made a master of the king's works and awarded some of the most important architectural commissions in the land.

So when, on 29th May 1349, Ramsey made out his will, it was a very significant inheritance that he left to Agnes, now wife of Robert Hubert. As the last words on the parchment were completed, a witness took a candle and dribbled some wax onto the folds. Ramsey reached forward and pressed his signet into the soft wax. Once removed, it left an exquisitely cut shield, containing a pair of compasses held between two rams' heads, with a gateway at the base. Even if his greatest works no longer stand, these arms – borne not by a knight or lord, but by a Norwich mason – attest to his achievement. With William Ramsey's death, the plague had brought a premature loss to English architecture; his passing was all the more tragic for the fact that, within days, the pestilence began to beat its retreat from the streets of London. It had by now, however, engulfed much of England.

7

Spring and Death

March–May 1349

It seem'd so hard and dismal thing,
Death, to mark them in the Spring.
Gerard Manley Hopkins, 'Spring and Death'[1]

At about a quarter to four o'clock on Friday, 13th March 1349, a still sleepy doorkeeper made his way in the early-morning gloom to Holy Trinity church. Unlocking the door, he entered and lit a taper. The young cleric did a circuit of the building, putting a flame to candles around the walls, enough to show the silhouette of the great pillars that held up the high roof of the nave. Then, hastening to the small room at the base of the tower, he untied the rope that dropped through a hole in the ceiling and pulled the cord vigorously, sounding a bell high up in the belfry. Within a few seconds, another bell could be heard, responding from the church of St Michael close by. For a few minutes the tolls came into time and then parted again, until the peal died gently away to silence and the morning birdsong could be heard once more. Coventry had been woken and the city began to stir.

The pickets that stopped up each of the roads coming into the city were removed, the night watch stood down, and within the hour traders started to arrive. The fish market in the Cross Cheaping opened at seven and was immediately busy: it was a fortnight into Lent, and fish was eaten on Fridays in any event. There was cod, haddock, ling, conger eel and plaice, as well as dried, smoked and salted herring, and one or other fishmonger may have brought in some salmon or trout. At nine, after Mass in St Michael's, the city's mayor, Nicholas Michel, walked about the fish market, inspecting the quality of the catch. Although the morning sales were reserved for citizens of the city there were already plenty of outsiders about, for Fridays was the biggest market day of the week, when the Drapery – the covered cloth market – opened up just to the south of St Michael's. Merchants from all over the Midlands came to the city, and every year their numbers increased. Coventry was now the most important centre for the textile trade outside London.[2]

Yet all was not as it should have been, this March morning, for pestilence had recently arrived. The hubbub was less intense, doleful faces were worn by all, and there were already gaps in the usual crowd. The merchant John Arthingworth, who would normally have been in the thick of the deal-making, was one of those missing. Nearly two weeks before,[i] John had signed over his property interests to two other Coventry citizens, with specific instructions as to what to do with his bequest. When he died shortly afterwards, leaving a wife and daughter, the executors immediately set about dealing with his estate. This Friday, they were huddled in a room with one of the beneficiaries, the guild of St Mary, a merchant institution closely linked to the city fathers who in 1345 had won the incorporation of Coventry as a self-governing city. John had bequeathed the guild three cottages and now the last details were being worked out. Fresh from his tour of the market, the mayor joined the party with the city's two bailiffs in order to witness the sealing.[ii]

Given that John was survived by a widow and child, handing over assets to the guild may seem a strange thing to have done, but it was in fact an ingenious act of estate planning. The provisions of the bequest ensured that John's direct heirs retained the benefit of the properties, even though the actual ownership rested with the guilds – in other words, the guild held them in trust. Should his wife and daughter die, however, which was a real possibility, then the guild would receive the rents and John's wealth would not be forfeit to the crown. John Arthingworth was not alone in this ruse – over sixty other citizens conveyed their lands to Coventry guilds. In John's case

---

[i] Sunday, 8th March 1349.
[ii] Only a week later they would repeat the exercise, the beneficiary this time being the guild of St John the Baptist, a religious confraternity set up to pay for priests to sing masses for the souls of its members.

it was a worthwhile precaution: on 14th April his daughter signed over her interest to her mother, presumably shortly before she too died. With no heir, John's cottages did indeed revert to St Mary's Guild. When, during the Dissolution, the guilds were stripped of their wealth, John Arthingworth's property holdings were added to the corporation of Coventry's estate, which its successor council still retains today.

The careful disposal of property by the moneyed men of Coventry was indicative of the ambition that possessed this fast-growing Midlands city. So great was Coventry's draw that by 1349 over half its inhabitants were immigrants, most of whom came from outside the surrounding county of Warwickshire (John Arthingworth, for instance, was from Northamptonshire). The majority had left densely populated manors in the east Midlands and Thames Valley, escaping the constrictions of the manorial economy. In lobbying for incorporation as a city, establishing guilds and fighting the prior of Coventry's influence within the town, these men were creating the structures which the community required in the absence of overarching manorial control. In many ways the guilds and the town council carried out the same functions as those performed by the feudal lord and the manor court – the regulation of life within the community, settling of grievances, arrangement of landholding and control of inheritances. The similarities go further still: the majority of larger towns were governed by an oligarchy of citizens, which was often almost as exclusive as the manor lordships from which they or their forefathers had fled. In the town, it was the citizens who were in control, not the lord and his officials. Their existence was not antipathetic to existing rural structures. Indeed, in providing a market for the produce of the feudal estates and catering to the demand for luxury and manufactured goods that flowed in large part from a nobility enriched by feudal tenure, medieval towns were very much part of the late-medieval feudal economy. There were, of course physical differences: towns were compact and densely populated; they relied upon constant immigration to sustain their populations; the range of occupations – even in the smallest towns – was far greater than in the largest manors. The greatest difference lay, however, in the opportunities towns promised to men and women who had not been born into privilege. In short, they came to embody aspiration and a sense of ambition quite distinct from that which could be found in even the most progressive manor.

Coventry did not grow in isolation. Like all towns and cities it lived on the raw products of the countryside around – grain for bread, cattle for meat, hides for shoes, wood and stone for building. Moreover, its emerging bourgeoisie demanded the kind of metals and luxuries – gold, spices and manufactured goods – which had to be imported from overseas. The town's success, however, was founded on the goods traded with other towns in England and abroad, principally cloth, a business that required the massive import of wool and export of finished product, which in turn relied upon good connections with the world around. Coventry was inland and its insignificant river, the Sherborne, was navigable only by shallow-bottomed boats, so there was no harbour with which to ship goods to the sea and beyond. Instead, Coventry reached its markets by road, trading through a system of highways that had evolved significantly over the previous 300 years. The remnants of the great Roman roads – Watling Street, Ermine Street, the Icknield and Foss Ways – remained, just as they had done in pre-Conquest times. Yet these routes linked garrisons and were built to facilitate the rapid movement of massed troops. Although several principal Roman towns had retained their pre-eminence (London, York), some had been reduced to villages (Silchester, Caistor), others were no longer important (Wroxeter, Colchester) and still more had been joined by powerful new neighbours (Bath, Gloucester and Cirencester were now easily eclipsed by Bristol, as was Leicester increasingly by Coventry). The Roman road system thus no longer met the requirements of trade, not least because of the proliferation of many smaller towns in between the larger cities, which had the effect of multiplying the number of routes between the same two places. So, on going from London to York, the traveller would take Ermine Street to just beyond Huntingdon, when the marshy Fens split the old Roman route into a number of medieval tracks, each one of which may have been preferable depending on the weather, flooding or the mode of transport – or indeed if the traveller wished to go north via either Stamford or Boston. For all their lack of organization, these roads constituted a discernible network, one that had London – then, as now – at its nodal centre. The majority of the most heavily used roads radiated out from London to the principal cities and towns in the provinces, the ancestors of the A road network still so much relied upon today.[iii]

William Langland's 'Truth' commands merchants to mend bad roads and broken bridges, so that they may 'abide in [Heaven's] bliss, body and soul for ever'.[3] This was not wishful thinking: the many bequests made by traders and their guilds all helped to maintain the principal arteries of trade both for the benefit of other traders and travellers and for the benefactor's own soul.[iv] In addition, the church had long promoted charitable giving directed at improving the ease and freedom of travel, preaching that such gifts would smooth the path of the benefactor in his own spiritual journey to salvation. Earlier in the fourteenth century, the bishop of Worcester commented that 'the ruin and damage of bridges is frequently of peril to souls and bodies', going on to describe their maintenance as a work of mercy greatly pleasing to God.[4] That this doctrine came about is not surprising: good roads promoted mobility (upon which an increasingly centralized church depended), facilitated pilgrimages (which generated considerable ecclesiastical income), encouraged the creation of wealth (in which the church had an interest as great as anyone else), impeded robbers (the scourge of the medieval traveller, many

---

[iii] From the capital major routes travelled south-east to Canterbury and Dover, and north-east into the major towns of East Anglia. There were several ways of reaching the Midlands towns of Leicester, Coventry and Lichfield, just as there were to York, Lancaster, Carlisle and the Scottish border. North Wales was reached from this north-west route; it was more easy to travel to south Wales from London via Oxford, the Severn crossing at Gloucester, Hereford and then Hay-on-Wye. The road to Bristol, which the modern A4 almost precisely follows, was the most travelled highway in England; the route to the south-west (taking in Guildford, Farnham, Winchester, Salisbury, Yeovil, Exeter, Launceston, Bodmin, all the way to the foot of Cornwall at Land's End) followed as many ancient droving tracks as it did portions of Roman road. There were other, equally important, routes which were not part of this radial pattern, like the road that ran north out of Bristol, crossed the London–Wales highway in Gloucester and then bifurcated at Worcester, the eastern branch going to Leicester and Coventry then on up to Doncaster, the western leg heading on from Worcester to Shrewsbury, Chester and Liverpool.

[iv] For example, the will of the corn-dealer Walter Neel, made out in 1351, gave money for the repair of the road from Wycombe to Newgate in London – a route heavily used by the traders who brought corn and other foodstuffs from the Berkshire, Buckinghamshire and south Oxfordshire manors to feed the metropolis. Neel had forborne the poor surface throughout his working life and now he was able to offer a remedy in death.

of whom were clerics), and helped to prevent accidents (which was to everyone's benefit). To be sure, the church was but one of the many parties whose involvement in the maintenance of roads attests to the central importance of road travel in late-medieval life. The upkeep of what could properly be called a transport infrastructure was a dispersed effort, shared through tradition, charter, statute and on an *ad hoc* basis by merchants, guilds, the king, municipal authorities and monastic institutions.[5]

The quality of a road largely depended on the destinations it served, the frequency of its use and the people it carried. Along most of their length, the main highways were kept wide enough to allow two carts to pass each other and were sufficiently gravelled to permit travel in all but the worst of conditions. Off the arterial routes ran a multitude of lesser tracks, connecting towns with villages, villages with one another and settlements with individual homesteads. Some had basic grading like the major roads, others more closely resembled a muddy footpath. Journeys were not quick by today's standards – a mounted traveller would average about twenty-five miles a day, whilst a walking journeyman might manage fifteen. Slow maybe, but serviceable: medieval roads facilitated the free movement of goods and people throughout the land. The inexorable growth in trade and effective centralization of royal administration at Westminster might be evidence enough of the extraordinary multiplication of roads in medieval England; for physical proofs one need look no further than the number of bridging points established through the Middle Ages. There were, for example, only three Roman bridges that crossed the Thames between Staines and Reading, a number doubled by the middle of the fourteenth century. Thus, within 200 years of the Conquest, a web of roads stretched across the country that – whilst unplanned – supported migration, the expansion of trade, the enrichment of towns and the most advanced bureaucracy in Europe. Remarkably, the road map of England would not be added to in any significant way until the advent of the iron bridge in the second half of the eighteenth century and the motorway in the latter part of the twentieth.

In 1342, Sir John Pulteney had founded a house of Carmelite friars. It was not in his adopted city of London, which already possessed a 'Whitefriars'. Nor was it in Leicester, which might have seemed the obvious choice given that Pulteney was originally from Leicestershire.

Sir John chose instead to give his endowment to Coventry, a place with which he had no native links. His familiarity with Coventry came through his extensive drapery business, which naturally gave him frequent reason to have dealings with the dyers and mercers of the newer Midlands town. That Pulteney, the archetype of a London merchant, might have such an association with Coventry shows well the breadth of exchange between English towns and cities – links created and energized by growing trade, increasing government and the ever-expanding activities of the church. These relationships depended upon constant and extended contacts, which in time created wider communities. None of these – church, trade, administration – were circumscribed, but were interconnected. While there was nothing new in all this, by 1300 these wider communities were more profuse, populous and deeply rooted than ever before. Just like the road network that facilitated it, the centre of this plexus was London. This was only to be expected: London was the trading centre of England and Westminster the hub of royal administration and government. Other towns enjoyed local prominence, however: there were the trading towns of Coventry, Leicester, Southampton, Norwich and Bristol; Oxford's university was internationally important and drew aspirant scholars from all over the country; the diocesan capitals of the larger bishoprics, like Winchester, Lincoln and Lichfield, may have been of minor economic consequence but they accommodated bureaucracies that had great local influence; likewise the Northern capital of York, which replicated many of the regional functions of London but for the far smaller market and population that lay north of the River Trent. The regular and heavy traffic that moved between these and several other towns, unhindered by the absence of those prohibitive internal tolls so prevalent on the Continent, increased the degree to which the urban centres of England operated within each other's orbit; indeed, the broadening of horizons and changing perception of distance that flowed from this further contributed to the ever-deepening relationship between towns that was being driven primarily by increased trade, administration and intellectual exchange. A simple comparison between Matthew Paris's map of c.1250 and the so-called Gough Map of c.1360 displays the extraordinary change that there had been, even in the course of a hundred years. The English had the greater measure of their country, because they were now travelling across it – between its towns and beyond – in greater numbers than ever before.

All the better to spread pestilence. English towns were primed for an epidemic explosion: they were packed with people, living close up against one another, and once inside, as elsewhere, plague spread voraciously. The only chance townsmen had of protecting themselves was to shut the gates and stop any kind of entry from outside. Gloucester, the first town to find itself in this unenviable situation, decided to screen entrants, turning away men from Bristol – who presented the greatest risk – before they could pass through the city gates. Such a tactic, however, amounted to self-imposed siege; unless the town were exceptionally well-prepared, it was a course that could only end in privation and ruin. So although other towns doubtless adopted similar measures to Gloucester, it was all to be in vain, for trade was the urban *raison d'être*, travel the means by which towns survived. Closing the gates, moreover, was useless against the many who appeared healthy but were in fact contagious, and selective entry untenable once London had become infected; for without trade and contact with London, trade and contact might as well cease. Indeed, within a couple of months of its infection, London was sending growing numbers of unwitting messengers of death both near and far. It was inevitable that as the great feast of Christmas came to an end trade resumed, gaining volume through the early months of the year as the daylight hours increased. As the weather improved, transport moved more easily and rural markets woke after their hibernation. So just as pestilence had followed the drover and grain-trader out into London's grain-supplying hinterland, it accompanied the merchant and the official to much more distant provincial towns, creeping from the out-villages of London into the countryside of Essex and Kent, when a hundred miles away and more it was showing itself in Oxford, Coventry and Leicester. Thus, before March was at an end, almost every English town south of Nottingham had succumbed to the epidemic.

In the days of the Angevin empire nearly 200 years before, when English possessions in France were larger than England itself, Oxford was a favoured place for holding parliaments and royal councils. English kings then ruled a realm that stretched from the Scottish border to the Pyrenees, so Oxford offered as convenient a place as any for meetings in England. Almost equidistant from Bristol and London, it also sat midway on the road from London to Gloucester and could be reached from Southampton with great ease; those same four sumps of plague ensured that Oxford was an early recipient of pestilential disease. But Oxford's citizens had feared plague's arrival long before it eventually appeared and the richer townsmen had started making their wills as early as October 1348, as soon as they heard the news of what was happening on the estuary of the Severn and then, shortly after, on the banks of the Thames.

Oxford had suffered something of a decline in the early part of the century. It no longer hosted royal assemblies and its merchants had been squeezed by the better-connected traders of London and Bristol. Business was now dominated by a small and close-knit group of traders – men like Richard Cary, a mayor in 1349, whose father-in-law, William Bicester, had been the mayor in 1311, whose wife in turn was the widow of the man who had been mayor the year before, in 1310. For all its shrinking fortunes, however, the old centre of business around the crossroads of Carfax was still bustling, with its butchery, drapery and vintnery, the fish, corn and spice markets, and ranges of shops accommodating mercers, goldsmiths, cordwainers and cooks. Here were all the usual enterprises that made up any reasonable urban community, serving in Oxford not only the town but also its famous university, whose members contributed perhaps a quarter of the population of the town.[6]

The plague came with an infected traveller who entered through one of the town gates early in the New Year. Most likely he came from London, through East Gate, straight into the university side of the town. The High Street here was crammed with shops selling academic paraphernalia: there were book-binders, parchment makers, copyists and scriveners, all offering their wares to the students and scholars of the university and the fellows of the colleges that were dotted around the east side of the town – Merton, University, Exeter, Oriel, and the most recent – Queen's.[v] The founder of this last was Robert Eglesfield, who had been chaplain to Queen Philippa – in whose honour he had named the college. It had a dual purpose: to

---

[v] Founded 18th January 1341.

provide education to clerics from Eglesfield's native Cumberland and neighbouring Westmorland, so as to improve the standard of clergy thereabouts, and to give out charitable doles to the blind, deaf and dumb of Oxford, whose indigence was the more apparent for all the advancement of learning that went on in the town. Yet Eglesfield perished in the plague, his foundation still incomplete. This was but one of the several losses endured by the university in 1349: the Mertonian natural philosopher John Dumbleton was probably a victim, and two chancellors died in succession, causing a 'tumultuous election' for a third, John Wylliot.[7] All was not lost, however: the celebrated mathematician Richard Swineshead not only participated in Wylliot's controversial election but continued writing his *Liber calculationum* while the pestilence raged through the town. Likewise, the logician William Heytesbury, one of Eglesfield's founding fellows at Queen's, also survived the epidemic. It seems that the majority of students were similarly lucky; like the townsmen they had heard the warnings early and many had escaped to the country. Students, who were mainly educated clerics, were a mobile group and thus best able to avoid the advancing epidemic. Something under 10 per cent of the theology faculty died in the plague year, a figure that might well be matched across the university. We must doubt that the townsmen were as fortunate: in April the mayor died, to be succeeded by Richard Cary, who in June followed his predecessor to the grave. By the time he fell ill, Cary had already buried his mother-in-law and brother-in-law, re-endowing the chantry that had been part of William Bicester's original bequest. Once again the pestilence had rendered nugatory the endeavours of an early survivor, striking a further blow to a town already in decline.

Coventry is almost fifty miles north of Oxford, yet the two were struck within weeks of each other; the pestilence was certainly also present in Coventry by late February 1349. It took another month before Leicester – its Midlands neighbour and competitor – was infected. Leicester had a long and eminent history. Like Gloucester, Chester and York, it still sat within its square Roman bounds, the streets roughly following the grid laid down 1,300 years before. Roman remnants were visible in the town walls and the ruins of the baths sat hard by the Anglo-Saxon church of St Nicholas. Yet Leicester was still thriving, however, despite Coventry's recent ascendance: the town had gained its own ordinances as recently as 1335, a sure reflection of its civic ambition and economic success. Here too the plague had the same devastating effect: the chronicler Henry Knighton, writing forty years after the Great Death, described how the disease 'spread every-where with the passage of the sun'.[8] There were nine parishes in the town, in just three of which Knighton claims there were nearly 1,500 deaths. A crude calculation would suggest that there were over 4,000 deaths across Leicester, which would be nearly three quarters of the population of the town.[9]

Henry Knighton was an Augustinian canon,[vi] whose house had a sister foundation in Northampton – the abbey of St James. Canon Passelew, one of the canons there, had witnessed the decline of his town over the years, its cloth industry depressed by the growing power of Coventry, which was just over twenty-five miles away to the north. It was a mark of Northampton's problems that it succumbed to the plague so much later than did Coventry and Leicester, despite being closer to the capital and on the main road between London and Leicester. For while Coventry and Leicester were infected at the begin-ning and end of March respectively, Northampton was not infected until a month or even two months later. Even so, once infected, the mortality was just as severe: out of nine parishes, seven lost their vicars in 1349, one of which suffered a double loss during the year. A promi-nent victim was the Dominican Robert Holcot, one of England's great philosopher theologians, who had some years before moved from Oxford to his order's friary in Northampton, and it was there that he died while working on his *Commentary on Ecclesiasticus*. As elsewhere, the deaths of clerics must be taken as a proxy for more widespread mortality; for every priest and religious that died, many more lay townsmen – like Canon Passelew's relative John, a butcher – perished.[vii] In this way, the Great Death dealt a further blow to Northampton, already eclipsed by its more-successful neighbours, who could hope for better times. It is telling that even in the middle of the plague year,

---

[vi] A religious order that sought to lead a simple life modelled on the eremitic commu-nities of the early church, following the fifth-century Rule of St Augustine. By the fourteenth century there were more Augustinian (or 'Austin') houses than any other order in England, although typically they were small and their members generally uninfluential.

[vii] He bequeathed a chest to the abbey and his seal to his kinsman.

the Franciscan friars petitioned the king to be able to purchase a house in Leicester, so that they could enlarge their friary. No doubt it had been previously owned by a victim of the pestilence. That the Leicester friars were preparing for an increase in their number even in the midst of such a catastrophe showed their confidence in the eventual recovery of the town.

> *Lenten is come with love to toune,*[viii]
> *With blosmen and with briddes roune,*
> *That all this blisse bringeth.*
> *Dayeseyes in this dales,*
> *Notes swete of nightegales,*
> *Uch fowl song singeth.*
> *The threstelcok him threteth oo.*
> *Away is huere winter wo*
> *When woderofe springeth.*
> *This fowles singeth ferly fele,*
> *And wliteth on huere wynne wele,*
> *That all the wode ringeth.*[10]

This anonymous poet, writing at the turn of the fourteenth century, gives a vivid depiction of springtime joyously dispelling wearisome winter. Spring was a familiar trope in medieval literature, employed variously to evoke love, new life, unalloyed happiness and sexual abandon. The year was in its youth; indeed, it was a time, as John Lydgate had it, of *misspent* youth. Much of this was the romancing of an elite, yet it would be foolish to dismiss the sentiments of the poets for that reason. Every Christian grasped the synonymity of Lent and spring, when food was still sparse but the warming sun encouraged hope for the plenty to come. The coupling of spring and procreation was real for this predominantly rural people, from the early lambing of February to the ravishing chorus of the songbirds, singing

---

[viii] Lent is come with love to town, / With blossom and birdsong, / That all this bliss brings. / Daisies in these dales, / Notes sweet of nightingales. / Each bird sings song. / The song thrush makes his noisy dispute too. / Away is their winter woe / When the woodruff [a white woodland flower] springs. / These many birds sing fairly, / And warble in their abundant joy, / That all the wood rings.

for new mates in March. The poets' literary treatment was not simply an empty device: spring brought clear evidence of new life, genuine joy and the fulfilled promise of rebirth. It was all the more appalling, therefore, that the arrival of spring further accelerated the spread of the Great Death.

With spring came movement. Rural peasants spent as much of the winter as they could indoors, sustaining themselves on root vegetables, stored grains, salted meat and any fruit that remained from autumn. There was nothing new to eat in March, for which reason the Lenten fast had a very practical application in preserving what food remained. However, preparations for the year had already begun: fields were being ploughed and seeded with spring crops, animals were taken out of the stalls and put out to pasture, and a few lambs were being fattened for Easter, the first feast of the New Year. Replacement tools had to be bought for the season to come, as well as new draught animals and, perhaps, extra seed-corn for the sowing ahead. So the many small local markets sprung back to life again, drawing villagers from round about once more. These were very local journeys but they were nonetheless significant: the capillaries of the countryside opened once more to the life-blood of trade, which flowed – within a few removes of the village – to and from the great urban organs and through the arterial routes in between. The pestilence, which by the end of March was ravaging the larger towns and cities of southern and central England, spread rapidly down the now busy roads and tracks that ran out into the countryside. Thus, during the spring of 1349, the epidemic exploded throughout central and southern England. The moments of chance infection multiplied, until the arithmetic progress of the disease – passing from one person to the next, city to city – became exponential, expanding through the urban population and bursting out into the surrounding villages and hamlets. South Oxfordshire in late March, mid-Hampshire in early April, Berkshire in May: now there was no discernable pattern, only the dismal serendipity of infection and consequential spread. It was as if England were drawn on blotting paper, ceaselessly flicked with ink, the many blotches enlarging towards each other until the whole had been stained one black. The plague was predictable in one way only: sooner or later it would arrive and, once present, would kill.

Cornwall was already cut off from the rest of the country by a great front of the disease, stretching from the Severn estuary to the south Devon coast. At first, the pace of the plague's progression westwards followed the familiar winter crawl, coming over the county border at Rillaton, in a dell to the east of Bodmin Moor, where the reeve died on 12th March.[11] The rate of mortality was as high here as everywhere else: indeed, in the village of Calstock, 60–70 per cent of the people died. Within just a month the epidemic had made its way right to the other end of the county. Helston, in the cleft of the cloven toe of Cornwall, was nearly a hundred miles from Exeter and fifty from Bodmin Moor, yet on 11th April 1349 the manor's bailiff perished.[12] Helston was a stannary town, where Cornish tin was tested for purity and taxed. There were long-established coastal and international trading links for marketing tin (so long in fact that it was claimed that the Phoenicians had come to Cornwall to buy the metal). Here – as on the Dorset coast and along the Severn estuary – the disease had probably been brought first by boat, up the Helford River to Helston. It killed in Cornwall until late summer, when it faded away. The trouble caused at Bodmin Priory shows how much destruction it wrought: all but two of the canons died, forcing them to write to Bishop Grandison for help. (He had to ask the neighbouring monastery at Launceston to send a new prior.) The effect of such mortality on the tin mines was severe. The Prince of Wales's estates in Cornwall derived much of their income from tin; the immediate and precipitous falling-off in revenues, probably from the collapse of production as there were so few men left to go down the mines, was an indicator of how profound the impact of the pestilence had already been.[ix] It would be hard to find replacements quickly, since tin mining was tough, fraught with danger. Men cooped up together in narrow seams, near naked because of the heat. It is no wonder that the infection spread so quickly amongst them.

Just as it reached the western tip of England, so too the epidemic silently spread east. The whole of Hampshire had now succumbed, invaded from Wiltshire and Dorset in the west, Southampton and Titchfield in the south, London and Surrey in the east, and Winchester at its centre. Cheriton, one of the many manors in the county owned

<hr/>

ix The Duchy of Cornwall had been created in 1337 for the benefit of the Prince of Wales.

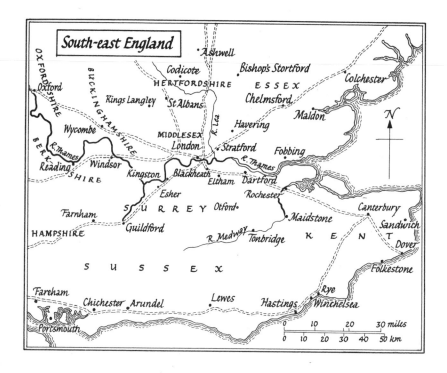

by the bishop of Winchester, started losing tenants around Easter.[x] Over the course of the following months, the village lost seventy-nine of its tenants, nearly two thirds of the total number. (Incredibly, Cheriton may have fared comparatively well: a sample of the bishop's manors in Hampshire suggests that on average about three quarters of the tenants died.) Such extraordinary mortality had an immediate impact on landholding. The piecemeal partition of land at Cheriton that had been the result of centuries of population growth was already being reversed as a result of the Great Death: John Creech, one of the few tenants to survive, immediately acquired a small plot of land that had been split off from his family virgate at some time in the previous century. At Alverstoke near Fareham, two women were the unexpected beneficiaries of William Rolf who, in the absence of any direct kin (most likely because they had all died), passed his land to his two aunts, Gillian and Agnes. On the other side of Winchester in the village of Crawley, Richard Kirkby, who had already lost his father

[x] Easter Sunday fell on 12th April in 1349.

in the pestilence, saw his grandfather go to the grave too; this young man, who was not more than twenty, thereby inherited a not inconsiderable holding, land that the father had long waited for but which now passed straight to the son.

Over the Solent on the Isle of Wight there were several cases in which mere infants succeeded to lands left empty by plague. At Gatcombe, in the middle of the island, Joan, widow of John de Insula of Gatcombe and the only remaining parent of their son John, died in July, leaving all her lands to the orphaned six-year-old. A few miles to the east the pestilence had brought about a similar succession in the manor of Compton.[xi] The lord of the manor, John de Compton, is lost to the records about this time, leaving a son – Richard – who was aged only four.[xii] John was by no means a model lord. Even before he had reached his majority, he had been dragged from his home by three local knights and forced to marry a woman against his will (we can only assume that he had got the girl pregnant and was now being forced to do the decent thing). In 1345, John was named as a debtor of the king, owing the large sum of £16 10s. 0d.[xiii] in fines and was threatened with arrest if he did not provide security for their payment. Nonetheless the sheriff did not need to wait long to get the errant John in chains: the following year an order for his imprisonment went out following the death of a certain William, whom John had fatally wounded in a fight. The manor tenants must have been glad to be rid of their unpleasant master: no doubt the pestilence had accomplished what many had on occasion considered doing themselves.

Not that there can have been many left to rejoice at John de Compton's passing. Elsewhere on the island, in the village of Shide, so many tenants had died that the lord of the manor, the keeper of the abbey of St Cross,[xiv] was having to find room for the thirty oxen and a cow it had received by way of death duties (heriots). It

---

[xi] Part of the village of Arreton.

[xii] On 15th April 1349, John de Compton's mother, Margery, died, leaving Richard as her heir, suggesting that Richard's father and her son – John – were already dead. He had volunteered to fight for the king in France in the 1346–7 campaign.

[xiii] i.e. £16.50.

[xiv] St Cross was a French alien abbey (i.e. it owed its allegiance to a mother house abroad – in this case Tiron in France) and was obliged to make additional payments to the Exchequer in time of war. It was in default of these payments and so the crown had appointed a keeper, Henry le Muleward, to manage its affairs.

was an unparalleled situation – a surfeit of draught animals and no tenants to drive them. Truly the world had been turned on its head.

The officials at Farnham in Surrey, a large manor owned by the bishop of Winchester, were having similar difficulties. There may have been an early outbreak here before Christmas; if not, the plague was most certainly present by late spring.[13] Farnham's reeve was one of the early victims and it fell to his successor, John Runwick, to bring some order out of the chaos the pestilence had created. His most pressing problem was dealing with all the animals he had received as heriots paid out on the deaths of tenants. Typically, the surviving family would be obliged to give their best beast to the lord, which the reeve would sell for cash, use on the demesne or slaughter for the lord's stores. In most years only a couple of heriots would be paid, but by the year running from October 1348 to September 1349 Runwick received a foal, a bull, nine wethers (castrated rams), 26 sheep, 26 bullocks, 54 cows, 26 horses, and 57 oxen. This was not the windfall it might seem. Other reeves were having to deal with a similar glut of heriots. At Cheriton the reeve had received 61 animals, at Hambledon there were 50. The first instinct of manorial managers was to sell but the markets were soon crowded with unwanted stock. Compounding the problem, the buyers who would normally wander between the stalls on market day were a much-diminished band. Supply boomed. Demand dwindled. Prices crashed. High-value animals such as horses and cattle now fetched less than a third of their price only a year before.

John Runwick, Farnham's new reeve, did what he could in the circumstances. He sold off the sheep and calves, which took more maintenance than they were worth. Next he enlarged the demesne stables to house the horses. It had to be quickly done: he paid two workmen and a lad to complete the structure in only five days, supplying them himself with two hinges, a lock and 600 nails. Additional meadows were used for pasture to accommodate the stock and a couple of boys were employed to watch over them. The herdsman and shepherd were kept on until the summer. The hope was that prices would eventually pick up. When they did not, John ordered a general slaughter of the cattle, sheep and pigs, sending the carcases to Bishop William's larder for storage. It seems, therefore, that despite all the deaths, John Runwick coped with the extraordinary burden that was placed on him during the plague year. Even with so massive a disruption, the manor still continued to operate. The ponds in the park were dredged, the demesne plough and carts were maintained, the fields sown and harvest were reaped – even a bucket that had fallen into the well was replaced, at a cost of 4*d*.[xv] This was much to Runwick's credit and to the benefit of his lord. Because of the heriots and the considerable income from entry fines charged to those inheriting tenements, the manor turned a considerable profit. Runwick must have known, however, that it was a short-term gain. There were too many heriots but the superabundance in this year only promised dearth in the next. By the end of 1349, fifty-two tenements still remained unlet, a worrying indicator for manorial incomes in times to come.

John Runwick was not just having difficulty finding buyers for animals. No potters' clay was sold through the whole of 1349, a sure sign of problems elsewhere in Surrey. The county had a significant pottery industry, helped by the ample clay to be found below the topsoil. This too was a seasonal industry. The frosts and low temperatures of the winter months made the curing of pots and setting of bricks impossible. Once spring came, the kilns were fired up and production began again. Carts soon started rolling to London, a two-day journey from Farnham. The counties around London supported many similar industries – crafts that required space and created noise and smell, but depended nonetheless on the pull of a strong urban market. There were the felt fulling mills in Wandsworth, the cutlers of Thaxted in Essex, the glaziers of Middlesex and Kent, the salt panners and iron founders of Sussex. This last county – thickly wooded and otherwise quite isolated from London – also had a considerable timber trade, which ensured its continued contact with the plague-ridden capital (although the evidence of early infection in the south of the county suggests that here, as in so many other places on the south coast, the pestilence was introduced by boat). At the small village of Wartling, overlooking the Pevensey Levels where William the Conqueror had landed in 1066, there were already twelve villeins and freemen dead by March 1349.

The mortality figures are mixed from these parts. At Apuldram, just outside Chichester, the villeins were reduced from 234 to 168 –

[xv] £0.02.

a decline of under a third; however, on the manors of the Bilsham family at Arundel only twelve miles away, every last villein was killed. Likewise at Fareham, over the Hampshire border, only nine tenants died, whereas at Gosport next door, all forty-eight of the tenants died. This variance in the incidence of tenant deaths need not indicate a corresponding variance in overall mortality, merely a difference in who died in which village. What is abundantly clear is that in south Sussex, as everywhere else that the pestilence had so far touched, the reduction in the population was profound; 50 per cent is normal, a figure above half not uncommon. None of this, however, comes close to describing the shock to families, almost every one of which lost members through the disease. There was the St George family for instance, minor landowners in Westhampnett on the other side of Chichester from Apuldram: William St George, his two brothers John and Roger, and two of his sisters – Joan and Agatha – all perished. Only one sister, Isabel St George, survived.

The misery brought by plague was near uniform. The fate of the family of Sir Thomas Dene, a knight of Ospringe in north Kent, was very similar to that of the St Georges. Sir Thomas and his wife Martha had four small children – Benedicta, who was aged five, Margaret aged four, and Martha and Joan, who were both younger still. Sir Thomas died first, on 18th May 1349 – it is likely that he picked the disease up on his travels, bringing it into his home. Martha was dead by 8th July and her two youngest girls perished by the end of the month. One cannot help feeling that this young family had been a happy one, yet by August only Benedicta and Margaret were left, now orphaned and deprived of their little sisters. William Dene, a monk in the Benedictine cathedral priory at Rochester, a few miles east up Watling Street from Ospringe, described how family tragedies like this were being played out in every village, everywhere that the pestilence had struck. 'Alas,' he wrote, 'this mortality devoured such a multitude of both sexes that no one could be found to carry the bodies of the dead to burial, but men and women carried the bodies of their own little ones to church on their shoulders and threw them into mass graves, from which arose such a stink that it was barely possible for anyone to go past the churchyard.'[14] This was not the hyperbole of an excitable monk: at Sandwich, on the east Kent coast, the cemetery filled so quickly that in June the earl of Huntingdon donated an additional piece of land in order that more bodies might be accommodated. The ageing bishop of Rochester, Hamo Hethe, whose diocese covered the western part of Kent, survived this hell, most probably because (like his episcopal confrères Ralph Shrewsbury and John Grandison) he secluded himself in his country hall, at Trottiscliffe. Nonetheless, the experience still took its toll on the old prelate, who was made progressively 'ill and miserable by the sudden change in the world'.[15]

On the other side of the Thames, the disease crept out of London to the city's agricultural hinterland, into the towns and villages of Middlesex and Essex. The epidemic progressed beyond Stepney, which had been hit before the New Year, to Stratford, where the abbot was struck down. At Blackmore, on the way to Chelmsford, the court held on 23rd March heard that already twelve tenants had died; the number of cases was on the increase as many more were sick. Colchester was hit early and hard: 111 wills were proved in the plague year, when normally the mayor's court would see only two or three.

The villagers of Great Waltham just north of Chelmsford were suffering similar problems. On 1st April they were obliged to attend the manor court, at Pleshey Castle, a couple of miles away. In the morning they set off early, walking across the meadows that straddled the brook which ran between village and castle. The Essex landscape here is fairly flat and there was a good view from the castle motte, so any sentries on guard will have been able to make out the throng of villagers when they were still some way off. The tenants would have been dressed like any others of the time, the men wearing long tunics girdled by a cord, from which a pouch (or 'gypcière') hung, serving as a large pocket. As the group neared, it became clear that there were also quite a few women amongst them, in long gowns, covered with a smocked apron. Both men and women wore wooden clogs and their heads were covered in hoods, tied under the chin. They were admitted to the castle hall as soon as they arrived, where they waited with apprehension for John Benington, the constable of their lord – Humphrey de Bohun, earl of Essex and Hereford. As Benington entered the room, he too will have immediately appreciated that much had changed at Great Waltham: not only were there more women than usual but many young men too, taking the place of several familiar faces who were missing. One by one they stood up to declare that so-and-so had died and that their tenement was vacant. Each time

Benington asked if anyone wished to enter the tenement. Several stepped forward: a widow, son, cousin or friend, all prepared to pay the entry fine and take on the land; but there were almost as many silences, a general shaking of heads and then the scratch of a pen as the manor clerk noted that the land was to remain in the earl's hands, unlet.

Then, when Constable Benington thought that all the court's miserable business was done, one of the villagers, Roger Andrew, stood up and stated that he wished to make a request. One can imagine the collective sigh that went round the room, for the weary villagers knew well the tale into which Andrew was about to tell – it had exercised him for some time and the village was all too aware of his complaint. Five years ago, Roger explained, his father had died and a horse had been seized from his land by way of a heriot. The peasant told how this was an injustice, as his father had held the land through rent and not through service and that therefore no heriot at death was due. There was no way he was able to prove this however, as a long time ago Richard's father's house had been burnt down and the land deeds been lost in the fire. The constable asked the senior members of the village to swear on oath that this was so, which they did, before John Benington pronounced his verdict, giving his reasons so forcefully that that the clerk felt the need to make a note of it: 'it seemed . . . that the taking of the horse as heriot had been wrong; and so, his conscience moved by the deaths and the pestilence which there then was, he paid Roger Andrew 18s.[xvi] as recompense for the horse. This halts the action concerning the taking of the heriot from the aforesaid tenements.'[16] So terrible had been the impact of the plague that John Benington, this forbidding constable, this imposing representative of the earl, had shown sympathy for a humble peasant. As Roger Andrew left the castle hall, he must have been content that a wrong long felt had at last been redressed. Several others in the throng of peasants that returned to Great Waltham had good reason to feel satisfied too but for reasons more material than moral: they were proud new tenants, inheritors of their own little estate. The plague had only just arrived, however, so between this April Fool's Day and the end of summer, almost half the men of the village would die, a proportion most probably equalled among the women and children too.

[xvi] £0.90.

Some of those leaving with a favourable result from Pleshey Castle will not have enjoyed it for long. Roger Andrew may well have been amongst them.

For the firmly rooted communities that stood in its way, the advance of the pestilence was proving irresistible; for the footloose, however, it was not inescapable. Most could do nothing in the face of the disease: they had land and animals to tend, family to care for and in the case of villeins (such as those at Great Waltham) were legally obliged to stay put. A very few, however, like the scholars of Oxford, were mobile enough to be able to flee the epidemic as soon as it threatened. Likewise, the magnates – men like Humphrey de Bohun – could afford to travel far, do so rapidly and take their households with them. Most nobles had many places to which they could flee; de Bohun, for instance, had houses and castles in his two earldoms of Essex and Hereford, and indeed elsewhere. Judging that Pleshey would be more vulnerable to the contagion, the earl sent orders to his steward in Brecon Castle to prepare for his arrival and a possible lengthy stay. The de Bohun lordship of Brecon was a natural fastness bounded by the Black Mountains to the east, the Brecon Beacons in the south, and further west the utterly remote Cambrian Mountains that form the central spine of Wales: it was a wild region that had, for centuries, been a place of refuge for the de Bohuns in times of crisis. On this occasion, however, it was not from a king or noble enemy that the earl fled, but plague, which, before long, reached even into Brecon.

The epidemic had spread beyond Gloucestershire, into Monmouthshire as far as Abergavenny, south-east of Brecon, by March 1349. Local manor accounts give a clear idea of the mortality: later in the year the steward of the lordship of Abergavenny could only take a third of the normal rents from the villages surrounding the town and at Wernrheolydd the scribe noted that 'there used to be rents . . . of £13 10s. 3½d.[xvii] and now remain £1 14s. 6d.[xviii] because of mortality.'[17] It was not long before the infection appeared to the west of Brecon, brought in from the sea: about the end of March the Prince of Wales's borough of Carmarthen lost both its customs officials and in the nearby

[xvii] £13.51.
[xviii] £1.73.

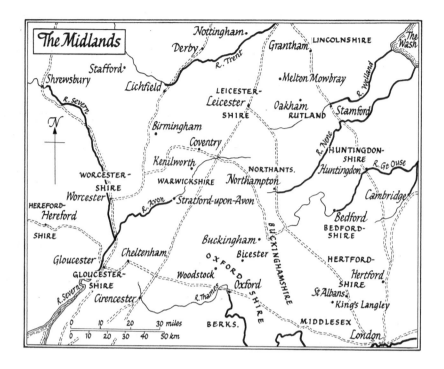

manor of Llanllwch all the serfs[xix] died and their lands reverted to the lord. It was not long before de Bohun's citadel was itself threatened. By April all the land south of Brecon was plague-ridden, while the disease was travelling up the road from Carmarthen and nudging the English border to the east. Whether Humphrey de Bohun would survive remained to be seen: his chances were not high. As John of Reading, a monk of Westminster, would later comment: 'there was in those days . . . flight without escape. How many who fled from the face of the pestilence were already infected and did not escape the slaughter.'[18]

By the end of March, the pestilential epidemic stretched from Essex and Kent in the east to Cornwall and south Wales in the west. In only three months it had sprung out of its winter reservoir of Dorset, Bristol and London, taken over the main towns of southern and central England and then, with the coming of spring, engulfed much of the countryside in between. Lent was soon to arrive at its

---

[xix] Called 'gabularii' in Wales. Serfdom, which had largely fallen into desuetude in England still persisted to some extent on the more traditional Anglo-Welsh manors.

much longed-for end: the great feast of Easter. Every man, woman and child would cram the churches for the elaborate ceremonies of Holy Week. This communal observance of the Easter mysteries did much to spread the disease. By May, there were few villages in the southernmost counties which had not yet been infected; a little further north, villages close to towns and major roads would be the first to be visited by the pestilence. Inkpen, for example, was a small village in west Berkshire, just off the main Bristol to London road, which was infected by March 1349. Cuxham, a similar distance from the London to Oxford road, was one of the first villages in Oxfordshire to be struck down: it could as well have caught the disease from Oxford (just twelve miles away) as from a chance encounter with a traveller making their way on the main road nearby.[19] It is almost always impossible to account for the precise cause of infection: in neighbouring Brightwell-cum-Sotwell, infection might have arisen from the journeys some tenants were obliged to make to Winchester, carrying with them chickens and grain, any one of which could have exposed them to the disease. Not only did they then spread infection in the villages they passed through on their return but, once back in Brightwell, they would soon infect their families and neighbours. In Iffley, just a mile and a half to the south of Oxford itself, it is possible to see the plague travelling from door to door: two villeins – Liripin and Herny – lived just two cottages apart in Hockmere Street and both died during the plague; tellingly, one of the houses in between them, which was owned by a freeman, changed hands during the year as well. Nor were the rich immune. The lord of Iffley, Grace FitzNiel, also died in 1349, leaving the village and land to Robert her son. Unfortunately, Robert had lost his memory, so royal custodians were appointed to look after the estate for him. It may have been a blessing in disguise: Robert had not only lost his mother but two of his three brothers as well. One person at least was able to forget the horrors that they had seen.

Across Oxfordshire the plague killed just as it had elsewhere, taking half or more of each village to the grave.[20] As in south Wales, the manor accounts give telling glimpses of the catastrophe that had been wrought. The corn at Duns Tew was left standing in the fields after the harvest of summer 1349, as there was simply no one left to wield the sickle. At Middleton Stoney, owned by the Shropshire knight Roger Le Strange of Knockin, some of the freely held tenements were 'lying untilled and uncultivated and worth nothing', the freemen tenants having perished in the plague, as had 'certain villeins who also died in the same pestilence' and whose lands and tenements were likewise lying 'uncultivated and in common'. The manor court, which had returned a profit of 24s.[xx] in 1328, was now only worth 6s.[xxi] 'and not more in these days on account of the aforesaid pestilence'. Roger Le Strange did not have to worry about the mess – he too died in 1349.

Several of the villages in this corner of Oxfordshire around Bicester had seen their number of tenants dip in the first half of the four-teenth century, either as a result of the Great Famine or because land was being agglomerated by the more wealthy among them. Some, like Tusmore, were completely finished off by the pestilence. However, there were other hamlets nearby that appeared to be in reasonable health before the epidemic struck but were abandoned during or imme-diately after the Great Death. Cote and Tilgarsley, on the other side of Oxford, were two such places. It is likely that Nicholas Upton, the abbot of Eynsham Abbey and lord of both manors, decided to move the few tenants that remained into larger settlements nearby.[21] Abbot Nicholas seems to have had a good relationship with at least some of his tenants: in 1344 they had helped him regain his position after it was usurped by the bishop of Lincoln.[22] It was probably with an eye to their welfare, therefore, that the abbot enforced the abandonment of Tilgarsley and Cote, villages which – other than the small hamlet of Quob in Hampshire, not far from Titchfield and the early outbreak in the Meon Valley – were among the very few settlements that vanished in the immediate aftermath of the Great Death. As the evidence from Oxfordshire suggests, the almost complete lack of aban-donment had nothing to do with low death rates. Indeed, the good fortune of Brightwell, where only nineteen of the sixty-six tenants, died, was not – unfortunately – repeated in many other villages else-where.

As was becoming clear, the economic impact of the loss of so many peasants posed a serious problem for landlords. As William Dene explained, 'the shortage of labourers and of workers in every kind of craft and occupation was then so acute that more than a third of the land throughout the kingdom remained uncultivated' – just as had

[xx] £1.20.
[xxi] £0.30.

been reported at Middleton Stoney.[23] The impact on manor finances was devastating and immediate, as was shown by the accounts from a small group of villages around Newbury in west Berkshire. At Crookham, owned by the countess of Salisbury (who died in late 1349), a manor that had been worth £10 per annum was by September 1349 worth nothing, as all the tenants were dead and all their holdings in the lord's hands useless and uncultivated. Likewise at Padworth, five miles away, the lord died in May 1349, his widow in June, leaving a manor that returned nothing 'because all the men are dead'.[24] In Newbury the fulling mill, which had been so busy before the Great Death that even a twelfth share of it was valued at 26s. 8d.,[xxii] was after the pestilence worth nothing 'on account of it'.[25] Newbury, like other small towns, suffered as markets declined and local trade fell off. At Bicester in Oxfordshire, of similar size to Newbury, the tolls from the market were said to be 'no more than 30s. on account of the pestilence'.[26] At West Wycombe in Buckinghamshire, there were forty defaults on rent listed in just the one manor, whilst not far away on the manor of Sladen the mill was by August 1349 worth nothing as there were no tenants to bring corn and no miller to grind it, all 'because of the mortality'.[27] That is, if the corn could be harvested in the first place. At Ham in Gloucestershire, so much land had escheated to the lord that it would take 1,144 man-days to reap and gather the harvest – labour that would either have to be bought in or else the crops would be left to rot where they stood.

Everywhere around there was evidence of the devastating effects of the great mortality – and not just the unkempt fields and untended crops, abandoned homes and near-empty villages, the untravelled roads and silent mills. As Henry Knighton later recalled:

> sheep and cattle wandered through the fields and amongst the crops, and there was none to seek them, or round them up, and they perished in out-of-the-way places amongst the furrows and under hedges, for want of a keeper, in numbers beyond reckoning throughout the land, for there was such a shortage of hands and servants that no one knew what ought to be done.[28]

[xxii] £1.33.

There were many, however, willing to try. At Englefield, midway between Newbury and Reading, over 50 per cent of the tenants died but had been replaced by incomers, perhaps because the lord offered very attractive terms. Remarkably, very nearly a third of their number – twenty-one out of sixty-seven – were women. The quiet efforts of the survivors to start anew were less dramatic than the chroniclers' reminiscence of devastation; but it was just as real and – to the observant landlord – it offered a glimmer of hope that they might rebuild their manors and recover the incomes that until recently they had enjoyed.

Just as the pestilence had sprung from Bristol and London to Coventry and Leicester, leaving for a while the towns in between, so too the first outbreaks of plague in Warwickshire and Leicestershire came well before anything was seen of the disease in Worcestershire, Northamptonshire and Bedfordshire. The same pattern obtained, however – it started in the towns and spread out to the countryside – and the results were precisely as they had been further south: the death recorded of a rector in Kenilworth in Warwickshire; forty-two deaths accounted for by the end of April in Kibworth Harcourt, in Leicestershire. The fulling mill lay idle and the dovecote ruined at Lord Wake's manor of Stevington in Bedfordshire; at Milbrook the lord of the manor died, as did his son, as did every one of the bondmen; at Whissendine in Rutland, approximately 450 acres were worth precisely 'nothing' because 'all the tenants are dead'.[29] Yet even amidst all this death, all this misery, a miracle of sorts was still possible. For in Oakham, a couple of miles to the south of Whissendine, Geoffrey Cockerel, lately convicted of larceny and false accusation, was hanged and his body cut down from the gallows and carried to Oakham church-yard for burial. On arrival at the cemetery, however, Geoffrey gasped for breath, sprung back to life and disappeared inside the church to find sanctuary from the law. Recognizing, perhaps, that a greater judge-ment had been passed on Geoffrey's case than he was capable of, the king pardoned the knave and let him go free. The letter of remission was sent out from Westminster on 2nd April 1349, just as the plague took hold in Rutland; it can only be hoped that Geoffrey, in cheating the gallows, avoided the plague as it went through his community.

The extraordinary number of heads of monasteries in Northamp-tonshire who died demonstrates well how pervasive was the mortality:

Katherine Knyvet, the abbess of the Cluniac abbey of Delapré; Dionysia, the prioress of the Cistercian priory of Sewardsley; Thomas of Higham, the prior of the Augustinian priory of Canons Ashby; William of Radeford, the master of the tiny hermitage of Grafton Regis; Amicia of Navesby, the old prioress of the Augustinian nunnery of Rothwell; Walter of Eketon, the master of the hospital for the poor and sick of Armston; Robert de Tadmarton, master of the hospital of St James and St John in aid of the sick at Brackley; William of Piddington, master of the hospital for the infirm of Northampton, dedicated to St John Baptist and St John Evangelist; William of Walcote, the provost of the chantry college of Cotterstock. All of these religious women and men, in just one county, perished, together – it must be assumed – with half or more of their sisters and brothers.[30]

The great abbey of St Alban's, in Hertfordshire, suffered an especially grievous loss. Owing to its closeness to London, the plague had arrived in this county fairly early in 1349, and by the end of Lent had got inside the abbey community. The abbot, Michael Mentmore, first showed symptoms of the disease on Maundy Thursday.[xxiii] Considered to be a paragon of monastic virtue, Mentmore would in his final days prove the truth of this reputation. Despite his suffering, the abbot performed this memorial of the Last Supper. In a repetition of Jesus' actions, Mentmore celebrated Mass and then washed the feet of the poor and his brother monks in a ritualized act of humility. The next day, with the plague now fully upon him, the abbot was unable to leave his bed. There he prepared himself for the end, making his confession and receiving the last rites. At around three o'clock on Easter Day, after the Resurrection had been proclaimed, Mentmore slipped from semi-consciousness to death. There was much grieving at this premature end: the St Alban's chronicler said that the 'fabric of his life was cut short when it seemed that the weaver had only just begun the cloth.'[31] Yet there were few left to mourn the good man: forty-six other St Alban's monks died in the plague, nearly three quarters of the strength of the monastery.[32]

Empty seats in the conventual stalls of St Alban's marked the dead monks' absence, a sight to be seen in religious houses across southern

[xxiii] Thursday, 9th April 1349.

England, Wales and the Midlands. These losses were not just to the detriment of the monasteries, taking many who were 'outstanding in religion';[33] they also threatened a restriction of doles, spiritual succour and charitable care. The curtailment of their ministrations to the communities around caused both hardship and resentment. Worse still were the arguments that erupted when monks attempted to assert their rights. In an almost exact repetition of the disturbances in Winchester, the monks and townsmen of Worcester clashed in a riot, the latter storming the cathedral priory with bows and arrows and other arms, setting fire to some of the buildings as they went, thereby achieving what the burghers of Winchester had only threatened to do. The cause of the dispute was most likely the same: the rights the priory claimed to bury all residents of the city, a right for which they charged a fee. Clearly this was a problem for those who were burying the third or fourth victim of the pestilence within the family. Unlike the residents of Bristol, who had been able to purchase land for a new cemetery without hindrance,[34] the people of Worcester were compelled to use the cathedral graveyard, whether they liked it or not. The violence that was unleashed as a result was serious enough to force the bishop, Wulstan de Bransford, to act. On 18th April, not even a week after Easter, Bransford – who had been bishop now for twenty years and knew the temper of his flock well – ordained that the burial ground of the leper hospital of St Oswald, outside the city walls, should be used as an overflow for the cathedral ground. The ordinance is couched in words of accommodation, expressing 'heart-felt anxiety' for the 'dangerous and (alas) too numerous burials in the churchyard of our cathedral church of Worcester, which have griev-ously increased in recent times because of the unprecedented numbers of deaths now occurring', wishing to come to the 'best remedy' not just for the priory monks but also 'the citizens and other residents of the city'. The bishop's sense of danger was clearly twofold: not just the risk of fighting but also the danger of infection from 'the decom-posing bodies'. Unfortunately, it seems that the master of St Oswald's was himself a victim – perhaps as a result of the same decomposing bodies now being outside his hospital, rather than in the cathedral cemetery. He was not alone. As in every other diocese, the deaths amongst the clergy were severe. Amongst their number was Wulstan de Bransford himself.[35] He had promised in his letter to 'devise some other solution to the problem' of burials in Worcester; it may well be that it was in the course of this that he was infected.[36]

The tales of death and desolation, lists of human losses and economic deficits, could be continued at great length. It would be unnecessary to do so, for the point, surely, is made: everywhere the Great Death killed in great numbers, often in excess of half the measured population. It caused grave problems to lords and the manorial economy. Even if the records were sufficient to allow comparisons between counties and regions, which they are not, it is likely that such an exercise would be fruitless. For record after record shows the mortality to be broadly the same in every town and every village: half the population of the place would, by the time the epidemic passed on, have perished – sometimes less, but very often considerably more. The only real variable was the date in which the epidemic arrived amidst a community, a point largely determined by the relative proximity of a town or village to wider networks of exchange and areas of contagion. In the end, however, it mattered not when the pestilence arrived nor what the fine difference in percentage mortality was: its human effect was always the same. As Geoffrey le Baker succinctly put it, 'people who had one day been full of happiness, on the next were found dead.'[37] Spring had been blackened by death.

By Christmas 1348 almost half the tenants of Thornbury manor, on the banks of the Severn, had died and by the time the pestilence had burnt itself out in early spring, very nearly two thirds had perished – 144 out of a previous total of 230. The land left vacant by dead tenants presented a considerable opportunity for ambitious survivors. John Fish – who had already taken on the land of Isabel Lynch at the end of November 1348 at a knock-down price – came before the court on 21st April to state that he would marry Agnes Gibbs, whose husband John had also died in November. For 2s.[xxiv] he gained the required licence to marry,[xxv] allowing him to assume control of Agnes's land as well. Thus, in the course of five months Fish had assembled a little holding of over ten acres, with a house and cottage to boot.

[xxiv] £0.10.

[xxv] 'merchet'.

Accumulators like Fish were helped by the fall in the value of rents which resulted from the glut of land. John Cole, a fisherman who had previously only sublet some small tenements from other villeins, had given 2s. on 15th December 1348 to marry a widow (whose husband's death had been announced at the same court), taking on her house and three acres; on 3rd March 1349, he paid a further 2s. to enter the twenty-one acres and house that had belonged to his late father.[xxvi] In both transactions, 2s. was paid, yet in the second it bought seven times the amount of land as in the first. Without such a dramatic fall in the cost of land, it is doubtful whether John Cole could have accumulated the twenty-four acres and two houses he managed in these months, which made him at a stroke one of the larger peasant landowners in Thornbury.

While this was good for John Cole, it was clearly bad for their lord, Sir Ralph Stafford. For although his officials recorded a massive increase in receipts from people marrying and entering newly vacant tenements, the total was offset by the fall in the unit value of an entry fine. This was not, however, a binary result – good for peasant, bad for lord: amongst the villagers there was wide variation in individual fortunes and even some of those who had done well out of the plague did not live to enjoy their sudden improvement for long. Thomas Wilcox, who had snapped up the just-widowed Matilda Thatcher at the end of November 1348, was himself dead by the beginning of July 1349, quite possibly from an affliction other than plague. Sadder still was the tale of Matilda Uphill, who entered her father's tenement on 5th January, making her the first daughter in the history of the manor to assume a parent's landholding. Plucky Matilda was dead within a month, however, so her novel succession was short-lived.

Thus, even within the course of the epidemic, the common and inescapable experience of death produced very different results in people's lives, changes that were often only fleeting because of the unremitting mortality. It was probably for precisely this reason that in Thornbury so many deaths and immediate remarriages were announced at the same court. Certainly there must have been a number of previous understandings and affections; on the whole, however, it seems that families waited until the pestilence had worked itself

---

[xxvi] i.e. £0.10.

through the household and then went to the manorial court to declare all their news and business at once. This not only avoided repeat visits but also reduced the chance of infecting others in the public hearings. Waiting to go to court also helps to explain why tenements were taken up with such surprising speed, given the chaos that pestilence undoubtedly brought. Of one hundred holdings made vacant in the plague year, seventy-nine were re-entered at the same court as the causative death was announced. Six were taken up later and only fifteen were still unlet by the end of the summer. In the majority of cases the land remained within the family: in sixty-seven of these hundred vacancies, the land was taken on by an heir within the family or by a widow's new husband. However, there was nonetheless a significant fall in the entries by family heirs compared with former times. Normally, a quarter of deceased villeins were succeeded by a son 'of full age'; in the plague year that proportion fell to a seventh. Likewise, on average about half of entries were by widows either in their own right or as a result of a remarriage; in the plague year it was about a third.

At Thornbury, then, there was even by Christmas and certainly by Easter a realization that the pestilence had been suffered in common, had been endured with some level of continuity, but had been survived with a significant degree of change. The vicar, John Enefield, had survived, so had not troubled the diocesan authorities with a vacancy to fill; here there was complete continuity. Similarly, the lord of the manor lived and his administration continued, despite the deaths of a clerk, a reeve and two beadles; here too there was continuity, despite the mortality. However, revenues were artificially high and unit income was depressed. At the level of individual landholdings the whole manor had more or less been rearranged and the underlying pattern of inheritance had been altered. Many had died, perhaps the majority: but, for a considerable number of those that remained, their lives had already been radically and irrevocably changed.

8

Cadwallader's Curse, Plantagenet Pride

April–May 1349

Alas for the Red Dragon, for its end is near.
Geoffrey of Monmouth, *History of the Kings of Britain*[1]

Edward III had been free to pursue his ambitions in France in part because his grandfather, Edward I, had so successfully subdued another of England's traditional enemies: the Welsh. Indeed, the first Edward's achievement was arguably greater than the third's fugacious victory at Crécy. It was not an achievement made by half measures: the army Edward I led out of Chester in July 1277 was the largest ever seen in medieval Britain, while the border had been secured by the marcher barons, thereby allowing the king to cross the Dee with his back protected. It was a perilous expedition nonetheless, through forbidding terrain, with near-impenetrable forests and mountains to the south and the sea to the north, the two separated only by a narrow foreshore of treacherous quicksands.[2] The threat of ambush from the Welsh, who with appropriate contumely had rejected the overlordship of the English king, was considerable – indeed it was amidst these trees that Edward's great-grandfather, Henry II, had been mauled in his first campaign against the ever-problematic native princes of Wales.[i] So Edward took no chances, proceeding with both overwhelming strength and great caution. In the vanguard were 4,000 axemen and labourers, who cut and levelled a road through the forest over which his great army and the supply caravan that followed could march. With so great a force, however, victory was almost assured: within only three months Edward had forced his enemy to capitulate. He buttressed his conquest

[i] 1157.

with a number of new castles, built to keep the Welsh in check; Flint and Rhuddlan alone were completed in only three years.

Edward's work was not yet finished, however. A rebellion brought the king back to Chester in late 1282, where he repeated the exercise all over again, forcing a final surrender by the following spring. This time he was determined that there would be no further challenge to the authority of the English crown. Even before the last rebels had lain down their arms, the construction of yet more castles had begun. At Conwy and Harlech thousands of men worked every daylight hour, realizing the designs of the finest military engineers that could be found in Europe. Completing this crown of stone, which would now bear down on Wales – quite literally – from above, was the great citadel of Caernarfon. With massive polygonal towers, topped by imperial eagles and spaced by walls striped in coloured stone, this castle imitated the fortifications that emperor Theodosius had built around Constantinople nearly 900 years earlier. There was nothing accidental in this: Welsh legend claimed Constantine as one of their own,[3] and when the footings of the castle were being dug the bones of the emperor were duly 'discovered'. Edward's statement was very clear: Wales was now an addition to his own empire. The classical references were grandiloquent but fitting, as the full resources of the king's huge realm had been used to complete his conquest – Gascon crossbowmen, cash from Ireland, English masons and foot soldiers from south Wales. Yet Edward had still not drained the well of historical allusion. The matrix of the seal of Llywelyn ap Gruffudd, the last native Prince of Wales, was melted down to forge a chalice – an Edwardian grail that the king presented to his new Cistercian foundation of Vale Royal. Then, with the conquest finally complete, Edward called his knights to the site of the Welsh court at Nefyn, to participate in an Arthurian round table.[ii] No doubt Edward wore the diadem – just looted – that was said to have rested once on King Arthur's head. These theatrics not only appealed to Edward I's sense of romance; they proclaimed none too subtle a message to conquered Wales. Cambrian prophets had for a long time promised that Arthur would return to free the Welsh from the Saxon yoke – now a Plantagenet king had appropriated the name and title for himself.

[ii] July 1284.

Edward I understood that the subjection of the Welsh would not be achieved without a substantial and permanent English presence. Towns were established around his new castles and Englishmen enticed to populate them with the promise of generous burghal rights. By the turn of the century, new English boroughs circumscribed north Wales: Flint, Rhuddlan, Conwy, Caernarfon, Harlech and Aberystwyth, all of which depended on the massive military complexes that Edward had established. Elsewhere, the existing Welsh towns of Criccieth and Denbigh were emptied of their Welsh inhabitants and converted into English boroughs. Welsh townsmen and the peasants who farmed the fields around were forced up into the less fertile lower slopes of the mountains inland, a further humiliation that was to cause very considerable resentment, only magnified by the generous rights granted to the new English immigrants who took their place. However, the bitterness of the vanquished was rarely allowed to boil over into rebellion, in part because of the firm control the English maintained over the country. Whilst additional lands were granted to the marcher lords – who had many generations of experience in the ruthless super-intendence of Welsh bordermen – the vast majority of Gwynedd and Ceredigion was retained as the direct property of the crown. This giant patrimony was, in 1301, handed to the king's first son and heir – Edward of Caernarfon – as the principality of Wales. The crown lands were divided into shires, fitted with all the accoutrements of English shrieval administration and taken within the dominion of English criminal law. (Sensibly, Edward I retained traditional Welsh land and inheritance law, in recognition of the very significant cultural differences that remained between the two nations.)

Beyond the fertile southern littoral and borderlands of the March, which had long ago been divided into Anglo-Norman lordships, most of the Welsh still lived in dispersed upland communities, bound together by customary ties of kinship and dependence. The way of life of this Celtic people – in terms of diet, matrimony, agriculture, law, religion and local government – more closely resembled the customs of the native Irish than the alien systems of their English conquerors. There the similarity ended, however, for by 1349, when the new ascendancy was still only sixty-six years old, English authority in Wales was gaining strength. In part this was because some Welshmen, especially in the March, where there had always been a

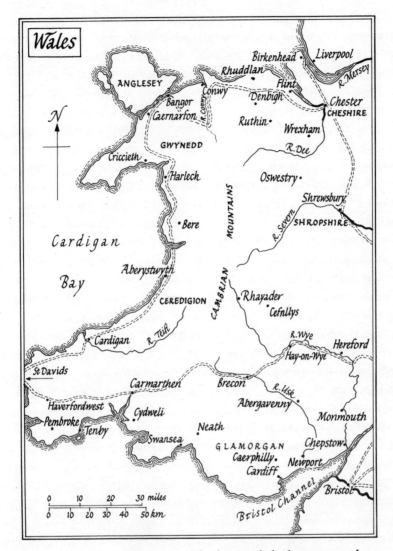

strong incentive to collaborate with the English, began to adopt an Anglo-Norman way of life – even Anglo-Norman names. Acculturation was not a one-way process: some Englishmen took on Welsh aliases, others married Welsh brides. Thus the sons of Gruffudd ap Gwenwynwyn became the de la Poles of Powys, whilst the plainly Anglo-Norman Almeric de Marreys called his son Llywelyn. Gruffudd ap David Holland, despite the confusion of his name, was described as 'an Englishman and an English tenant' of Denbigh. It was all quite unlike the situation on the other side of the Irish Sea, where racial and cultural distinctions were becoming more, not less, obvious and the crown's grip on its territories was becoming correspondingly loose. The manner in which the Great Death entered and progressed through Wales goes some way to explain how the differing fortunes of the two colonies came about.

The pestilence had entered south Wales in early spring 1349, quickly advancing north to Abergavenny and west – by sea – to Carmarthen. Although the land between these two towns, with the Pembroke promontory beyond, had for two centuries been largely pacified and turned into something approaching the Anglo-Norman model of manors and market towns, it was still relatively backward. The settlements were tiny: Cardiff, Abergavenny, Carmarthen, Haverfordwest, Pembroke, even the cathedral city of St David's had no more than a thousand inhabitants. The land was not very productive and was some distance from major markets. Consequently, although the towns did grow in the course of the thirteenth century, they were only locally important as centres of exchange and irrelevant to the wider economy of the British Isles. In England, the rise of strong towns and decline of their competitors reflected dynamic rural markets and a growing sense of urban ambition; in south Wales, urban stasis mirrored malaise in the rural hinterland. Part of the problem lay in the large tracts of land owned by Benedictine and Cistercian monasteries. Many of these were, by the early fourteenth century, heavily indebted, largely as a result of a drop in wool revenues and a falling-off in endowments. They also seemed to have suffered from that perennial enemy of monastic houses – poor management – which led to annual deficits and thence inexorably to debt. The common response among these monasteries was to give up trying to manage their more remote and infertile lands, leasing them instead to laymen farmers – something not yet attempted on any scale over the border in England. At the Cistercian abbey of Margam, for instance, demesnes were progressively leased between 1291 and 1336, none of which prevented the monks having to forfeit lands in 1337 because of their non-payment of rent. By the same year, the priory of Goldcliff, despite being the richest (or least poor) of the Benedictine houses of south Wales, had farmed out all of its manors bar two.[4] For the reluctant monks, this was a difficult transition to make: direct cultivation reaffirmed the monastic community's place in the natural order, retained a physical link between the monastery and its landed endowment, and appealed to the prayerful simplicity of manual labour that St Benedict had prescribed in the Rule.[iii] That these increasingly distressed monastic communities were willing to countenance the worldly compromise of leasing was an indication of how serious their impoverishment – both physical and spiritual – had become. Nonetheless, the land was still cultivated, flocks of sheep were still pastured, spring fleeces still carted to western English markets. There remained all the opportunities for exchange that would bring early infection from the plague-riddled towns and villages across the Severn Estuary, Bristol Channel and indeed the Irish Sea.

The poverty of the monks of south Wales stood in stark contrast to the prosperity of the marcher barons, whose lordships straddled the English border with Wales from Monmouthshire in the south to the Palatinate of Chester in the north. These territories had originally been granted to the early Norman barons, who were given considerable freedoms in return for their efforts to police the frontier with Wales. The lordships soon evolved into mini-principalities, independent of royal jurisdiction and enjoying liberties that landowners elsewhere did not possess. The king's writ famously stopped short of the Welsh March; inevitably, therefore, the marcher lordships came to serve as remote powerbases from which restless barons could manoeuvre against – or for – the king and, when things went wrong, as places of refuge to which the errant lords could flee. Unsurprisingly, these baronies were at the centre of almost every instance of baronial unrest in the Middle Ages. The March had been the nexus of turmoil during the reign of Edward II (led in part by Humphrey de Bohun's ancestor) and it was to Edward III's great credit that he managed early in his reign to bring stability to this area.[iv] The peaceful coexistence of the marcher lords – both with each other and with the crown – had borne considerable economic fruit. Land was enclosed (in what were some of the earliest instances to found in the British Isles) and sheep were farmed extensively. Tenants were milked for rent whilst the revenues

---

[iii] Ch. 42 of the Rule of St Benedict. St Benedict's most famous saying is 'orare est laborare, laborare est orare' ('to pray is to work, to work is to pray').

[iv] One tactic was to grant lands back to families that had opposed each other in his father's reign: reinstalling the disinherited almost guaranteed the loyalty of grateful heirs. Indeed, this was how Humphrey de Bohun had come to hold Brecon.

from justice and taxation – which here were the property of the lord and not the king – were extracted from the local populations with little mercy.[v] The earl of Gloucester stated his policy simply: he organized his March holdings 'ad maximum detrimentum possidentium'.[5]

Continuing peace and agricultural improvement inevitably increased the porosity of the March frontier and the frequency of contacts that the lordships maintained with other parts of England. Thus, as the pestilence made its way up through the western counties of England, it moved swiftly into the March and without hindrance across the border into Wales. Herefordshire was infected from Gloucestershire to the south and Worcestershire to the east; the disease had crossed the Malvern Hills by Easter[6] and by the end of April a rash of clerical vacancies suggest that much of south Herefordshire was infected. The preparations made by the bishop of Hereford, John Trillek, reveal not only the fear of those who stood in its path but also their pragmatism. Only days after he had received the king's mandate for prayer in October 1348, the bishop banned the playing of games in Ledbury church, ordering the priests there to focus the minds of their congregation on holier things. In March he had ordained fifty-eight new priests in preparation for the many deaths that news from further south had led him to expect, adding a further thirty-five the following month. It was a wise precaution: of those candidates for the diaconate ordained at the same time,[vi] more than half subsequently disappeared, never to complete their progression to the priesthood.[7] In Hereford itself work on the new chapter house ceased. Perhaps the masons swapped their chisels for spades: eleven years later one parishioner of St Peter's church in Hereford recalled seeing twenty bodies being buried every day in that churchyard alone.[8]

From his castle, Humphrey de Bohun, earl of Hereford, will have heard of the fast-approaching pestilence – the same that he had gone to Brecon to avoid. Certainly by late April his lordship had been surrounded: Abergavenny to the south had been desolated, Carmarthen in the south-west, at the end of the Brecon road, had been hit, and now Herefordshire to the east was infected. The border with England

---

[v] Some of the lordships produced well in excess of £1,000 a year, a figure sufficient to fund the household of any self-respecting marcher magnate, which was more often than not income received in addition to the receipts from extensive lands held elsewhere.

[vi] From mid-April to the end of September 1349.

was crossed at Grosmont and Skenfrith, just north of Monmouth, and no doubt Hay-on-Wye was soon infected as well; so it cannot have been long before Brecon itself succumbed. The deaths of tenants incurred massive arrears: the earl's steward took in 568 head of live-stock from the earl's Brecon tenants in lieu of debts, while 167 oxen and steers were bought from the sale of debtors' goods.[vii] Yet only a fraction of this was of use to the de Bohun household in Brecon, so twenty surviving tenants were ordered to drive more than 400 of the beasts all the way to Pleshy. Even in the midst of such a crisis, there-fore, the produce of the lordship was nonetheless expropriated for consumption elsewhere. Still holed up in Brecon Castle, Humphrey de Bohun could look forward to returning to Essex, where his table would be amply victualled by the surplus cattle so recently transferred from the foothills of his Welsh estates – once, that is, pestilence had passed and he was able to leave his March retreat, whose high walls kept the earl safe while plague raged all around.

Shropshire was infected from the east before the plague moved over the Herefordshire border from the south; it was certainly present in Quatt, just two miles from the Worcestershire border, by late April 1349.[9] The contagion spread slowly but surely, peaking several months after the epidemic reached its height in Coventry and the west Midlands, which were as far north from the original infection as were the rolling Shropshire hills. Although this was one of the more remote parts of England,[10] the effects of pestilence were equally devastating. Sir Robert Harleigh, who owned lands not ten miles from Quatt, was an early victim: he died on 16th May. Harleigh's wife, Margaret, died two months later and the whole estate passed to their son. It was an unexpected inheritance, yet one whose worth was now uncertain: a jury convened a fortnight later was unable to give a value to fields on Wenlock Edge, as the pestilence had killed so many that no one was left to describe who owed what in services to the lord.[11]

To the north of Shropshire was the palatinate of Chester, the prop-erty of Edward of Woodstock, Prince of Wales – the young hero of Crécy who would later be known by the sobriquet 'The Black Prince'.[viii]

[vii] The major render paid by the tenants of Brecon was in the form of a biennial cow-tribute (commorth).

[viii] Prince Edward had held the principality of Wales since 1343, a title that was now accompanied by the earldom of Chester.

The county palatine enjoyed even greater independence from the crown than did other marcher baronies, and indeed possessed its own parliament – a privilege that was never bestowed on the Welsh. Chester itself was a busy little port, with perhaps four or five thousand inhabitants. Long gone were the days when it was a springboard for the Welsh campaigns but it had adapted well: now it sent forth fish from the Dee and imported corn from Ireland to the English settlers of north Wales. In return it traded lead from Holywell, coal from Ewloe and timber from the same forests that had caused such difficulties to Henry II and Edward I. It was in many senses the northern mirror of Gloucester, which served the southern March. Indeed, like Gloucester, it is conceivable that Chester was infected by boat via the Dee, coming in from Drogheda or Malahide across the Irish Sea; yet it is impossible to be sure, for Chester sat on the conjunction of the Dee and several important roads, including the road from Gloucester, which met others from London and the Midlands, the North via Warrington, and Birkenhead – where a ferry took people and goods across the Mersey to Liverpool. It was no surprise, therefore, that this confluence of so much traffic contracted the plague somewhat earlier than did Shropshire to the south.

Two villages – Sandbach and Middlewich – sat six miles apart on the busy London to Chester road. Middlewich had only a chapel for the parishioners and therefore possessed no graveyard of its own. The villagers would normally take their dead to the mother church at Sandbach for burial, but in these difficult times there was no one willing to make the day's trip there and back, so corpses were simply dumped by the side of the road and left to rot in the early summer heat. Hazards such as these can only have accelerated the spread of plague throughout the Cheshire countryside.[12] At Frodsham,[13] midway between Chester and Warrington, there is yet more evidence of a mortality rate of at least 50 per cent and the county town suffered in like kind: both the abbot and prioress of the two Benedictine establishments in the town were killed, whilst business declined as trade collapsed. As a result, the value of the large corn mill on the river Dee, which ground corn brought in from both Cheshire and Ireland, dropped by a third,[14] presenting a bargain that the then mayor of Chester, Bartholomew Northenden, could not miss – he snapped up the mill at a considerable discount, despite the apocalyptic horrors all around. Unfortunately, although Bartholomew survived the plague, he had clearly upset some of his fellow burghers and was murdered before his year of office was out.

Thus, by mid-summer 1349, the pestilence stretched right up the March, from Gloucester to Chester, killing people throughout the border lordships that lay in between, while the southern coastal plain of Wales had been infected since late spring. From these two fronts the disease moved round the lowlands that followed, more or less, the entire shoreline of Wales. On the route from Chester into northern Wales, the plague travelled the very track, now well-trodden, made by Edward I seventy-two years earlier. At Holywell in the county of Flint many of the lead miners died and the survivors refused to work; no doubt – like the tin miners of Cornwall – they were more attracted to the safer jobs now available elsewhere. Ruthin, a little further on, was infected by mid-June: seventy-seven of the English inhabitants died within the next fortnight, as did some of the Welsh serfs resident there. The plague quickly spread further out and was at a peak in the surrounding lordship of Dyffryn Clwyd in August, by which time it had overtaken Deganwy, on the opposite side of the river from Conwy, where the demesne manor was emptied of tenants, either through flight or contagion. It is clear from records made in following years that every part of this northern shore was badly affected by plague, which should tell us something about the fate of those communities that sat on the road further round the coastal rim of Wales, between Caernarfon and Aberystwyth.

From Aberystwyth the coastal road continued south, riding the ever more vertiginous cliffs until Cardigan was reached. Easily reached from Carmarthen, this little town was probably infected from the south rather than the north. Whatever the direction of infection, the native settlements[ix] were ravaged over the summer, making it almost impossible to find replacement officials to take over from the beadle, reeve and serjeant, all of whom had died; nearby St Dogmael's Abbey was said to have lost a very great number of its monks. From the monastery the road continued south to the ecclesiastical capital and westernmost settlement in Wales – St David's. This minuscule city yields a crumb of information about the mortality in the Cambrian highlands, inland, much of which was ministered to by the bishop of St David's. The current incumbent, Bishop Brian, was abroad and so his energetic archdeacon, Gruffudd

ix commotes.

ap Rhys, led ordinands all the way to Hereford to be priested by Bishop John Trillek. During 1349, 108 ordinations were performed by the English bishop, four or five times the number of candidates put forward in a normal year. The large numbers of new ordinands for this diocese, which normally had only a small cadre of priests, strongly suggests that the disease managed to penetrate the Cambrian highlands, reaching up through the valleys to the uplands beyond.

Sixty per cent of Wales lies above 150 metres, a quarter above 300 metres – almost all of which forms the central massif that runs north–south down the middle of Wales. It was amongst these time-tempered mountains that what was left of the native Welsh nation was forced to live. They persevered quietly, causing little trouble and subsisting much as they had done for hundreds of years. The highest ground was snow-covered in winter and inhospitable for much of the rest of the year, so their mere survival dictated that the inhabitants practise transhumant agriculture: in the summer they camped out on temporary upland pastures, coming down to their semi-nucleated lowland villages as soon as the autumn rains began to fall. It was at this point, most probably, that the native Welsh picked up the disease from the more static coastal communities, trading the milk, cheese, meat and hides that were the staples of the native Welsh economy and diet; for it was probably only by the late summer of 1349 that the pestilence completed its journey up the March, through north and south Wales and round the coastal rim, completing the encirclement of infection that, at some point or other, was certain to close in on the native Welsh.[15] It was the same demonic halo that had enforced the cruel containment of the Welsh for over sixty years, a feat of conquest that the medieval English never accomplished during their time in Ireland.[x] In 1282, when the independent Welsh nation was at

---

[x] As in Ireland too, colonization was defined primarily in agricultural terms, with Anglo-Norman manors imposed on colonized lands, and more informal agriculture and transhumance practised in native Celtic regions. It is no coincidence that in Wales the native Welsh were encircled not only by English castles but by English manors, dominating the more fertile land. In medieval Ireland no such encirclement – neither agricultural nor military – was achieved. It is also important to note that in both nations the colonization of better land by the English further retarded the development of the native Celtic people, who were forced to continue with semi-nomadic subsistence farming, which was inimical to the emergence of strong markets and urban centres.

its end, native bards despairingly asked: 'is it the end of the world?', 'do you not see that the whole world is in danger?'[16] What the Welsh would later call *Y Farwolaeth Fawr* – the Great Mortality – provided them with an elegiac reply: their infection had been hastened, if not achieved, because of their subjugation by the English.

The Welsh will soon have found ways to comprehend the tragedy. They were great lovers of bardic prophecy, which no doubt styled a response quite different from that of the more prosaic English.[17] Indeed, for the Welsh there was historical precedent for the pestilence, one repeated in the *History of the Kings of Britain* by the twelfth-century cleric and historian Geoffrey of Monmouth. Although some doubted the historical accuracy of the *History* early on,[18] it was a hugely popular work that reflected the patriotic spirit of Geoffrey's native Welsh. Britain, Geoffrey claimed, had been founded by Brutus, the great-grandson of Aeneas, the hero of Troy. His arrival on this island presaged 1,800 years of British rule, broken only by the Roman invasion of Julius Caesar. The British were resurgent, however, under glorious Arthur, whose court Geoffrey placed at Caerleon-on-Usk, near Newport. Nevertheless, not long after, Britain was harried by war, famine and plague. Evoking the familiar trinity of the Apocalypse, Geoffrey described how the Britons first quarrelled amongst themselves, falling into a vicious civil war. Then there was a terrible famine, 'grievous and long-remembered'. Finally Britain was visited by a 'pestilent and deadly plague [which] killed off such a vast number of the population that the living could not bury them'.[19] These vexations forced the last king of the Britons – Cadwallader – to flee to Brittany, leaving only a few Britons, 'living precariously in Wales, in the remote recesses of the woods'. These remnants of the British nation 'were given the name of Welsh', much of the rest of the island now largely filled by marauding Angles and Saxons. Cadwallader wished to return to Britain and rule once again but an Angelic Voice warned him off. He could not go back, the Voice said, until the prophecies of Merlin to Arthur, which comprised the usual vatic ambiguities, had been fulfilled.[20] Thus Cadwallader would never see his land, 'the best of islands', again.[21] His people – the Britons, now called the Welsh – were condemned to wait for future deliverance. Although dedicated to his Norman masters, in whose favour the text could be read, Geoffrey's real intent was to remind the Welsh of their past glories and give them promise of better times to come. For the Welshmen of the middle of the fourteenth century – oppressed in part through their own division, pushed to the margins of existence and now racked by plague – the clear echoes in this familiar mythic theme will not have gone unmissed. It proved, if any proof were needed, that Edward the Conqueror's claim to Arthur's crown had been fraudulent. The Welsh had still to wait for Arthur's true heir to come and regain what Cadwallader had been forced to leave behind.

Edward I was not alone in aspiring to sit on Arthur's throne; his grandson held the same ambition. In 1344, before he had won any significant battle, Edward III held his very own Round Table, in clear emulation of the Arthurian ideal.[xi] Yet this was a different Arthur, not the king of Cambrian prophetic myth but a creation of French chivalric romance. The changed provenance is instructive, for whereas Edward I had expended much effort and treasure across the March in Wales, Edward III had sought a far larger prize in France. Yet whatever his intentions after the triumph of Crécy and the capture of Calais, they were to be reshaped by events beyond his control. The death of Princess Joan in July 1348 had nullified the Castilian alliance, which had been concluded in order to secure the southern frontier of English Bordeaux. Little Prince William of Windsor's death later in the summer had drawn a pall over the celebrations that had occupied Edward and his court since their return just under a year earlier; no more jousts would be held for over seven months. With his captains disbanded and returned to their estates, Edward had – despite the shenanigans that had filled the autumn – stepped down from a war footing, for the time being at least. Then, in the flush of his diplomatic coup in Flanders, Edward had summoned parliament for a session first thing in the New Year. Once again, his motives are unclear: Edward had already been granted a three-year subsidy in spring 1348 and given the reticence of the Commons in that parliament when invited to comment on the king's successes in France, it seems unlikely that Edward trusted the assembly to make bellicose noises before peace negotiations with the French resumed in March (although it was a tactic he had tried before and may well have intended to employ again). Perhaps he planned

[xi] 19th January 1344.

to introduce measures against papal interference in clerical appointments and court decisions, calls for which had been growing in recent
years. The pope, who was French and whose French sympathies were
well-known, had not replied to Edward's requests for help in coming
to a negotiated peace with France, from which he inferred that Clement
had been leant on by Philip VI. A threat to papal rights – Edward
might have reasoned – would encourage the pope to withstand the
pressure being exerted by the French king.

Whatever Edward's plans, the news coming out of London in the
last fortnight of December – whilst the king and his family were celebrating Christmas at the archbishop of Canterbury's palace at Otford
– made it quite clear that holding parliament in the capital in January
would now be wholly impractical. Many would decline to attend
through fear for their lives and those that did would be at risk, principal among them being the king himself. So, on 1st January 1349, he
prorogued parliament until 27th April, to coincide with the first day
of government business following Easter.[xii] Although the session would
no longer be a prelude to discussions with the French, it would now
immediately follow any agreement made with the enemy and Edward
could, therefore, put the terms of the truce to a grateful parliament.
Furthermore, as it was likely that the pope would still be made arbiter
of any agreement reached, suitable legislation that would prompt the
pope to act favourably could still be introduced. Quite apart from
these schemes, the delay indicated that the king expected the pestilence to pass, at the very least, by the end of April. So Edward hunkered
down, ready to sit it out. Over Epiphany at Merton the court indulged
in more 'games',[xiii] then stole away to the king's manor at King's
Langley in Hertfordshire. This was a favourite Plantagenet palace:
bones recently found in the wine cellar show a prodigious consumption of lamb, rabbit and venison, goose and pheasant, crab and all
manner of fish. There may even have been carp, an exotic species
brought to England from the East – much like the plague which, by
the time the royal family had arrived at Langley, had made it to London
but not yet Hertfordshire. Edward was nonetheless unwilling to take
any risks, sending for his relics so that he and his family might enjoy

[xii] Hocktide, the second Monday after Easter and the first day of the administrative
Easter Term.
[xiii] Epiphany fell on Tuesday, 6th January 1349.

their protection should the plague burst out of the capital into the countryside around.

Back at Westminster, the wheels of government continued to turn – albeit slowly – in the king's absence. Most of the king's principal ministers had also left the capital: the treasurer, Edington, had gone to his Surrey manors of Farnham and Esher; the chancellor, Ufford, remained at Otford; whilst the justices of the King's Bench, the principal criminal court, were due to spend their first term of the year in York, well away from the plague.[xiv] Westminster Hall was far from empty, however, as the clerks to the various departments of state continued to go about their work. This building, despite being two and a half centuries old, was still the largest roofed secular space in Europe. There were the same massive side walls, enclosing a giant rectangle with entrances on all sides, a row of pillars down the middle of the building holding up the double span of the heavy Norman roof. The space was at the same time cavernous and, owing to the many stone piers, labyrinthine. The high windows admitted only a poor light, leaving the dimness below to be lit by flares which sent plumes of sooty smoke up to the blackened beams.

The Stygian gloom of Westminster Hall made it a dismal and forbidding home for the apparatus of royal government, grown large through the many increments in administration and its centralization in London (itself a function of its increased size and the improvement in communications). Every office of state had its own designated area, each furnished with chests and tables, and lit by tallow candles. Between partitions put between the many stone pillars clerks worked quietly, kept apart from the lawyers, petitioners and officials who milled in the spaces in between. In one corner was the Chancery, the official secretariat of royal government. This was the largest single component of the administration, employing about a hundred full-time clerks, who issued formal letters of instruction and charters conferring rights. Next door were the two royal courts of justice – the Common Pleas (the highest civil court in the land) and, when it was in London, the King's Bench (which heard criminal cases). Through a side door in its own annex was the Exchequer – the second-largest office in Edward's administration, employing

---

[xiv] Hilary Term, in 1349 from Tuesday, 20th January, to about Tuesday, 10th February.

about sixty clerks, who supervised the receipt of taxes and other royal revenues, and undertook the audit of sheriffs' and other royal accounts. Instructions to all these departments – the courts, Chancery and Exchequer – were processed via the office of the Privy Seal, which acted as the conduit by which the king's wishes were communicated to the relevant part of his administration. It was a correspondingly small bureau, having only a dozen or so officials. However, much of the day-to-day running of government was not by official command of the king but through his chief ministers, the chancellor (who oversaw the Chancery), the treasurer (the Exchequer) and the justices of the courts. These met *ad hoc* as the royal council, often in the absence of the king, and issued uncontroversial instructions in his name. Thus Westminster Hall held within its walls an impressive bureaucracy, the result of several centuries of administrative growth and judicial innovation. Across Europe, it was the most advanced government machine of the time. However, this was no modern government, nor a modern state. The extent to which this administration gave Edward control over his subjects would be exposed in the months to come.

Despite the prorogation of parliament at the beginning of January, Edward anticipated that the core of his administration would be able to continue to operate. That expectation was soon to be challenged. By the end of the month he had heard from the Exchequer that the audit of a sheriff's accounts had been adjourned, as the county officers feared for their lives in the capital and refused to attend. These hearings had legal standing so their postponement required a good excuse. Clearly the situation was now serious. Edward promptly sent a letter from King's Langley to the justices of the Common Pleas in London, who were now the only senior officials left in the capital, advising them to adjourn their hearings until after Easter.[xv] Never mind that they were almost a week into their sittings – the king was worried for their health, 'on account of the mortality due to the terrible plague chiefly in the city of London and neighbouring parts, whereby the justices, the clerks, serjeants and other ministers of the Bench and the people suing their affairs, would incur great danger'.[22] However, court cases (especially in the Common Pleas) were extremely lucrative,

[xv] Monday, 26th January 1349.

so the judges and attorneys had good reason to stay and they disregarded the king's advice. The royal clerks, who formed the *corps administratif*, had less choice in the matter and were obliged to carry on working.

The absence from London of the king and his chief ministers mattered little: the administration was now well-trained in functioning effectively during the king's prolonged campaigns abroad. During these early months of 1349 Edward and his chief ministers were never more than sixty miles away, so it was possible to send bundles of papers for information or decision out from Westminster to the country in full expectation of a speedy return. Thus, after the early splutter, the machinery of royal bureaucracy soon ran smoothly again. Chancery, Exchequer and offices of the royal household continued to operate, just as they were used to before the onset of the plague. The diligence of the administration, despite the perils and problems posed by the disease, was impressive. There was no active response to the epidemic; nor can its presence be easily identified within the reams of records that survive from the early months of 1349. However, if the officials did not react to the plague itself, they also ensured that the plague did not allow the everyday business of royal government to slip. This was not a conscious or collective act of resistance: it was simply a reflection of the fact that the administrative duties of royal government, in matters small and great, did not cease.

So royal government carried on, sending out and receiving instructions, accepting petitions and registering transactions. There can be no doubt that all this communication added to the transmission of the plague. Take the case of Richard Large, who came up to London from Winchelsea in late February, specifically to deliver a remaindered cargo to Westminster Hall. In order to cross the river he will have had to negotiate the streets of London, clogged with rakers pushing diseased bodies to and from Smithfield. At Westminster Hall he was received by Thomas Clopton, one of the Chancery clerks. Clopton sent a report of the seizure to Edward's staff, who were with him at King's Langley; Richard Large, meanwhile, returned to Winchelsea – which had not yet contracted the plague, but was soon to do so. Whether Richard carried the disease back from infected London it is impossible to tell, but the many hundreds of journeys such as his all helped to spread the disease around. Indeed, it was precisely because of the risk of infection that the king had removed himself from the capital. Other than the issue of the occasional mandate, there was little evidence of active rule. Given Edward's usual hyperactivity, this quietude suggests that the royal court had gone into self-imposed isolation. It is probable that access to the monarch, his family and privy advisers was strictly controlled to prevent their infection. Thus it was as much out of self-interest as consideration for others that on 10th March the king prorogued parliament, already postponed until April, once again. The plague had utterly engulfed London and was by now breaking out all over the south-east, so any hope of holding the assembly had, for the time being, to be abandoned, simply because 'the assembling of magnates and other lieges there would be too dangerous'.[23] This time the delay was indefinite, an admission that no one was willing even to guess when the epidemic would cease. Whatever Edward's plans for parliament, they would have to wait for another day.

Yet, other matters were still pressing, prime among them the nego-tiations to create a permanent peace with France. Both Edward and Philip knew these to be a sham; both also needed, however, to assuage domestic concern and, perhaps, salve their own consciences that an effort had been made. So the talks that had been agreed back in the autumn went ahead. On Thursday, 12th March, two days after parlia-ment had been cancelled, William Bateman, the bishop of Norwich, was despatched once again for the Continent. He crossed the channel by the end of the month, leaving his peaceful diocese behind. The bishop was joined by Humphrey de Bohun's brother William, the earl of Northampton, Sir William de Clinton, the earl of Huntingdon, and Sir Walter Manny, who only a few days before had been at the dedication of the enlarged cemetery he had helped purchase in Smithfield. All three had seen the horrors of London first-hand and, on arriving at Calais, they found a scene of familiar desolation. The English citadel had been infected in the late summer of the previous year and the plague had taken, in its course, the captain of the town's garrison – Sir John Montgomery – whose body had been shipped back to London for interment in the Carmelite friary there. We cannot be surprised that he did not want to be buried in conquered Calais, which was an unnatural place at the best of times. Shorn of its French citizens, replete with English soldiers, still bearing the scars of the recent – most terrible – siege: it lacked all the signs of organic urban life. The town was isolated, marooned on a vast salt-marsh, an English enclave in France physically and politically separated from the rest of the Continent. Yet in this cheerless place, now ravaged by plague, there was a new sign of hope: as Calais had few outside contacts with which the momentum of infection could be maintained, it is probable that the disease had already begun to burn itself out. Here was evidence that the plague might indeed, at some point, come to an end.

The mock-talks commenced at the now traditional meeting place, in the village of Guînes, on the edge of the Calais bog. Bishop Bateman's delegation was soon sending reports back to England, describing the progress that had been made. No doubt he also mentioned the situation in Calais: how the town had been denuded of people, was desolate but had at least managed to throw off the plague. It is the most likely explanation for the sudden improvement in Edward's mood, for now the king was making plans for a tournament, the first of the year. Believing that the threat of pestilence was at last receding, he considered that an assembly of 'magnates and other lieges' might no longer be quite so 'dangerous'.[24] This would be no ordinary jousting competition, however. With little to do during his self-imposed isolation of early 1349, Edward had whiled away the time embellishing his idea for an order of chivalry. As the 1344 Round Table showed, the idea for a chivalric fraternity, taking as its model the Arthurian court, had been around for some time.[xvi] Only the previous summer Edward had founded a collegiate chapel in Windsor dedicated to St George, whom he clearly envisaged as patron of his new order.[xvii] Now he was in receipt of such promising news from Calais, it suddenly seemed not so outlandish to commemorate St George's Day, the perfect occasion to inaugurate this confraternity with its first assembly of member knights. As he pondered the risks, the reasons for going ahead only multiplied. It would be a welcome moment of relief from the *ennui* of enforced winter retreat, not least for the royal family, who were still at King's Langley over Easter. It was, moreover, a long-overdue opportunity for Edward – ever-conscious of the need to keep key magnates close to him – to gather his lieutenants together. In their pursuit of the nimble

[xvi] Indeed, there was probably a loose companionship in existence by the time of the fabulous celebrations for the birth of Prince William on 24th June 1348.
[xvii] Wednesday, 6th August 1348.

lance and sturdy seat, they would send a suitably belligerent signal to Philip (who would inevitably hear of the festivities) that the plague had not purged the English or their king of martial purpose.[xviii]

Thus, on 23rd April 1349, Edward and his family emerged for the first time since the pestilence had forced them into hiding. The celebrations, which were held at Windsor, were magnificent. The king, Prince of Wales and twenty-four other inaugural members were there. The initiates included some of Edward's greatest commanders, among them Sir Ralph Stafford and the earl of Lancaster. There were some conspicuous absentees, however: Humphrey de Bohun was still trapped in his bolthole of Brecon, while Walter Manny and the earl of Huntingdon were in France with Bishop Bateman, detained on the king's business. Thus, while his diplomats treated with the French, the royal party indulged in play-battles 120 miles away in Windsor. Around the armoured thigh of each jousting knight was a garter, bound by a buckle emblazoned with a motto: *Honi soit qui mal y pense* – 'evil to him that thinks evil of it'. This was the new order's device, after which it would become known, worn by king and his fellow warriors revelling in the pretence of battle but in preparation for the resumption of the real thing. The whole *mise en scène* – motto and monarch, the clash of arms and the cries of 'St George!' – was a none-too-subtle celebration of Edward's claims and intentions in France. It gave the lie to the charade underway across the Channel at Guînes. Avalon had been invoked once again, its name debased by yet another Plantagenet king.

[xviii] Especially as the pestilence had prevented the king from sending that exact message via parliament.

9

Uses and Abuses

May–June 1349

Prosperity doth best discover vice, but adversity doth best discover virtue.

Francis Bacon[1]

If Edward had wished his St George's Day pageant to herald the end of the pestilence, he was to be disappointed. Whatever the reports from Calais, the epidemic was far from over. No sooner had the debris of the feast been cleared away than Edward was told of fresh problems back at Westminster.

After a brief hiatus, the business of the royal administration had continued in the face of pestilence. When the London fish merchant William Greyland, executor of so many wills, had attended Chancery in March, the clerks had processed the land transfers he brought in the normal way, as if nothing had been untoward, while in the week after Easter, as pestilence still raged all around, the Council had convened in an attempt to clear up the mess left by the collapse of Chiriton's customs company.[i] To this end they had met a delegation of London merchants, despite the clear dangers of doing so, in order to discuss what to do.[ii] We may suspect that some limited measures must have been introduced, at least to ensure that officials and visitors congregating in Westminster Hall kept their distance, one from another; whatever the reason, it was believed to be safe enough to allow the courts to return to work, as was normal, after their

---

[i] See Ch. 5, p. 111.

[ii] As a result, on Tuesday, 21st April 1349, just two days before Edward's extravaganza at Windsor, orders were sent out from Westminster transferring Chiriton's rights and assets to royal administrators.

Easter break.[iii] The Court of the Common Pleas met in its usual place in Westminster Hall; the Court of the King's Bench (which, in an innovation introduced the previous year, was holding assizes around the country) continued its peregrination, transferring from York to Lincoln.

York had thus far been free from plague but pestilence had broken out in Lincoln only three weeks before, and so for the first time the King's Bench, with its judges, attorneys and clerks, entered an infected area.[2] Yet back at Westminster, which was in constant contact with the travelling court, the extent of the spread of the epidemic north was not precisely known. Perhaps messengers from the King's Bench coming south from Lincoln were received in Westminster Hall in the belief that they travelled from a disease-free region, so none of the precautions devised for visitors from areas known to be infected were used. For it is a striking coincidence that the movement of the King's Bench from York to Lincoln immediately preceded the outbreak of plague at the centre of royal administration, which had thus far remained unaffected despite the widespread epidemic in London and all the countryside around: as April rolled into May, some of the recording clerks in Westminster began to show signs of the disease and were soon dead, their absence marked by the uncharacteristic muddles in the records that followed their demise. Ominously, the king's physician – who may well have attended to the stricken clerks – was also an early victim; an auditor of the royal household, Nicholas Buckland, perished shortly afterwards. Within weeks, on Wednesday 20th May, the head of the entire administration, the chancellor – Archbishop John Ufford – died at Tottenham.[3] Three days later William Bret, the sheriff for Essex and Hertfordshire – where the king had only lately been – was struck down. This was enough for Edward, who had already gone back into seclusion, this time even further away, at his palace of Woodstock in Oxfordshire: fearing that the very means of government were now threatened, he summoned his privy office from Westminster to be with him so that he could keep his main instrument of rule close by. On his orders, the Trinity sessions of the Common Pleas and King's Bench, scheduled to begin on 15th June, were both abandoned.[iv]

[iii] On Monday, 27th April 1349.
[iv] Trinity Term, in 1349 from Monday, 15th June, to Tuesday, 14th July.

Edward's celebrations were thus shown to have been premature: he had surfaced at the first hint that the epidemic had abated but within the space of a month, between the Garter celebrations and the death of Sheriff Bret, his confidence had been dashed. Pestilence had not only started killing officials but now affected the routines of those that remained. Edward may have been able to escape the contagion but he could not now avoid the consequences of plague.

William Dene, the Rochester monk and chronicler, did not give 'Archbishop Ufford a complimentary obituary. He had 'borrowed a great sum of money from all sides to give to the pope', Dene claimed, 'but he might as well have not bothered for he died soon after and thereby lost the lot', which was to 'the ruin of a great many creditors, who were reduced to poverty'.[4] Another whom Dene fingers was the bishop of Ely, Thomas Lisle. A Dominican friar, Lisle had spent some time in the mid-1340s at Avignon, where he had become accustomed to the pleasures of the papal court. Consequently, he sought an English bishopric that would allow him to live in appropriate style and in 1345, having paid a handsome sum, secured the diocese of Ely by the pope's appointment. Although this ancient diocese was wealthy, Lisle had to extract every penny in order to pay off the huge loans he had taken out to purchase the office, bringing financial ruin to his see and the censure of several contemporary observers. Unlike others, Lisle did not compensate for this profligacy by giving assiduous attention to his flock.

It was true to this prelate's past form, therefore, that as the plague threatened in the autumn of 1348[5] he thought it the moment to set off for Rome. His excuse was the Jubilee celebrations planned for 1350; the return journey to the Eternal City was a long one but in no way required a year, let alone the eighteen months that Lisle had allowed.[6] The bishop certainly knew what he was leaving behind, as he appointed a full five vicars-general to act in his absence – a significant allowance for wastage.[7] It was six months before he heard news, in the spring warmth of Avignon (a convenient stop en route to Rome), that plague had reached his diocese.[8] So, on 9th April, Lisle issued a personal order, appointing a further three vicars-general, 'because the epidemic, even in our own diocese, wondrously increases, as we have heard not long ago from go-betweens'.[9] Amongst them was Edmund Gonville, who was now rector of the village of Terrington St Clement,[10] four miles west of Lynn.[v] In this mandate the bishop set out a strict hierarchy of succession, should any of the vicars-general die, whilst relaxing the rules concerning the institution of clergy to vacant parishes to make their task a little easier. It is a mark of the sheer scale of mortality and the administrative workload that the bishop felt obliged to appoint eight representatives in his stead. He was not, however, going to get involved himself. Thomas continued to enjoy Provençal heat and the comforts of Avignon, waiting the year out before he travelled on to Rome.

The absent bishop had not been idle, however. On 10th March the curia sent out a dispensation to his nephew, Robert Michel, permitting him to hold a benefice even though he was neither ordained nor over the legal age of twenty-one (the boy was still only nineteen). Young Robert spent the next few months making great use of his new position, swapping benefices one for the another, making a tidy profit on each transaction. For as clergy started dying from the plague, more and more benefices became vacant, waiting for Lisle's vicars-general to appoint a new priest. Those who arranged the appointments (the bishop's staff) and those personally close to the bishop (like Robert) could manipulate the distribution of these positions to their advantage: a vacant parish could be taken on, its accrued title income extracted and then resigned in favour of someone new. If an ambitious cleric kept his eyes and ears open, he would be able to do this several times, making money whilst not staying long enough to have to organize any costly pastoral coverage. Robert's example is typical. A few miles west of Gonville's parish was the little village of Newton, which lay – like Terrington St Clement – on a silt bank that formed a fertile levee between the salty Wash and the barren Fens. Sometime in late March, the rector of Newton died and on 10th April Robert was appointed his successor. He would have possession for only 103 days, as on 21st July he gained the larger rectory of the neighbouring village of Tydd St Giles. This trade in benefices certainly enriched the priest-trader, in Robert's case earning him £2 during this short period; however, whilst not illegal, the practice was frowned upon and offenders were called 'chop-churches', a double-meaning that was

[v] Renamed King's Lynn by Henry VIII.

clearly intended. For what made benefice swapping particularly egregious was the destabilizing effect it had on parishioners, whose rector changed from one month to the next and would often fail to minister to his congregation, an offence made that much more grave given their present dire need.

This was but one of several tactics employed by worldly clerics to squeeze money from their cures. Most parishes were served by a rector. A number of these chose to take the income from the parish tithes and fees and use a portion to pay a vicar to look after the pastoral work, keeping the remainder as profit. This was an accepted practice, not least because it was the means by which the clerks in the ecclesiastical and civil administrations were paid; indeed, most of the officials in Westminster Hall were nominally rectors of one parish or other, sometimes many miles from London. However, the holding of multiple (or plural) benefices – 'farming' them out for income – was considered a gross abuse, as was nepotism (showing favour to a relative), absenteeism, and simony (the purchase of ecclesiastical office). The decentralized administration of the church meant that prevention and punishment of abuses required the constant vigilance of strong and principled bishops. Thomas Lisle, it must be said, was not one of these. Indeed, his own example was appalling: he had purchased his bishopric, promoted the interests of his nephew and was for long periods of time absent from his see. It is no wonder, therefore, that standards in the diocese soon slipped. The principal offenders were members of Lisle's household. While some could make the excuse that they had been seconded to the bishop's diocesan office, others were only profiting from the surfeit of vacant benefices, vacancies they chose to fill in their favour rather than in the interest of those in their spiritual care.

All the while the diocese of Ely was being laid waste by plague. It arrived – as in the Midlands and East Anglia – in late spring. At Soham, five miles to the south-east of Ely, two thirds of the tenantry (and most likely a similar proportion of the village) was dead, by early June.[11] In the clutch of villages to the north of Cambridge, a dozen miles to the south of Ely, the mortality was as severe as in central England. At Cottenham at least thirty-three of the fifty-eight tenants (57 per cent) died; at Chesterton there were probably almost seventy deaths in the year, whereas normally the villagers could expect fewer than ten.[12]

None of this – the arrival of the Great Death, the fear and disruption, not even his duties as one of Lisle's vicars-general – kept Edmund Gonville from his founding work in Cambridge, where his hall of scholars was halfway to fruition. His refusal to countenance a delay was all the more remarkable given the problems the disease was making in the university town. His persistence was typical of this academic colony, which, at little more than a century old, was still in its infancy. Before the scholars came, the town had been a small market, on the way to nowhere of any importance, an inhospitable and unpromising place. The land was soggy, the wind from the flat Fens penetrating, the Cam often foul. With a defunct castle, tatty market square and a number of unremarkable houses, this place offered nothing to the scholarly immigrants, nothing except that which the scholars craved and which kept the merchants away: isolation. Just as the Benedictines had found such beneficial solitude in the Fenland edges, at their great abbeys of Crowland, Peterborough, Ramsey and Thorney, the scholars in Cambridge could get on with their study in peace, untouched by the troubles of outside life. The schools they established in the early thirteenth century soon formed a loose academic union, which then became a university in its own right. Cambridge being so small, the scholars soon achieved a predominance over the townsmen, endowing the place with an atmosphere of learning early on. As at Oxford, it had attracted some considerable benefactions in the previous two decades: King's Hall (founded by Edward II and reinstituted by Edward III), Clare Hall, and Pembroke Hall, which – like Clare – had a noblewoman as its foundress.[13] Now there was to be Gonville Hall. Gonville had managed to secure accommodation for his scholars by the end of 1348 and on 4th June 1349 he made out the deed of foundation, naming John Colton as the first master of the college.

Colton would have been wise to hold off taking up his position, for the isolation of Cambridge had not prevented the arrival of plague. Between April and August sixteen of the forty scholars lodged at King's Hall died, whilst the neighbouring hospital of St John the Evangelist (which had nothing to do with the university) went through four masters in three months. The first, Alexander, died at the end of April, to be replaced by a Brother Robert on 2nd May, voted in by his fellow brothers Alan, William, Roger and Richard. Robert died almost

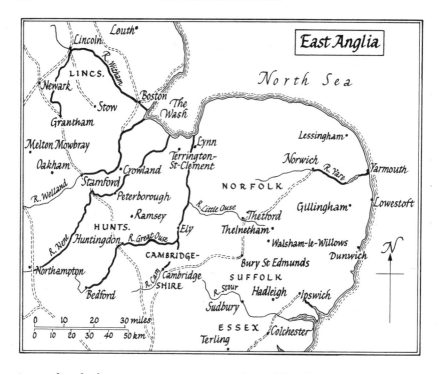

immediately, however, so Roger was elected by the remaining three. He died within a month, to be replaced on 28th June by Brother William, after an election in which only Brother Richard was left from the original complement of six; now, after the recent arrival of a new entrant, the community numbered only three. The hospital was important locally and its travails were to the further disadvantage of the sick of Cambridge, so Brother William was installed by the chancellor of the diocese with utmost haste, anxious at 'how much danger threatens the hospital through lack of a master'.[14] The pestilence was not an unmitigated tragedy for Cambridge, however: some were able to use the events to further their own ends. The clerical society of Michaelhouse, for example, finding opportunity in disaster, was able to purchase new buildings, no doubt as a result of their desuetude caused by the plague. Michaelhouse and the adjacent King's Hall would later be joined to make Trinity College, opposite whose gatehouse the school of divinity would be built in the nineteenth century. As the Victorian workmen dug deep to lay their foundations, they uncovered a pit of bodies, the skeletons lying just as they had been thrown in. Perhaps these were the victims of these months – the scholars of King's Hall entangled in death with the patients and brothers of St John's Hospital.

Cambridgeshire was most probably infected by travellers coming from Hertfordshire or London to the south. However, it is possible that the disease came via Norfolk, as a road ran between Cambridge and Norwich, where the pestilence had been present since the New Year. We shall never know: the progress of the disease had, by late spring, become so rapid and widespread that it is impossible to discern a definite line of infection. A similar problem obtains further east, in the two counties of Norfolk and Suffolk that made up ancient East Anglia and the medieval diocese of Norwich. At Little Cornard, which sits in the Stour Valley just outside Sudbury, the plague was probably present by late March and had killed many tenants by the end of April. Yet just as the disease was creeping from Essex into Suffolk, it was already spreading over Norfolk – not only from Norwich but from the ports of Lynn and Yarmouth too.[15] Two events, on the same day, make this clear. At Heacham, near Lynn on the eastern shore of the Wash, a dispute was heard at the manor court on Tuesday, 28th April. It was a marital feud between Reginald Goscelin and his wife Emma, the question being a matter of dower. With steward and jury assembled, only Emma appeared. It transpired that not only had all of her witnesses died the previous day but her husband had too, so the case no longer needed to be heard. The very same Tuesday, at Yarmouth on the other side of the county, the wills of two prominent burghers – Charles Bennett and Simon Hall – were granted probate. Simon gave £7 0s. 2d.[vi] in religious bequests, some of which no doubt was intended for the rebuilding work then in progress on the west end of St Nicholas's church. It was not to be used for some while, however: the plague – had forced the work to stop, no doubt because so many workmen had died.

This was the chaotic scene that greeted Bishop William Bateman on his return from the Continent. Like Thomas Lisle, Bateman had been away from his see during April and May, when the plague had spread through both their dioceses. Unlike the wily Lisle, however, Bateman's absence was not of his choosing, he having been sent at the king's bidding to France at the end of March to negotiate a truce

---

[vi] £7.01.

with the French. In terms of a permanent peace it had been a fruit-less exercise, since both parties were eager to return to battle: Philip wished to regain his lost territory, Edward wanted to make use of his advantage. However, the Great Death was causing havoc in France, just as it was devastating England, so for six weeks the ambassadors danced the waltz of concord and then agreed an extension to the truce to extend from 1st September 1349 to 1st May 1350. It was the ideal outcome: this synthetic peace allowed the kings to salve their consciences and buy themselves time to sit out the plague. Nonetheless, it was still possible for the parties to resume hostilities before the truce's end, given that some incident or other – real, imagined or confected – would with ease excuse a return to arms.

His mission accomplished, Bateman sailed for home. From his correspondence with his officials in Norwich, the bishop knew already that the epidemic had by now spread beyond the city.[16] Bateman's vicar-general, Thomas Methwold, had dealt with matters as best he could, managing the mounting crisis from Norwich in the bishop's absence. By the beginning of May, however, Bateman had arrived back in England and was staying at his manor of Terling, in Essex. Between them, Bateman and Methwold made seventy-three institutions and other appointments in May alone (a total of fifty-three had been made in the first four months of 1349). Then, at the beginning of June, just as the plague was reaching its peak in Suffolk, Bateman made a circuitous route through the east of the county to Yarmouth, where he was able to see the town's problems for himself – the spread of the contagion, the great losses suffered so far, the halting of the rebuilding work at St Nicholas's church, the deaths of the burghers Bennett, Hall and Reed – some of whom Bateman must surely have known.[17] Yet almost as soon as he had arrived, the bishop received the news of the death of his brother, Sir Bartholomew Bateman, at Gillingham, but fifteen miles away; he rode there immediately to console his brother's widow, Petronilla. His visit produced at least one positive piece of news, for the parson's position – only recently made vacant – had already been filled,[18] a heartening sign that his vicar-general had been doing his job.

Bateman did not stay long: he made for Norwich, where he conferred with Methwold and his other harassed officials for only one day, before heading south towards London in order to report to the king on the treaty he had just made with the French. As he travelled once more through Suffolk, Bishop Bateman cannot have failed to be shocked by the depopulation that had been the first effect of the pestilence, nor by the unkempt fields and wandering animals that had been its result. Everywhere there was evidence of the progress of the Great Death. It was said that half the monks of the abbey of Bury St Edmunds had died; certainly their manors had fared no better.[19] At Walsham-le-Willows 110 tenants had perished between 6th March and 15th June, the very point at which Bateman passed by. Perhaps 700 in this large village had perished by the end of the summer – more than half the whole community. Individual tragedies abound, yet there was the odd miracle among the long lists of deaths that extended the manorial roll. John Robhood was among the luckiest: not only did both he and his wife survive but so did their six children.

Theirs was a remarkable tale, for almost every other family was ruined by plague during these months and as many marriages dissolved – including that of Lady Rose de Saxham, whose husband had been lord of the manor. As her three sons were also dead she – like so many of her peasant tenants – was now left quite alone to manage the estate; the heir, her grandson Thomas, was probably still a minor. At Lessingham in Norfolk (as in Thornbury) the deaths of husbands were a spur to better marriages for ambitious widows: Egidia Burt lost her husband Edward and immediately remarried another Edward, in so doing repudiating a debt of 30s.[vii] owed by her late husband to one Margery Brown. (Margery took her to court and won: Egidia – now Bunting – had to honour the debt, despite her new name.) There existed ladies even more brazen than Egidia in Lessingham, however: Alice Foghal got through three husbands in these pestilential months. Perhaps by the third the village had no more grooms to offer, as the last was an outsider to the village and had to pay extra in order to take her down the aisle.

Bateman will have been well aware of this proliferation of widows, as more and more were named as patrons of churches requiring a replacement priest (his sister-in-law included). In the twenty days since the bishop had been in Gillingham, a hundred clergy had been presented to vacant cures, of which fifteen had been under the

vii £1.50.

patronage of a widow. The allocation of these men consumed much
of his time and the efforts of his administration. Every candidate had
to undergo examination, most of them at the diocesan office in
Norwich. Passing first through the city, they came to the precinct of
the cathedral priory. It was a peaceful space, separated from the bustle
of the streets and markets by a wall that ran between two bends in
the River Wensum, which flowed in a loop behind the cathedral,
marking the remainder of the priory's perimeter. A gate in the wall
allowed entry from the west. From here the clerics crossed the northern
close, with the cathedral on the right and the bishop's palace on the
other side. This close had for many years contained the cemetery
where departed monks lay at rest. Normally grassed over, the soil was
now exposed, rough earth scarring the open sward. Walking between
the freshly covered graves, these applicant priests must have been
reminded, if any reminder were needed, of the fearful ordeal on which
they were about to be sent. Yet it was not through an act of courage
that they did not stop and turn round, although there were undoubtedly many brave men among them. For what else could they do? Flight
was no option, as there was now nowhere that they could get to that
was free of the plague. So they carried on, these dozens and hundreds
of priests, just as their bishop had insisted on fulfilling his duties in
the diocese before leaving for London to confer with the king. As
Robert Michel of Ely had shown, the plague could certainly encourage
abuses; indeed, there were some, like his bishop-uncle, Thomas Lisle,
who failed their flock. Most, however, were stoics. Necessity and
example made them so.

Some time towards the end of June, a new grave was dug in the
monks' cemetery, ready to receive the body of the priory infirmarer,
Ralph Swanton.[20] On the other side of the cathedral nave lay his
former domain – the infirmary.[21] It was here that Swanton[22] had cared
for infirm monks and the sick of the wider monastery community,
and here too that he most probably caught the disease that killed him.
His patients occupied beds set out in two long rows, projecting from
the walls. The windows on one side had a good view of the infirmary
garden, where Ralph had grown herbs and medicinal plants, which
formed the base feedstock for his many treatments. The produce of
this physic garden – rhubarb, peonies, fennel, squills and the opium

poppy – was supplemented by exotic species, which had to be imported from abroad: liquorice, aniseed, turbit (a cathartic drug), dragon's blood (a bright red resin used in the treatment of wounds, diarrhoea and fevers), agaric (a fungus), mace, cloves, pepper, nutmeg, as well as foodstuffs with well-known medicinal properties such as almonds, dates, figs, pomegranates and cane sugar. Swanton had been expert in mixing these ingredients, according to their different pharmacological qualities, to create remedies for his patients. By modern standards, some of these preparations were extremely crude; they could be effective, however. It is clear, for instance, that infirmarers were able to mix potent – if sometimes extremely toxic – analgesic preparations.

This knowledge was derived from the collective experience of healers, amassed over many hundreds of years, much of it with origins in ancient folk medicine and magic. In the main it was a tradition quite separate from that which informed the medieval system of diagnosis, which had come down from Galen, a Greek doctor practising in the second century, who drew upon the medical philosophy of Hippocrates (c.460–c.370 BC). An amalgam of these two systems, Gallenic and Hippocratic, given an Aristotelian gloss, constituted the theoretical corpus of medieval medicine. In simple, this proposed that the human body was governed by the four chief fluids of the human body – blood, yellow bile, black bile and phlegm, which corresponded with the four elements – air, fire, earth and water, the intrinsic components of the created universe. The balance of the humours in the body determined both the physical and psychological disposition of a person, a predominance of one or other humour creating a dominant 'temperament', in turn sanguine, choleric, melancholic and phlegmatic. The elements, humours and temperaments, together with each of the four seasons, shared pairs of qualities, or 'opposites', with one another: warm and moist (air, blood, sanguine, spring), warm and dry (fire, yellow bile, choleric, summer), cold and dry (earth, black bile, melancholic, autumn), cold and moist (water, phlegm, phlegmatic, winter). If the humours were balanced within the body, then the body would show itself to be healthy. Conversely, ill-health was taken as evidence of an imbalance in the humours, although an individual's predisposition might make them susceptible to particular illnesses; a phlegmatic person, for instance, would be vulnerable to cold and moist ailments, such as colds.

As disease was understood to be caused by a surfeit or deficit in one of the humours, it followed that an illness could be diagnosed by identifying which humour was out of balance. The humours were regularly 'expelled' from the body, so doctors could rely almost entirely on extrinsic assessments to conduct their diagnoses. The careful examination of a patient's skin colour, vomit, urine or pulse allowed a physician to ascertain the precise nature of the disequilibrium, whether in presence (surfeit) or absence (deficit), that was causing the imbalance and sickness to occur. Treatments sought to re-establish the balance by restoring the bodily equilibrium. In a case of humeral excess, it was necessary to 'draw out' the harmful humour from the body. Some diagnoses demanded that this be done physically: the presence of blood in urine, for example, would be attributed to an excess of blood in the body, which might be treated by the application of leeches to draw the surplus away. Likewise, emetics would be administered to induce vomiting to expel phlegm. Non-physical interventions relied on the application of a poultice or fabric with 'similar' qualities, which was believed to attract the excess humour through the skin in a process akin to osmosis: yellow flowers such as dandelion were pressed to the skin to treat jaundice, which was believed to be caused by too much yellow bile in the liver.[23] In the rarer case of a humoral deficit, a restorative would be administered: cane sugar, for instance, was thought to restore moistness and would be used, therefore, to treat conditions reflecting an insufficiency of blood or phlegm.

The neatness of this system made it very attractive, not least because it had the appearance of logic. (Indeed, it is surely much less far-fetched than many alternative therapies touted today.) Neither was it an exclusive theory, unable to operate in the presence of other ideas. It easily accommodated native medical knowledge and the use of indigenous plants that had not been known to the Greeks. Most importantly, although Galen was a pagan, his theories – as transformed by medieval doctors and glossators – permitted space for a Christian interpretation of illness. Galenic medicine relied on the observation of 'natural' phenomena, all of which might happily coexist with 'supernatural' forces, from witchcraft and the influence of the planets to the will and works of God Himself. While a doctor might be able to diagnose an imbalance in the temperaments of his patient, a priest might also determine that it had been God that had caused the imbalance to arise. In turn this allowed the church to teach that ill health was none other than a symptom of spiritual sickness. For some time, therefore, the church had instructed physicians to tell their patients to seek the healer of souls before resorting to human medical intervention. Fundamental to this view was the understanding that, whilst medicine was a human intervention, both instrument and outcome relied upon God's power. As the medical faculty of Paris University stated in the plague year, 'although God alone cures the sick, he does so through the medicine which in his generosity he provided.'[24] For this reason the church could claim that the healing of the soul would serve to increase the efficacy of medication, for 'when the cause is removed the effect will pass away'.[25] Thus was the medieval Galenic system almost infinitely flexible and capable of free adaptation. It was the principal reason why, in this pre-scientific age, this interpretation of the physical world and explanation of the biology of man enjoyed such widespread acceptance and would receive no serious intellectual challenge for many hundreds of years, not even from Arabic commentators, who, in mathematics and other fields, had already succeeded in subverting the prevailing Western orthodoxy.

Whilst Ralph Swanton had worked within the Galenic tradition, he had been no more qualified than a common apothecary. This placed him somewhere in the middle of the hierarchy of medieval healers, the lowest of whom – the barber surgeons – were concerned only with the treatment of open wounds and those ailments that had an obvious surgical cure. This was not medicine: surgery was considered to be a craft and its practitioners skilled craftsmen. Nonetheless, some surgeons gained a considerable reputation, none more so than John Arderne, who had made his name through his perfection of a procedure to remove a type of anal abscess caused by extended periods spent in the saddle. Physicians, on the other hand, were specialists in the art of medicine, in which they had a university degree. John Gaddesden, a former fellow of Merton and cleric attached to St Paul's Cathedral in London, was the most famous of these 'doctors of physic'.

Gaddesden managed to acquire a reputation that long outlived him, largely because – like Arderne – he was neither modest not ashamed of self-promotion: he declared his great treatise, the *Rosa Anglica*, to be the supreme achievement of all medicine. To modern eyes, it is certainly one of the more eccentric: for the loss of memory he prescribed the eating of a nightingale's heart and to cure epileptic fits he recommended hanging the head of a cuckoo round the neck, to draw the fits away from the victim. There is much, however, of interest and value in Gaddesden's *Rosa*, not least the schema by which the treatments are ordered. His rationale is simple (and self-serving) but no less perceptive for that. Just as the rose (that best of all flowers) has five petals, he would divide his treatise (which excelled all previous works) into five separate disciplines – fevers, hygiene, injuries, diet and drugs. It is a familiar and sensible system, one that showed that Gaddesden, for all his ludicrous and speculative cures, possessed insight too. It was not for nothing that Gaddesden could boast esteemed clients (Edward II, the Black Prince and Princess Joan were among his patients) and insist on highly lucrative fees.

These hundreds of years later, Gaddesden is still an ambiguous figure: a man who – for all the whiff of a fraudster – deserves recognition for his insight and talent. It was a view shared by contemporaries as well. There is little doubt that Geoffrey Chaucer had the boastful doctor in mind when he penned his portrait of the 'Doctour of Physik'. Although his Doctour was 'a verray, parfit, praktisour', with an ability to read the stars and interpret the four humours that was second to none, he also 'lovede gold'. Here is a paradox, one that reflected a contemporary ambivalence to which all medical practitioners, whether they be physicians or village herbalists, were subject: these healers enjoyed continuing and widespread popularity, for all their quackery and fraud. Thus, even though it was well-accepted that 'gold in phisik is a cordial', people – rich, middling and poor – continued to hand it over, knowing that there was a possibility of recovery that would make the outlay worthwhile.[26] For those unable to afford a physician, there were potions devised by apothecaries such as those of Ralph Swanton, or the nostra provided by old village spinsters, who all too often received brutal punishment when things went wrong. More than the false refuge of the superstitious and desperate, the resort to medicine strongly suggests that practitioners were able, on occasion, to provide relief from pain and sometimes a primitive cure, even if success owed more to experience than to the theories used to explain its cause.

Medical treatment, like medieval death, was expected to take place at home, where care and sustenance could be provided by the patient's family. For some, however, this was neither suitable nor possible. The very poor might be unable to afford to feed an unproductive mouth; the leper was an outcast, not just from their community but from their family too; it was often impossible to care for the insane and the blind in the cramped confines of the peasant cottage; neither the indigent nor the poor traveller could rely on the help of their kin. The usual recourse for all these people was the hospital, funded and staffed by a charitable and – most usually – religious foundation. In Ireland the Celtic tradition of hospitality had propagated a multitude of small hospitals for the poor pilgrim and impoverished traveller, while the religious orders – both closed and mendicant – offered accommodation for the sick in some of the larger towns. In England the monastic infirmary was the model for ever-expanding numbers of urban hospitals (indeed, in Ireland especially, some of the larger monasteries admitted patients from outside the monastery community for care). Most hospitals specified the group of people they intended to serve. (This definition was sometimes very precise: the hospital of Clyst Gabriel outside Exeter, for instance, cared for aged and infirm priests – laymen had to look elsewhere.) The monastery also provided the format by which hospitals were ruled and administered. The establishment would be staffed by brothers, who would dress, like monks, in a habit; where inmates were expected to stay for some time, they too would don a uniform. This was not mere appearance: hospital communities lived and prayed by a pared down version of the monastic rule, not only because healing was understood to be a spiritual as well as physical process, one which required prayer as much as medication, but because it was expected that the brothers should pray for the souls of the foundation's benefactor. A hospital was, therefore, a popular form of pious endowment and so by the middle of the fourteenth century there were well over 400 across the country.

Unlike monasteries, hospitals were predominantly urban institutions, largely because the ills with which they dealt were the unfortunate but inevitable consequences of urban living. Even leper houses, which made up the majority of early foundations, were as much a result of municipal legislation as a charitable response to what was believed to be a highly contagious disease. In Bristol, for example, lepers – like prostitutes – were not permitted in the town, so were forced to find refuge in one of the leper houses that lay outside the town boundary. Lepers were just one of the several classes of urban dispossessed, and were significantly outnumbered by the vagrant poor. These, too, merited care and increasingly foundations were set up in their aid. Indeed, by the middle of the fourteenth century, many more hospitals had been established to care for the vagrant poor and leprous than for the sick. In Berkshire, for instance, seven towns[27] were served by no fewer than six hospitals for the poor, five leper houses (two of which were solely for women) but just one dedicated solely to the sick. In Norwich the provision for the sick was even more limited – among the six hospitals in the city, other than the priory infirmary, there were three for the poor, one for lepers and none at all for the infirm.

The predominance of institutions serving the urban poor reflected the fact that in the towns there was little in the way of those extended family and community structures that provided a safety-net for the vulnerable – especially those unable to work through incapacity or old age – out in the villages. It was to this class of dispossessed, there-fore, that the majority of hospitals ministered. The large Midlands institutions were typical: the hospital of St John Baptist in Coventry looked after the poor who were sick and old, just as the foundation in Warwick of the same name cared for poor wayfarers, as well as local paupers and the impoverished infirm. The greatest of all was the ancient hospital of St Leonard in York, an Anglo-Saxon founda-tion whose wealth and pedigree had no equal. Whilst in 1339 the hospital only had nine chaplain-brethren, the staff was considerably larger, as its huge responsibilities attest: the house was obliged to care for no fewer than 206 poor sick and infirm people.[28] If they recovered, patients were not to be discharged until they had convalesced and were capable of work; those that wished to remain could do so, so long as they lived and worked as a lay member of the brethren. Caring for the poor sick was but one part of St Leonard's charitable work. Alms (food and clothing) were to be distributed daily to thirty paupers at the hospital gates, whilst the brethren were also expected to supply provi-sions to prisoners in the city gaols and to lepers who were accom-modated in a number of other hospitals across the city.[29] It was an impressive operation, suitable in every way for so great a city.

The majority of hospitals can have played little role in the unfolding tragedy of the pestilence; nor should they have been expected to do so – for the function of most medieval hospitals was not the provision of a general facility for the diseased and dying. That so many hospital masters died during the years of the Great Death strongly suggests that these institutions remained open during this time and persisted in what their founders had intended them to do. This was certainly the case in Newcastle in 1349 when, while plague was either imminent or already present, Margery de Denome fled her home dressed only in a night-gown, desperate to escape her violent and adulterous husband. It was to the hospital of St Mary the Virgin that she ran for refuge.

The surest sign that hospitals, of whatever purpose, continued in their work, was that they escaped the telling censure of contemporaries. The same could not be said of doctors, who had opprobrium heaped upon them. In a description that sounds unerringly close to a commonplace, Chaucer tells how his 'Doctour' was very careful in what he spent, saving all that he made in times of pestilence. The implication was clear: doctors profited from the desperation of sick people in times of plague. Some, it has to be said, were more scrupulous: John Arderne would later state that hopeless cases, like plague victims, should not be accepted, lest the doctor lose his reputation, or worse be accused of poisoning. Boccaccio too seemed resigned to the futility of medicine, although he does nothing to impugn the motives or efforts of exasperated Florentine doctors:

> Against these maladies, it seemed that all the advice of physicians and all the power of medicine were profitless and unavailing. Perhaps the nature of the illness was such that it allowed no remedy; or perhaps those people who were treating the illness (whose numbers had increased enormously because the ranks of the qualified were invaded by people, both men and women, who had never received any training in medicine), being ignorant of its causes, were not prescribing the appropriate cure.[30]

If anything, the abject failure of doctors, both famed and unknown, served to confirm the widely held conviction that their skills were limited. Incapable of healing others, no doubt many – like Ralph Swanton – followed their patients to an early grave. The greatest among them may well have been a victim too, for John Gaddesden was dead by the middle of 1349.[31] Those who heard the news no doubt wryly recalled the Hebrew proverb repeated by Christ: 'Physician, heal thyself!'[32]

John Arderne was to learn the limit of his abilities early on. He had been in practice in Newark, Nottinghamshire, for only a couple of years when the Great Death arrived, in mid-spring 1349. The town was on a junction, between one of England's most heavily used roads and one of its busiest rivers. The main road from London to the North passed through, following the route, more or less, of today's A1. The town was distinguished by its great castle, the property of the bishop of Lincoln (even though the town was actually in the archdiocese of York), which watched over the slow-flowing Trent. This great river, with the Thames, Severn and Ouse, was one of the most important of England's inland waterways. Here goods were unloaded from wagons arriving from the south, placed on barges and transported north. Once the cargo was afloat, a journey north from Newark to York, via the Trent, Humber and Ouse, was several times more rapid (and in winter less vulnerable to poor weather) than if the trip had been attempted by road. Thus Newark was among the first places to be infected in the plague's relentless journey north, finding victims some time before villages in Warwickshire and Leicestershire, to the south, had received the disease from Coventry and Leicester. The situation was so bad that by the end of April the small churchyard was close to filling up. If nothing were done quickly, there would be no consecrated soil in which to bury the dead, to the immortal peril of their souls. So the vicar of Newark seized the initiative, found a suitable plot and wrote immediately to the bishop asking him to license it for burial. The petition found archbishop Zouche at his country palace of Cawood. His reply, sent out on 15th May, was to the point but did not spare on bureaucratic form:

> The care of the pastoral office pressing on us, urges and leads us to give, with God's help, all possible support to the just desires of our subjects, particularly when they concern the health of souls. A peti-

tion put before us on your behalf has shown that the mortality of plague which has been afflicting various parts of the world began to attack the townspeople of Newark some time ago, and has carried off numerous residents and inhabitants of the town, and is daily gaining in strength there, with the result that the burial ground of the church, because it is small and has no room to expand, is not adequate for the burial of the dead. With all this in mind, you have purchased, at your own expense, a certain plot or piece of land, which is walled and lies in the street called Apiltongate in Newark aforesaid, between the tenements of Peter Swafield on one side and Marin Sadler on the other. With the approval of all those who have an interest in the matter you have petitioned that we should deign to grant a licence and give our authority for the burial of the bodies of the dead there.[33]

Thus Newark got its new cemetery. Sadly, this town was not the first nor the only place to encounter such problems.

On 31st May, the townsmen of Newark, Arderne most probably among them, saw a small procession of horses enter their town and head for the castle. It was not an uncommon sight: the bishop of Lincoln, John Gynewell, had come to stay. With him was a small staff – the archdeacon perhaps, a rural dean, his chaplain, a few clerks and a registrar. This new bishop had been busy, for he was still conducting the visitation of his vast diocese, a journey that he had embarked upon more than eighteen months before. It was now almost a year since he had issued his proclamation ordering processions and prayers in anticipation of the pestilence, a plague that had now arrived and had just touched his own see.[34] One month earlier, he had had to write to the vicar of Melton Mowbray in Leicestershire, to demand that the fee be paid for the consecration of the new churchyard there.[35] Some parishioners had refused to pay, no doubt objecting because of the extraordinary circumstances of their original request. Five days later, on Monday, 4th May, Gynewell had made the short journey from his manor at Lyddington in Rutland to the little village of Great Easton in Leicestershire, where the parishioners had requested that they be permitted to bury their dead in the grounds of the chapel there, as that of Bringhurst – a mile away – had little space left. The plague was again the reason, yet the bishop was not afraid to do what needed to be done. Having got the approval of Peterborough Abbey, the parish patron, he had gone personally to the chapel and dedicated a temporary burial ground there, stating that it could be used for as long as 'there increases among you, as in other places in our diocese, a mortality of men such as has not been seen or heard aforetime from the beginning of the world, so that the old graveyard of your church is not sufficient to receive the bodies of the dead.'[36] On returning to his manor house, the bishop had determined that further action was required. So he sent out instructions to his rural deans in south Lincolnshire, enquiring into the number of parishes that had no priest and the speed with which wills were being proved by church officials, in preparation for his imminent visit. This was little notice for the hard-pressed clerics, as Gynewell had soon set off for Lincolnshire, where he undertook a five-day tour. Then he made for Peterborough, where half the monks died during the pestilence, before heading towards St Ives in Huntingdonshire – the easternmost part of his diocese, which neighboured Thomas Lisle's see of Ely. There he rested, but only for only two days, as he had returned to south Lincolnshire by 21st May, where he stayed for a week, all the while travelling, checking, visiting and ensuring that the church was performing as it should – in parish, monastery and administration. When this was done the bishop went west, stopping off in disease-stripped Leicester for only as long as he needed, before making fast for his castle at Newark on 31st May, Whit Sunday. He had been on the road for half the month, travelling over 210 miles as the crow flies, a figure that must have been at least half as great again when one takes account of the twists, turns and deviations that the country tracks forced him to make. He had not avoided the plague but neither had he confronted it. The bishop had simply continued his energetic and assiduous visitation, all the while making sure that he dealt with the problems created by the pestilence as he went on. It was a remarkable, even heroic, example – one that must have given inspiration not just to his priests but to the many in his flock that saw him as he rode through their plague-ridden towns and villages.

John Gynewell's work was far from done. He stayed at Newark for just a week, time in part employed arranging for new priests to fill the shoes of those rectors who had caught the disease, died or resigned in anticipation of death.[37] In the year from 25th March 1349 the bishop made over a thousand appointments of this kind, which meant that at least half the parishes in his diocese had their priest replaced during the plague year.[38] Then, on 6th June, keen to get on with his visitation, the bishop set off once again, heading into south Lincolnshire, just as he had warned his local officials. He arrived at Grantham in the afternoon, where he intended to stay the night. Grantham was but ten miles from the edge of the Lincolnshire Fens, a large band of marsh that ran almost to the sea. The wind had been howling all day, blowing off the North Sea, unchecked by the reeds and shaking the roofs of the buildings inland. Then it began to rain. By the time the sun started to set, the inundation was so great that the streets of Grantham ran like streams. It was a noisy and uncomfortable night. For the monks and nuns of Sempringham, who lived just at the point where the land disappeared into the Fen, it must have been terrifying.[39] The storm coincided with a high tide out at sea, forcing seawater up the River Welland, behind the ancient silt banks that separated the Fenland from the sea. The ensuing flood was unforgiving: it rose as high as the capitals that topped the pillars in the cloister next to the church, submerging the priory six feet deep in muddy saltwater. Many books in the library – the prize assets of any monastery – were destroyed, and eighteen sacks of wool with them. Floods like these came only once or twice every century; it was the poor luck of the Sempringham brethren to be hit just as they had to contend with the plague. Yet, despite the flooding, Gynewell continued with his tour: two days later he was at Hougham, five miles due north, where he consecrated a further fourteen new incumbents, who had come to seek his blessing from all over this huge diocese; the next day he was in the tiny village of Stragglethorpe, but five miles north of Hougham, east of Newark on the flat low land between the tributary fingers of the river Brant. Here too the villagers had had difficulties burying their dead, which the recent storms had only served to exacerbate. On arriving in the village, the bishop saw the problem for himself and heard the petitions of the rector and leading villagers:

> In our personal visitation of the archdeaconry of Lincoln, humble
> supplication was made to us on the part of the parishioners of the
> chapel of Stragglethorpe ... that on account of the deep floods of
> waters which have taken place during this pestilence and in other years
> as well, the bodies of the dead of the aforesaid hamlet have oftentimes
> for three days and more been unable to be borne to the mother church
> of Beckingham [three miles away], and so long have rested above earth
> unburied to the infection of the living.[40]

Gynewell ordered that the villagers should have a churchyard of
their own. The next day he was off again, making for Lincoln to
the north, leaving the soothed villagers of Stragglethorpe behind.
Only a few years before, the rector,[41] like Edmund Gonville, had
paid for new aisles to be added to his parish church at Beckingham,
to relieve the increasing press of people in the decades before the
Great Death. These new aisles, like those at Thelnetham, would not
now be required, for everywhere the population had been cut in
half. Yet why did the disease not kill everyone? Somehow, in each
place that it possessed, pestilence came to an end, usually leaving a
remnant of the former community to carry on in its wake. Some
just seemed to be resistant to this most infectious of epidemics. John
Gynewell was surely among them, despite his daily ministrations in
the midst of the disease. Indeed, it almost seemed as if a miracle
had been reserved for this pious man, whose outstanding example
must have brought comfort to the terrified and troubled people of
his Lincoln see.[42]

Catastrophes create the conditions in which great acts of heroism
can take place; they also bring close the anarchy that permits baser
enterprise. Back in Lessingham, one lady – Alice Wakeman – inherited a plot of land from a recently deceased relative. No doubt grief-
stricken, Alice was glad to be offered help by Henry Anneys, who
said that he could help her avoid the payment of a heriot, if only
she were to give him a cow. Alice agreed to the offer but, unbeknownst to her, she had been sold a pup, as no heriot was payable
on the land in any event. Even if she did not know the terms of her
ownership, her fellow villagers did, and they were quick to point out
the trick to the steward at the next manorial court. Henry was

ordered to return the cow and was given a heavy fine. Next up at the same court were a husband and wife, who had cleared an acre and a half of someone else's oats. Doubtless the crop was growing adjacent to their land; doubtless too they knew that its owner was dead. On the other side of Norwich at Bunwell, meanwhile, William Sigge had stolen so much, including pots, pans and even the lead from one dead man's roof, that the court clerk did not bother to list all the items.

It would be wrong to claim that these thefts were much out of the ordinary, as crime had been rife before the pestilence and would continue to be so afterwards; yet it is likely that the epidemic at least sharpened the many possible motives to steal: the confusion made detection even less likely and the mass mortality allowed people to discount the consequences of getting caught. For some, pestilence provided good cover, or at least a further excuse, to right an unforgotten injustice or repay some ancient vendetta. Thomas Walsingham claimed that the villagers of Barnet exploited the situation by tampering with the manor rolls. One can detect a similar motivation in the case of two Welshmen of Ruthin – Madoc and Kenwric ap Ririd – who on one pestilential night crept into the house of Aylmar (an Englishman) and took his basin, pitcher and some old iron. In Rhiw, up the road, they took six head of cattle from John Parker (also an Englishman). How they must have congratulated themselves afterwards, Madoc and his brother Kenwric, at getting one up on their oppressor neighbours – that is, until they were caught. Yet the mainspring of crime was, as ever, poverty, which led some people to do extraordinary things. Gilbert Henry, from Tibenham, in south Norfolk, had gone to the house of John Smith, who had recently died, intending to steal some malt and barley. He left, however, with more than he had come to take, for on finding Smith's corpse prostate on the bed, he helped himself to the coat and waistcoat as well, stripping them off the decaying body. Careless about infection, Gilbert was careless too about evasion, as he was promptly caught and ordered to pay the value of the clothes he had taken.[viii] A less shocking crime in the fourteenth century, perhaps, it was also probably quite common: in nearby Bunwell a woman was charged with precisely the same offence.

[viii] 6d. each, or £0.05 in total.

If robbing the dead was as frequent as these two adjacent crimes suggest, then there must have been a widespread disregard for the risks of getting so close to a plague corpse, risks which from Italy to Ireland were already well-known. It was perhaps a measure of the indigence of these thieves that they were prepared to ignore what all common sense told them they should not do.

It was not only desperate peasants who made use of plague: there were opportunists in far more prosperous circles too, as one extra-ordinary case in London demonstrated well. Although the precise details are uncertain, all the ingredients of a great fraud were there. The target was no less than the capital's royal mint, located in the most secure building in the country – the Tower of London. One of those implicated was Adam Walpol, a former warden of the Gold-smith's Company, whose family's status can easily be gauged by the fact that his brother John had owned a tenement neighbouring Sir John Pulteney's mansion of Coldharbour. Shortly after Walpol's death, in the summer of 1349, an extremely suspect arrangement with the Master of the King's Mint began to unravel. It transpired that the Master owed a considerable sum to the Exchequer, a debt in which Adam Walpol had become entangled and consequently (it was alleged) he had benefited from the money left owing to the king.[43] It seems that a serious lapse in oversight had occurred, opening up the oppor-tunity for a swindle, something to which the confusion and mortality that resulted from plague must have contributed.[44] As soon as the Exchequer uncovered what had happened, they seized property from Adam's executors and rented them out in an effort to recover their costs.[45] Luckily for the Master of the Mint and his estimable accom-plice, neither was alive to answer for what had happened, and so the crown recording clerks treated the whole episode with the grace that its late perpetrators were thought to deserve. It seems likely, nonethe-less, that Adam Walpol of London was as guilty of making base use of the pestilence as was Gilbert Henry of Tibenham – both charged, in their different ways, with seeking to profit from the torrid circum-stances of plague.

*   *   *

Thanne I schel flutte[ix]
From bedde to flore,
From flore to here,
From here to bere,
From bere to putte,
At te putt fordut.[46]

The medieval funeral rite, so simply described by an anonymous thirteenth-century poet, is the recognizable ancestor of modern Western custom. Our inherited ceremony, however, has become a vessel, emptied of the religious and social significance with which it was once filled. There was nothing contrived about the medieval ritual. The urgency with which communities sought out a bishop to consecrate new burial ground during the Great Death attested to the fact that, no matter what horrors they faced, the correct interment of the deceased was of immediate and real importance to those that were left behind. Not that there was anything odd in this – the obsequies given to the dead are one of the defining communal acts of the living, no more or less for the men and women of fourteenth-century England. Medieval people shared much of their lives within the embrace of their community: in the manor court, in the fields at harvest, in leisure, and – most frequently and importantly – in the festivals of the church. The majority of these, such as feast days and the Sunday Mass, were regular, creating rhythm within the year. Others, funerals among them, marked key moments within the life of an individual and their family, in turn involving the wider groups to which they belonged. In a village, where work and life were shared by one and the same people, the funeral would involve most of the population. In this sacral ceremony was found much that was descriptive of medieval society, of its profound sense of community and of its all-encompassing faith.

A corpse's journey from deathbed to grave offered the living a last chance to attain salvation for their dead. The body was traditionally prepared and clothed in a shroud by women: a symmetrical act to swaddling the newly born and a conscious imitation of the actions

---

[ix] Then I shall pass from bed to floor, from floor to shroud, from shroud to bier, from bier to grave, and the grave will be closed up.

of Mary and Mary Magdalene following the removal of Jesus' body from the Cross. The body had finished the trial of mortality; it was now to be made ready for the tomb, in expectation of rebirth into eternal life. The wealthy sought dignity in a coffin, hired or purchased for the event. Increasingly, they also requested the Office of the Dead, a litany originally sung by monks on the death of a brother but a privilege now extended to priests and those laymen who could afford the additional cost. The ritual was heavy with significance. The night before burial, flanked by torchbearers, the body was taken to the church on a bier. Then it passed through the church door and was borne down the dark and empty nave. Beyond, light escaped from the chancel, separated from the nave by the roodscreen. The deceased was then carried across this threshold, under the Passion statuary of the rood. This entrance to the most holy sanctum was a journey denied to the layman during his life. The corpse was laid at the sanctuary steps, before the stone altar. Candles were all around, principal among them the lamp before the pyx which contained the consecrated Host.

Surrounded by clergy, the Office began. The prayers consisted of elements taken from the liturgical 'hours' of Vespers, Matins and Lauds which, in the ordinary Office, constituted the daily liturgical routine of priests and monks alike. Vespers was the final service held in daylight, a conclusion to the day's labour, a remembrance of God's own works during the six days of the Creation and a meditation on His Incarnation. Matins, correctly observed, was sung in the middle of the night; thus it was largely left to monks to rise in the small hours and pray in dirge-like monotone for the world, while the world itself was still asleep. Then, as the sun began to rise, Lauds would be sung, in joyous Gregorian chant, to proclaim the new day. The Office for the Dead was a contracted version of these 'hours', encapsulating in sequence a life's work just completed, the long night now embarked upon, and the promise held out to every Christian of the new dawn of salvation.[47] Redemption was still not assured, however, so the final oration – Psalm 129[48] – was supplicatory:

> Out of the depths I cry to you, O Lord;
> O Lord, hear my voice. Let your ears be attentive to my cry for mercy.
> If you, O Lord, kept a record of sins, O Lord, who could stand?

But with you there is forgiveness; therefore you are feared.
I wait for the Lord, my soul waits, and in his word I put my hope.
My soul waits for the Lord more than watchmen wait for the morning,
more than watchmen wait for the morning.[49]

The Office of the Dead complete, the corpse was left overnight in the church, in final vigil before going to the grave.

The requiem Mass took place the next day, a communal rite of departure extended to every Christian after death. It was an extravagant scene. The church was packed full of people, for even had there been no material incentive to attend (which, indeed, there often was) there was a strong spiritual and social obligation to go. The bier was placed in front of the roodscreen, between the Paschal candle – lit once at baptism and now lit again in death – and the Passion scene above. Acolytes stood around holding long tapers (the richer the deceased, the greater the illuminations). Prayers were said, hymns sung. The liturgy was based on the ordinary Mass but with additional text inserted, some of which, like the *Dies Iræ*, were amongst the most powerful and beautiful in medieval literature.

The service finished, the body was carried out of the church to the graveside, followed in procession by the clergy and congregation: it was the deceased's last procession – that familiar response of a community in time of distress – a final reprise of the many processions that studded the ecclesiastical year. By the graveside the corpse was once again sprinkled with holy water. It was normal to be buried in the same church where baptism had taken place and a Christian life begun; this last blessing sanctified the completion of that life. Indeed, the ground itself had once been consecrated – blessed, as by Bishop Gynewell in the new graveyard at Stragglethorpe, with a prayer and a sprinkling of holy water. Thus was every new Christian cemetery sanctified – prepared for the reception of the baptized and communicate dead. In this place they would wait, silent, until summoned by the Seven Trumpets that heralded the Apocalypse – the end-time – which would conclude with God's Last Judgement.[50] So the corpse was now lowered face up, with the head facing west and the feet to the east, in order that on that final day, at the trumpet blast, the corpse would rise out of the ground – resurrected in body, just as Christ – facing the New Jerusalem. For the while, however, the body was returned

from whence humanity had originally come: the dust from which
Adam had been formed.

The funerary rites of the rich were more elaborate – there were
more candles, more masses, a choir and more clergy. There might
even be a more luxurious shroud: Thomas Lisle's sister-in-law, who
died in the plague year, rested in peace ensconced by no fewer than
eleven sheep pelts. These were superfluities, however, as the essen-
tials of the medieval funeral ritual were shared between rich and poor,
townsman and villager, noble and peasant. For every baptized and
communicating Christian should be given a Christian burial. In its
several parts this ceremony spoke of the homogeneity of medieval
Christian observance, its structured theology, the alloy of direct assertion and highly developed metaphor. The medieval Christian message,
in its intellectual coherence, its atavistic appeal, its emotional power
and – of course – its monopoly on belief, was both distilled and
exemplified in this liturgy of death, this final ritual of life.

May was a month of maintenance and merriment. Out in the fields,
the ploughing had been done and the sowing completed. Buildings
were repaired, hedges trimmed, ditches cleared and re-cut. Yet the
burden of work was light and there were hours to spare. Villagers
could enjoy this rare opportunity for leisure, a time for relaxation
before summer's hard labours began in earnest, midway through June.
Unsurprisingly, more censorious clergymen – who preached the value
of graft and the perils of idleness – regarded this prized month of
May with considerable suspicion. Now the restraining rigours of Lent
were undone, the sun had begun to shine, and women and men had
a moment to live at ease. Their disapproval only served to heighten
May's bucolic romance. For Chaucer, this was the only time of the
year when he could be tempted away from study and prayer, 'whan
that the month of May / Is comen, and that I here the foules synge,
/ And that the floures gynnen for to sprynge, / Farewel my bok and
my devocioun!'[51]

How different was this miserable month of May 1349. From the
Midlands to the south coast, the most easterly point of East Anglia
to the lowlands of south Wales, daily processions bore the dead from
home to church, church to graveyard, graveyard to graveside and graveside to burial. Now the time for merry-making was filled with grieving,

maintenance put off whilst relatives were cared for and friends interred. The burial of so many people was in itself a considerable challenge: many chroniclers repeat the line that there were hardly enough people living to bury the dead.[52] This was a well-worn turn of phrase, however – one that had been pressed into service in the description of many a crisis before the Great Death. Self-evidently the living – even if there were indeed 'hardly enough' – did not fail to honour their obligations to the dead. The numerous petitions for new churchyards and extensions to existing cemeteries, the riots that erupted around burial grounds, the complete absence of accounts of the dead being left to rot in their beds: all of these facts point to the continuation of the traditional customs of burial. Nonetheless, it must have been true that fear caused a partial deviation from normal family and community behaviour. Geoffrey le Baker and John Clyn told how many people refrained from visiting and caring for the sick. Yet, even admitting those instances of people benefiting from the deaths of those around them, there is nothing in the English accounts that suggests the heartless panic that Boccaccio described in Florence, where 'brothers abandoned brothers, uncles their nephews, sisters their brothers, and in many cases wives deserted their husbands, . . . even worse, and almost incredible, was the fact that fathers and mothers refused to nurse and assist their own children, as though they did not belong to them'. Deserted in death as in life, Florentines went to the grave without the 'funeral pomp of candles and dirges' and were lucky to have 'anyone at all to witness their going'.[53] Some of this must also have been true of English funerals too. The circumstances of mass urban burial, as seen at Smithfield and elsewhere, prevented an elaborate funeral. We can be sure, moreover, that some people – like the reluctant members of the Grocers' Guild in London – made their excuses and failed to turn up.[54] Others, perhaps, must have found the grief so overwhelming, the loss so great, that they simply lost the will to mourn. Yet in the absence of statements to the contrary, taken together with the evidence of the episcopal registers, it must be assumed that in general funerals continued and the graveside rituals were maintained. There would be the family that survived, the friends still living and the neighbours that had not yet been struck down. The reeve might be there or a town councillor; maybe fellow members of a local guild. By the time all these people had come together, they may well have consti-

tuted the larger part of the parish. Yet each procession told of a diminishing community, as with each funeral the turnout would be a little
smaller: one or two who had been there but a couple of days before,
following an earlier bier, were now confined to their beds, perhaps
already dead.

Doubtless the funerals themselves did much to propagate the
disease. With mourners stuffed into churches, walking in processions
in tight formation, there was no better environment in which the
pestilence might spread. A glancing remark by Thomas Burton, a monk
of Meaux Abbey in Yorkshire, points to this fact. 'God's providence',
he wrote, 'ensured that, in most places, chaplains survived unharmed
until the end of the pestilence in order to perform the exequies of
those who had died. But, after the funeral of the laymen, chaplains
were swallowed by death in great numbers, as others had been before.'[55]
The delay is easily explained, for the one person who was not amongst
the throng was the priest, separated as he was from the congregation
by the roodscreen that divided the nave (where the people stood)
from the chancel (where the funeral rite took place). Absent from the
contagious crush in the body of the church and reluctant as many
were to hear confessions,[56] a number of priests probably did escape
the initial surge of the disease, only to succumb later through some
unlucky encounter.[57] Yet nothing was learnt from this, for whilst there
was a widespread recognition that close contact with infected people
was dangerous, the peril posed by public gatherings was almost entirely
missed.[58] Besides, in the case of funerals, there was a good incentive
for a mourner to attend. At the conclusion of each burial it was the
custom to hand out gifts of food or money to those who had attended,
small bequests designed in part to ensure a good turnout at the end.
These 'doles' would normally constitute little more than a day's worth
of grain or a small memento mori; however, in these times of mass
mortality, of daily and twice-daily funerals and burial processions,
some could make half a living just from attending the exequies of the
dead. We may doubt that anyone recognized the risk in mixing with
so many seemingly healthy people; even if they had, the return was
clear to see – a free lunch or a gift of money that removed the need
for work that day. Some, unsurprisingly, viewed this semi-professional
mourning with dismay. William Dene claimed that 'because of the
doles handed out at funerals, those who had once had to work now

began to have time for idleness, thieving and other outrages'.[59] For this disapproving monk, it was as if the Great Death had permitted survivors to take one long, abominable holiday, or even worse.

Such moral indignation reflected a broader concern among the landowning classes. Although medieval people did not possess a modern concept of 'the economy', they had a clear understanding of the relationship between supply and demand, forces that applied both to prices and to the cost of labour. By these middle months of 1349, prices had already begun to fall: heriot-livestock crowded markets whilst grain stored since the harvest of 1348, originally intended for six million Englishmen, now had a market of several million fewer consumers. Tumbling prices were just one of several anxieties that beset landowners at this time – the effect of so many doles, and that wage-earners, in their reduced numbers, would make mischief out of the growing mismatch of demand for labour and its ever-diminishing supply. The trend in itself was not new: wages had been drifting upwards since the Great Famine. Before 1315–18 a carpenter, for example, could expect to earn 2½–2¾d. per day, but by 1347 his wage might be around 3d. per day, an increase of as much as 20 per cent. Nor was there anything new in peasants attempting to control wages: in 1324 the villagers of Standon in Hertfordshire had tried to limit itin-erant labour coming into the village in an attempt to enforce the 'closed shop' of local labour.[60] But these incremental movements in wages were slow and inter-generational; now it was feared that come the harvest season, in a few months' time, labourers would attempt to negotiate significantly higher rates of pay. This had already happened in some of the towns that the plague had passed through and it is probable that the mayor's council in London, which had issued local ordinances in January controlling the hire and payment of glovers' workers,[61] was vocal in its demands that something be done.

Despite this, there is little evidence that such an increase, during May and June, was underway in the countryside. At Farnham in Surrey, where the reeve, John Runwick, ran such a tight operation, grinding and winnowing the corn from the previous harvest cost the same as in previous years, as did the weeding and mowing of the fields that was already taking place in these first weeks of summer. To be sure, there will have been instances where tenants applied pressure, especially in those areas of the south-west and around London where the plague had started to burn itself out. Much of the country was still aflame with pestilence, however, and it seems unlikely that, given all the other things with which people had to contend, there was anything like a widespread demand for higher pay in these first six months of 1349.[62]

Nonetheless, the prospect of truculent peasant-labourers – bellies full with funeral doles, enjoying a life of indolence and vice, extorting exorbitant wages from helpless landowners – was for many lords too much to countenance. The very existence of feudal society, however fractured and contorted by the free market, relied upon the economic suzerainty of landlords and the maintenance of their feudal authority. For this conservative elite, whose wealth flowed from inherited power, such a challenge, however minor, threatened not only their incomes but their position in society too. The Rochester monk's exaggerated reports are evidence enough of these fears: 'thus the poor and servile have been enriched and the rich impoverished.'[63] The king, as the chief landowner, was under increasing pressure to act; by the end of May he was in a position to attempt a solution. Although it was only a couple of weeks since pestilence had shut the courts down, word had it that plague was finally leaving London.[64] Edward needed little encouragement to return: the Great Death was now raging across southern and central England, laying waste the counties where the royal family had hitherto found refuge. Now it looked as if London might be the safer place to be. So Edward made his way back over the Whit Sunday weekend.[65] He did not find Westminster as he had known it. The stench of death still lingered in the emptied streets. In the great hall there was none of the usual chatter – the many lawyers who, in any normal year, would have been preparing for the start of the Trinity term, were now nowhere to be seen. It was a desolate scene, yet one that was soon to be filled with renewed activity. The king was acutely conscious of how much needed to be done. The pestilence had detained him long enough: now it was time to take up the reins of government once again.

Edward called a meeting of the royal council for the middle of June. Before business could start, however, he had to appoint a new chancellor, a post now open because of Ufford's death. (The importance that Edward attached to the post was amply demonstrated by his command to the Chancery clerks not to issue any important documents during the current vacancy without his knowledge.) On 16th June, Edward appointed the bishop of St David's, John Thoresby, who had accompanied Edward as Keeper of the Privy Seal (his private secretary) during the most recent French campaign.[66] Now the full council – Edward, Thoresby, Edington, the chief justices and assorted nobles – could convene. There was much to discuss, not least the faltering truce with the French. On this little could be done, as Edward was awaiting a report from Bateman, at this point still making his way from France, via his East Anglian diocese. So the king and his councillors turned their attention to the pressing matter of prices and peasant wages. No doubt some felt that the king should seek to control prices, putting an artificial floor below which nothing could be sold. There was a good precedent for price controls, albeit against inflationary price-fixing – as civic authorities had for a long time sought to prevent prices in bread and other goods rising above a set rate.[67] But such a move would not address the root concern of the nobility, which was the feared shift in the balance of power from landowners to landworkers. So someone (it would be reasonable to assume that it was the treasurer, Edington) proposed a statutory ceiling on wages, to ensure that by the time harvest arrived landowners had a legal weapon to head off the wage demands that were now widely expected. Opinion fell to the latter option. It was, in the first instance, easier to control wages than prices, as wages – although influenced by external conditions – were ultimately set by landowners, whereas prices were made within the market. Besides, low prices had their own benefits, both for the rich and for the poor. Most importantly, wage controls with the force of law gave manorial lords the ability to enforce their will, even when the labour market was not in their favour.

Thus, on 18th June 1349, a proclamation was sent throughout England which sought to suppress wage inflation, both by expanding the supply of available labour and by stipulating maximum rates of pay. Subsequently named the Ordinance of Labourers, this was the first piece of national wage legislation that an English government had ever introduced. The preamble noted that the king had made his decision having 'discussed and considered the matter with our prelates and nobles and other learned men', 'mindful of the serious inconvenience *likely* to arise from this shortage [of workers], especially of agricultural labourers'. The ordinance was comprehensive. Every able man and woman under the age of sixty not already in employment was compelled to work, should work be offered them. When employed, wage-earners were not to be paid more than they had been prior to 1346 or, with studied vagueness, 'some other appropriate year five or six years ago'.[68] Employees should serve out their full terms of service, although lords were not compelled to pay them any more than the new wage rates even if their pay had been negotiated prior to the proclamation. Whilst the ordinance was aimed principally at wage-labourers, it also sought to control the demand side of the wage market as well: the lords themselves. It decreed that whilst lords should have first claim on their existing tenants, they were not – in a nod to the tightness of the labour market – to retain more than they needed. Any lord found to be paying more than the stated rates was to be prosecuted, just as the peasant was to be imprisoned for accepting improved wages. It seems that the townsmen had made complaints to the council, too, for the ordinance also covered urban tradesmen and the prices at which they sold products, thereby nationalizing the municipal controls that had been in place for many years across the country. Finally, in a further novel instruction, able-bodied beggars were ordered to stop taking alms and look for work, rather than 'spending their time in idleness and depravity . . . robberies and other crimes'.[69] In all, it was a radical but carefully formulated mandate, one that evinced an impressive and – for the age – precocious under-standing of basic economics (without a doubt, it had the fingerprints of William Edington all over it).[70] For the first time the apparatus of the state, on behalf of landowners, had been deployed in an attempt to compel people to work and to work at a national rate. It was a bold move, for the king and his ministers were doing no less than pitting royal authority against the invisible forces of the market. By the sanctions the ordinance imposed, it is clear that the king and his ministers already anticipated that the conflict would cause dissent.

Despatched in tandem with the ordinance was an instruction to the bishops, directing them to issue a similar mandate to the stipendiary clergy who, like vicars and chantry chaplains, worked for a wage. Bishop Hamo Hethe of Rochester was among the addressees and within a few days had dutifully sent out an order throughout his small diocese.[71] He started by explaining that the king had been forced to act, as those who refused work and demanded extortionate wages were causing 'great detriment of the state'. It was an argument the bishop was happy to extend to his own clergy. He had, he explained, a responsibility to exercise his ministry 'for the public weal' and in so far as greedy clergy hindered this, he would act. So henceforth, stipendiary clergy should work only for 'an appropriate salary'.[72] It was a powerful notice of intent: no matter what the circumstances, the episcopacy was determined to ensure that the clergy performed as they should. Despite the tribulations caused by plague and the temptation grasped by those unable to resist – whether they be Lisle's administrators or their more lowly stipendiary brethren – the hierarchy was, in the main, determined that right should be done. There was a degree of self-interest for the church in all this, as they like laymen had to contribute to the cost of wage-earning clerics. Yet Hethe's words show that the desire to curb the opportunism of the stipendiary clergy had solid pastoral ends too. It was a noble motivation, one that the magnates, eager to protect both their position and their wealth, certainly lacked.

IO

Northern March

June–October 1349

John Ufford's death left a vacancy not only in the chancellor's office but also at Canterbury, where the old man had been archbishop. It fell to the monks of Christchurch Priory there to find a successor, as it was their ancient right to choose the Primate of All England, the highest position in the English church.

The Canterbury monks had survived the pestilence almost unscathed by submitting themselves through the spring to self-imposed isolation. Now, only weeks after they had tentatively reopened the priory doors, they were besieged once again, not by epidemic disease but by a plague of visitors and messengers from London: officials and clerics all wishing to know their intentions and influence their decision. After a fortnight, they were ready to proceed to election. At close to nine o'clock on Thursday, 4th June,[1] the prior and monks filed from the cathedral quire, where they had just celebrated their morning Mass. Descending the great steps that led down to the nave, the monks turned towards the north transept, past the spot where Thomas Becket had been martyred, hacked to death for his defiance of the king.[2] Now they crossed the same floor that had been washed with the archbishop's blood, nearly 180 years before. It was a timely reminder – as they left the cathedral through a side door – of the importance of the decision that it was now their responsibility to take. Crossing the corner of the cloister, the prior followed his monks into the chapter house, whose echoes returned the sound of their shuffled entrance. This large hall, oblong and austere,[3] was amply filled by the convent, which still numbered more than seventy, every one of them a survivor from the Great Death. It had been less than a year since the monks had gone through this exact process; now they prayed, deliberated and voted all over again. The king had no doubt already indicated that this time around he would be prepared to accept Bradwardine, so it was little surprise that the prior and monks of Christchurch settled once again on the famous Mertonian scholar to sit in what had once been Becket's chair.[4]

Back in the autumn of 1348 – what must now have seemed an age away – it was Ufford who had been preferred by the king: given the trouble caused previously by Stratford, Edward wanted someone utterly dependable as archbishop and in Ufford – pliant, loyal, unremarkable – this is exactly what he had got. Now, however, Bradwardine's obvious qualities – his intellectual brilliance, devotion and rude health – seemed all the more appropriate to the circumstances and, therefore, desirable. That the new appointee wished to make straight for Avignon to receive the pope's consecration (a journey never attempted by John Ufford during his ten months in office) showed that he was not reluctant to take on the prelacy; indeed, he may even have lobbied for it himself. He decided to wait a few days before leaving, however, as by a happy coincidence an old friend had just arrived in the capital, one who planned to make the same journey himself.

The acquaintance was none other than Richard FitzRalph, archbishop of Armagh, who in March had denounced the Anglo-Irish colonists in Drogheda. It was in defence of his title that Richard FitzRalph had come to London. After his humiliating ejection from Dublin by crown officials a couple of months earlier, he had resolved to take his claim to the primacy of Ireland direct to Avignon, where he knew his arguments would be well-received, not least because Alexander Bicknor, the archbishop of Dublin, had fallen out with the papacy many years before when, amongst other transgressions, he had failed to repay papal loans. FitzRalph had a cynical motive too: as Bicknor was in no position to defend himself (for he was both very sick and – at eighty or more – very old), he recognized that now was his best chance of settling the dispute on his own terms and so had made straight for London in order to obtain the king's licence to travel abroad.

Although the king had little fondness for Bicknor, who had had a long-running wrangle with the Exchequer, Edward was not keen to allow FitzRalph a protracted absence abroad: the archbishop served an important role in Ireland and to lose him to vain lobbying in the papal court might do further damage to the colony.[5] However, he might do something useful on behalf of Edward while in Avignon. The king had lately been mulling over the problems posed by the pope's general indulgence, which promised the full remission of sins to every truly penitent man and woman who made the pilgrimage to Rome during the Jubilee year of 1350. With France in dangerous abeyance, the Scots restive without their king and the Gaelic-Irish as troublesome as ever, he did not want his dominions, already depleted through pestilence, to be further disabled by an exodus of pilgrims – in particular the noble warriors and city merchants on whom he depended – to the Eternal City. Moreover, he knew full well that many in the French nobility would wish to make the pilgrimage, leaving his great enemy all the more exposed to attack. So Edward ordered FitzRalph to put this petition to the pope: seeing that the Great Death had made the Jubilee indulgence all the more important, yet at the same time pestilence made the journey to Rome all the more hazardous, the pope should grant the Jubilee indulgence to the English without enforcing the corresponding obligation to go to Rome.

Thus was FitzRalph despatched, only a couple of days after Bradwardine had been made archbishop-elect.[6] In all likelihood the two friends boarded ship together, bound for Avignon, the Provençal city that for forty years had been the capital of Western Christendom.

Within the first three weeks of June, Edward had overseen the election of a new archbishop of Canterbury, sent messages to Rome with FitzRalph, appointed a new chancellor, presided over a meeting of the council, authorized the Ordinance of Labourers, and received a debriefing from Bishop Bateman on his recent embassy to France.[7] This surge of activity was only made possible by the waning of the pestilence in and around London; further north, however, the disease was still waxing strong. Westminster was well-aware of the fact: John Vaux, the sheriff and escheator of Nottingham and Derbyshire had written to the Exchequer to explain that most of his officials were either ill or dead and it would be difficult, therefore, for him to present his annual accounts. It would become impossible, for Vaux himself was soon dead.

The disease had spread into the north Midlands counties from the south, first taking towns like Newark and Lichfield, where it had interrupted the works that William Ramsey had designed for the

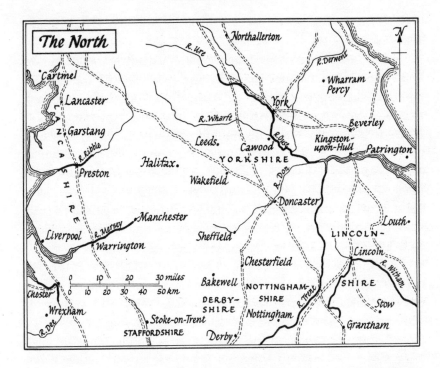

cathedral's east end. The Great Death was doing its work in Stafford-shire by late April, some time before it had emerged in neighbouring Shropshire and Derbyshire.[8] The Wakebridge family, knights and landowners of Derbyshire, had their manor house atop a hill just outside Crich, eleven miles north of Derby. In the church there was a record of the deaths in the family, to which no fewer than six additions were made in 1349. The head of the family, William Wakebridge, had already lost his brother, Nicholas, by the middle of May 1349;[9] later in June he also lost his sister-in-law and by the middle of August his father, his wife, two sisters and another brother as well. We must suspect that William was left to mourn alone. Clearly the epidemic was particularly virulent in these parts: at Pentrich, only a couple of miles from Crich, three priests left the vicarage feet-first, a sad succession that was over in just five weeks. Further north still, at Chesterfield, the Great Death claimed one of its few noble victims. For it was there on the night of 30th May that Thomas, Lord Wake of Liddel – cousin of the king and *châtelain* of Liddel Strength, the fortress stormed by the Scots on their rampage to Neville's Cross – died.[10] His body was placed on a wagon and taken to the Augustinian priory he had founded at Haltemprice, just outside Kingston-upon-Hull, in east Yorkshire.

Hull had so far been spared the plague. No doubt someone in Lord Wake's cortège would unwittingly bring the disease with them; if not, infection was sure to come from elsewhere soon, for the borough was midway between two old cities, where pestilence was raging with great force. Lincoln, across the Humber by ferry and thirty-five miles to the south, had been in the grip of the disease for several weeks, perhaps as early as Palm Sunday.[11] The toll was terrible: almost thirty years' worth of wills were proved in this single year of 1349. As in London (and so many manors)[12] some properties were passed on twice within the same day, such was the rate of mortality. The mayor had died (in addition to two of his predecessors), whilst almost every post in the cathedral administration had changed hands.[13] Yet Lincoln had been fighting a slump in business for some time, as traders had increasingly bypassed the city in favour of the flourishing Midlands towns. To this depression the epidemic added little but short-term chaos. Indeed, the very timing of the plague's arrival in Lincoln made plain its previous decline, for pestilence came to the city no earlier than to far humbler Newark, which was now the more popular transfer-point for travellers and traders heading for York and the North.

York: capital of the North since the Roman occupation and for 600 years the seat of England's second archbishop.[14] Both Norwich and Bristol now had larger populations but the great panorama of York's Roman walls, with its giant minster standing proud above the battlements, remained the more-impressive sight. The River Ouse pierced the surrounding wall, cutting the square city in two. At night, great chains were hauled up from the riverbed and secured between towers on either bank, thus maintaining the defensive line. The chains could not hold back the water, however – the rains had not seemed to cease since the middle of 1348 and by late autumn the boats that brought news of the plague's fatal progress further south sailed in on a swollen river. In November the archbishop had warned that the danger of plague, which he had first raised back in July, was now 'imminent' and that special masses – *pro mortalitate* – should be sung.[15] Although the city burghers could do nothing to contain the over-laden Ouse, against the plague they had at least one recourse: to shut the gates and raise the chains. Yet even if self-isolation *had* been imposed, it would not have lasted long, for on the last day of the year the Ouse finally burst over its banks and submerged the west side of the city. Any obstruction to the river – chains and all – would surely have been swept away. The city's cellars did not empty until Lent, two months later.

With or without the flood, the city would soon have had to open itself to the outside world, as like all other towns it could not survive long without trade. This basic urban instinct ensured that as the flood subsided and the riverine mud was shovelled away, a more deadly inundation would soon arrive. The boats moored at the quay-side came and went, from far and wide, some carrying wool via Hull and the Humber down the east coast and across the North Sea. (It was a trade that had made a fortune for several merchants, John Gold-beter – the some-time associate of the Chiriton company – among them.) Other vessels traded cargoes with the Midlands towns and counties, via the Trent. Either of these routes could have provided passage for the disease (although Newark's early infection suggests that the Trent might be the more likely). It is almost certain that the final leg of the journey was made along the Ouse, for when the pestilence eventually did arrive in York, at the end of May 1349, it did so without touching the countryside around.[16]

Archbishop Zouche needed no encouragement to heed the warnings given in his several plague letters: as soon as the pestilence was discovered in York, he fled his residence at Cawood for Ripon, a safe distance to the north-west.[17] There, on the very day the Ordinance of Labourers was issued in now plague-free London, he made out his will, stating 'that whilst death was certain for every human creature, the hour of death itself was uncertain'.[18] Back in York, the certainty of death could not have been more clear: the scale of mortality was as grievous as in the cities further south. In 1349, 208 new freemen were admitted to the town, whereas in the previous year only sixty had made the cut.[19] This fresh cohort represented over 50 different trades – including 8 skinners, 10 mariners, 12 mercers, 22 tailors and 33 shoemakers – all taking the place of established traders and craftsmen who had perished. Of 21 clergy for whom there are records, 17 did not see out the plague year. It is likely that the master of famous St Leonard's Hospital, John Giffard, was also a victim.[20] At last, by the final days of July, the short reign of pestilence in York came to an end.

The survivors seem not to have believed that the terror had gone, for when William Needler, a resident of Coppergate, died on Friday, 7th August, an inquest was called to ascertain whether his death was suspicious, and the coroner reported that William had died 'a natural and not a violent death by reason of the pestilence'.[21]

Brave as Zouche had been against the Scots, he was unwilling to face the plague, sending his suffragan, Hugh of Damascus, to do battle on his behalf.[22] In the neighbouring diocese of Lincoln, however, Bishop Gynewell continued to demonstrate true diligence in the care of his see. Having given the villagers of Stragglethorpe a new cemetery so that they could bury their dead, Gynewell kept up with his great visitation, embarking on a perambulation of Lincolnshire that saw him cover over 500 miles in less than two months.[23] By the middle of June, he was in the cathedral city, staying at his manor of Nettleham outside the city walls, well away from the mêlée of disease. He did not tarry long, however, for he was in Grimsby, in the north-eastern corner of his diocese, by the end of the month.[24]

Although Grimsby's haven was the natural first mooring for ships turning inland before Spurn Head, the port communicated not – as did Hull – with York, but with enfeebled Lincoln. Grimsby was in decline, therefore, its fortunes done further damage by the silt that choked the harbour. Consequently, the boats tied up to the quay were only small coastal fishing vessels, capable of no more than skimming for herring on the sandbanks just off the Humber mouth.[25] There was a flip-side to being cut-off from long-distance trade: there was as yet no sign of the awful evidence of the pestilence, even though York (to the north) and Lincoln (to the south) had been suffering for months.[26] Some unfortunate townsmen had already started the unwitting month-long journey to death, however, the disease having lately crept into the city with a traveller, unannounced; market day, on the third day of the bishop's visit, would ensure that the disease was further spread around.[27]

Even if it had not yet made itself known in Grimsby, only a little further south the epidemic was beginning to cover ground. Undeterred, Gynewell set off into its midst. After a short stay in the abbey at Louth, where the Great Death had just arrived, the bishop rode a great arc over Lincoln back to Newark; on one of the days he covered more than thirty miles – a demanding distance on horseback.[28] Despite the incredible mortality, he persisted in doing everything he could to soften the impact of the disease on his diocese. Every day he appointed priests to posts made vacant through death; on 14th July, whilst at Newark, no fewer than fifteen clerics were instituted to new benefices. The Great Death was throwing all that it could at John Gynewell yet he responded with vigour. When word came that Abbot Walter of Louth, who had received him a week before, had died but four days later, Gynewell turned on his heel and made once again for the abbey, in order to give the new abbot, Richard of Lincoln, his blessing.[29] Thus, in just eight days, Gynewell covered sixty or seventy miles: it was behaviour typical of a man obsessed. Well he might be, for Bishop Gynewell's simple piety informed him that this was not the moment to relax his ministry to his flock. As the Louth Abbey chronicler later declared, 'it was thought that so great a multitude of people were not killed in Noah's Flood',[30] a flood imposed by God, as the Book of Genesis describes it, to correct the 'wickedness of man'. Yet Noah had been saved because he was a 'just man'.[31] So this brave bishop, conscious of what was expected of him by both God and men, endeavoured to carry on. From his second stint in Louth, he made straight for Leicester, on the other side of his diocese, where he instituted a further thirty-eight priests; on Wednesday, 5th August, he returned to his manor of Lyddington in Rutland. It was three months since Gynewell had been here last.[32] In the interim he had ridden the best part of 900 miles, a punishing average of twenty-one miles for every day that he had been on the road.[33] On his way he had consecrated cemeteries and appointed hundreds of priests. More important still, he had provided hope, succour and support, both through his presence and through his actions, to a people laid low by plague.[34]

Around York and the East Riding of Yorkshire, the Great Death was now demonstrating its destructive force to the full. Hugh of Damascus commissioned a new churchyard at Beverley, a few miles north of Hull, on 26th June; it was certainly required, as was shown by the will of one of the citizens, which left property to a son but making provision lest the boy die too.[35] The prior of Haltemprice, in whose church Lord Wake had – only a couple of months before – been buried, was another casualty;[36] on 6th July an inquest adjudged income on the late lord's manor at Cottingham, north-west of Hull, to have fallen already on account of the pestilence. Thomas Sampson, the warden of the chapel at Sutton, on the other side of Hull, died in late June. Sampson came from an important local family and was an archdeacon and canon of York Minster, where he was buried; the date of his death suggests that it was in York that he died, not in his parish. His will, proved on 4th July, directed that the considerable sum of £20 should go towards rebuilding work planned for the choir. There was one condition attached: the works should start within one year, 'as I have often said to Thomas Loudham [the cleric in charge of the minster fabric] and Thomas Pacenham [the minster's master mason]'.[37] However, both Loudham and Pacenham died in the epidemic and the project was put on hold for lack of funds, although some limited setting-out work was started, probably just to ensure that the terms of Sampson's will were honoured.[38] The villagers of Patrington, however, had already embarked on the rebuilding of their great church – the final landmark on Holderness – and the aisles were half completed when the pestilence struck. With so many struck down, the villagers were unable to finish what they had begun and so the finely corbelled pillars were fitted with temporary wooden roofs, never to receive the stone-groined vaults that had been intended.

For all the disruption caused by the plague, it would be a mistake to think that all and everything descended into disarray. Thomas Sampson's brother, Sir John de Sutton, was showing the same persist-ence that had earned him a knighthood at the Siege of Calais. A couple of years earlier he and his brother had set up a new chantry college in Sampson's parish of Sutton. Now, in August 1349, the building was reaching its completion, just as the pestilence attained its full strength – at the Cistercian abbey of Meaux, not five miles from Sutton, more than half the brethren died during the month, including the abbot, who went to his grave with five other monks on the very same day.[39] As if the mortality were not trouble enough, the weather had not been kind, one particular deluge coinciding with a high tide and flooding the old port of Ravenser, not far away.[40] Unperturbed by weather, plague and the loss of his brother (who had been destined to become the college's first master), Sir John spurred his builders on. By the end of August, the building was ready for consecration. John fixed the date for Saturday, 12th September. He planned a great event: the restored and beautified church, with its oak screen, Lady Chapel and several altars, was something of which to be proud. Now, however, there was even more to celebrate: the plague, which had killed so many and ruined so much, was noticeably in retreat. So come the day, the whole remainder of the village turned out; more relieved than overjoyed, almost all were still in mourning. Yet the weather now conspired to bring a little hope, for happily it was warm and sunny.[41] Sir John de Sutton was there, with his family. Then, arriving in all his finery, appeared Archbishop Hugh (still standing in for the absent Zouche). He walked around the church, sprinkled holy water and uttered the dedication. That the ceremony was followed by a tremendous party is more than likely: everyone – peasant, knight and archbishop – would have been involved. Tellingly, when the villagers recalled the day many years later, they remembered Hugh of Damascus not as a prelate, but as a friar. It was a reassuring return to normality, even relieved informality – this brilliant, early-autumn day. The villagers of Sutton could be forgiven for making merry with more than usual enthusiasm, for they had survived many weeks of extraordinary misery, to emerge battered but nonetheless alive.

In the admonitory letters sent out by Zouche and other English bishops, in the tense months when plague threatened but had not, as yet, arrived, the pestilence was described simply as a punishment brought down by God on sinful and unrepentant Man. It was the interpretation given by John VI Kantakouzeunos, one of the first Europeans to witness the disease, and had been faithfully repeated ever since.[42] That this should be the first and automatic explanation for the plague was unsurprising – it was a hoary formula pressed into service by scholars and clerics to explain those things that otherwise appeared to be inexplicable. Yet therein lay an age-old problem: it was difficult to reconcile the terrors of nature – droughts, storms, floods and disease – with the New Testament God's unexceptionable benevolence. It took some neat deductive logic, therefore, to explain why God had willed this unprecedented epidemic into being: if God would never inflict undue suffering on Man, there must be justice in his torments; that there had been judgement assumed that Man had sinned; therefore the pestilence had been sent by a just God, creator of all, to punish him for that sin.

Before its arrival, when the pestilence remained unwitnessed and unknown, there was little attempt to expand on the bishops' reasoning;

when at last it came, people had better things to do than explain the terror with which they were at that moment afflicted. However, as the plague at last began to subside, it was natural that those who had survived should reflect further on what had befallen them. The first instinct was to look for portents: events that with hindsight seem to have augured impending disaster. The chronicler of the abbey of Meaux, Thomas Burton, told of an earthquake that hit the abbey during the daily vespers, at about five o'clock, on Friday, 27th March 1349.[43] Just as the monks were singing the words 'He hath put down the mighty from their seats',[44] the ground shook and the monks were thrown 'sprawling' to the floor. Burton was not so incautious as to make a direct connection between the earthquake and the ensuing mortality; however, that he included the two episodes within the same sentence suggests that he wished a connection to be made. Similarly, the old monk recalls the shameful behaviour of noble men and women 'before the pestilence came to dominate England', before proceeding to describe the appearance in Hull of a 'human monster', 'shortly before this time' – thereby fashioning a relationship between these separate events, as if they were harbingers of the calamity with which they coincided. Burton gives special attention to the Hull 'monster', which was clearly not one person but two – being conjoined twins, 'divided from the navel upwards . . . and joined in the lower part'.[45] 'When one ate, drank or spoke,' he remarked, 'the other could do something else if it wished'; together 'they used to sing . . . very sweetly.' When they were about eighteen one of the twins died and the other was left holding its dead sibling in its arms for three days, until that twin too passed away – 'a short time', Burton added, with an allusive flourish, 'before the pestilence began'.[46]

Although Thomas Burton wrote his account some four decades after the Great Death, he was committing a tradition to vellum that had its origins in the very weeks and months that followed the retreat of plague.[47] It was in this reflective aftermath that the recollection of phenomena was interpreted in an attempt to give shape and meaning to the unfathomable events that had just passed. In these local narratives, portents assumed a significance because they were seen to have been themselves part of the unfolding catastrophic drama. With a retrospective eye, such omens were viewed as evidence of a dangerous imbalance in nature, which was the prerequisite for some disastrous event. In this analysis, popular lore corresponded with the postulations of the astrologers. The planets, they claimed, were ruled by their four elements, just as the human body was governed by the four humours. The relationship between the two theories was not accidental, as it was believed that both elements and humours interacted with each other through their intrinsic qualities of hot, cold, wet and dry, maintaining a cosmological equilibrium within the body of the universe that was entirely analogous with that which existed within the body of a human being.[48] As portents were perversions of nature, they were held to be symptoms of some wider cosmic malaise. As the Creation was deemed to be perfect, such a disequilibrium in nature could only be the consequence of the malign and unsettling influence of human sin. Universal balance could thus be restored only through the intervention of the divine physician Himself. Through this formulation, the astrologers were able to reconcile the moral cause of the pestilence (as identified by the bishops in their assertion that the plague was a consequence of human sin) with the mechanics of the natural world. The star-gazers were not at odds, therefore, with the bishops' invocations on the necessity of prayer, as only God could remedy such universal corruption and He was bound to listen to the supplications of men.

Consensus did not stifle academic enquiry, however. As the respected astrologer Geoffrey of Meaux (not of Yorkshire, but France) made plain in the preface to his treatise on plague, written in Oxford just after the outbreak, there was real interest in precisely how the plague had come into being, for what reasons the epidemic had moved among men, and why it killed as it did:[49]

> I have been asked by some of my friends to write something about the cause of the general pestilence, showing its natural cause, and why it affected so many countries, and why it affected some countries more than others, and why within those countries it affected some cities and towns more than others, and why in one town it affected one street, and even one house, more than another, and why it affected nobles and gentry less than other people, and how long it will last.[50]

Geoffrey's search for an answer to these questions began, as was usual and appropriate, in the observation of the heavens. Whilst many,

Thomas Bradwardine among them, disputed the ability of astrologers to divine the future from the planets and the stars, all were in agreement that the celestial bodies influenced earthly affairs and could, therefore, be used to explain what had happened in the past. It was a view underpinned by the long-settled consensus in the Hellenistic astronomical model, in which the flat, fixed earth was circled by seven planets – Mercury, the moon, Venus, the sun, Mars, Jupiter and Saturn – revolving against the more distant stars which were arranged, like some great cosmological backdrop, into the twelve constellations of the Zodiac. These planets and zodiacal signs all had predominant qualities (just as did individual men and women), each influencing the earth and its inhabitants in different ways. Thus, just as the villagers of east Yorkshire sought portentous meaning in the phenomena of the recent past, Geoffrey of Meaux searched his astronomical charts for some planetary combination that could have caused the pestilence. He did not have to look too far back, for in mid-March 1345 there had been a conjunction of three planets – Saturn, Jupiter and Mars – in Aquarius, together with a lunar eclipse. The potency of this series of cosmological events had been recognized by astrologers at the time; now Geoffrey was to recast it as the first natural cause of the plague. He described how the combined powers of Saturn and Mars, which had a harmful influence, were increased both by their conjunction in Aquarius and by the eclipse of the moon (which otherwise might have had a balancing effect), a disastrous celestial conjunction that caused a corruption of the air on earth.

Geoffrey's main interest, however, was in the variation of its impact, which he attributed to the differing temperaments of people and places: as a result some individuals, towns and countries were especially susceptible to the corruption caused by the baleful conjunction of the planets, as their particular qualities were shared. It was an elegant thesis and it is likely that Geoffrey's friends (if it is they for whom the treatise was really intended) were happy with its conclusions. Yet these conclusions were not more than an adumbration of those given in Paris a few months before,[51] nor indeed those proposed by Jacme d'Agramont in Lerida a year previously.[52] That this should be so not only demonstrates the unity of Western scientific thought – the widely held hypotheses that provided the framework in which these very similar explanations of pestilence were made; it is also evidence of the celerity with which many in the European academic community – in Spain, in France and in England – arrived at such close agreement on the natural causes of this extraordinary plague.

For all their theorizing, the astrologers and physicians of Paris University still started from the premise that 'any pestilence proceeds from the divine will', a judgement with which no contemporary commentator disagreed.[53] The tragic conjunction of the planets was to these scholars the physical manifestation of that divine intent.[54] Not that scholars attempted to expand on what exactly that 'will' might ultimately be: the university masters may have perceived the origins of the pestilence, the bishops might have been clear as to its punitive purpose; neither group, however, was willing to speculate on the place that the Great Death had in God's plan for mankind, in the meta-history of salvation. Yet given the apocalyptic scale of the epidemic, it was only to be expected that many thought that the pestilence marked the beginning of a new epoch, perhaps even the first act of the final Revelation. It was to be expected, therefore, that stories of pestilence soon acquired the language and structure of the chiliastic legends so beloved by medieval Europeans. Normally the stock-in-trade of wandering preachers and eccentric friars, these well-worn fables were now repeated by educated men, even if they were reluctant to give open credence to some of the wilder claims going around. Shocked and bewildered by the ferocity of the plague, otherwise right-thinking people were now much less certain about what they should believe and what they could dismiss. John Clyn, in the final pages of his chronicle, affords space for the lengthy retelling of a legend that had been doing the rounds, in one form or other, for nearly a century. The story went that a Cistercian monk in Syrian Tripoli had been interrupted in the middle of Mass by a phantom hand that proceeded to write a prophecy on the corporal cloth predicting, amongst other things, the fall of Tripoli and Acre, the turmoil and eventual triumph of the church, battles, famine and pestilence, all followed by a period of peace before the coming of the Antichrist. The fable had been widely circulated since the end of the previous century, as it was said to have foretold the fall of Tripoli to the Mamluks in 1289 and Acre to the same in 1291. Clyn's version, however, had become mangled in its journey over the Irish Sea, not least because in his account the mystery hand episode occurred in 1347, making manifest nonsense of the Levantine prophesies that were so central to the authenticity of the other calamities foretold. Perhaps he recognized this, for Clyn repeated the account as reported speech. Any doubts notwithstanding, it was a mark of the uncertainty created by the pestilence that Clyn thought it worth recording the story just as he had heard it.

Likewise, when William Blofield, a Carmelite friar in Cambridge, wrote to a Dominican friend in Norwich about rumours that had travelled over from Rome, he did not refrain – despite his own caveat – from repeating them at length.[55] Well he might, for it was a riveting tale: the Antichrist was alive and aged ten. Indeed, he was a very beautiful child and supremely well-educated. There was another boy too, who was twelve years old and living amongst the Tartars, although he had been brought up a Christian. This second youth would come to destroy the Saracens and rule over all Christendom, inaugurating a period of peace and reform within the papacy. Despite revolutions, he would only suffer defeat at the hands of the Antichrist. Here was a conflation of the old tale of Prester John (a mythical Christian king in the distant East) with the widely accepted figure of the Emperor of the Last Days, whose reign would anticipate the end-time. Both these legends, Blofield's and Clyn's, share a familiar millenarian topos, a common redaction of the Apocalypse, into which chronology the recent pestilence seemed to fit so well. That the Great Death had arrived from the East (a fact repeated, tellingly, by almost every chronicler) only made it seem more likely that the pestilence corresponded with some great – possibly final – divine plan. For in the East was to be found the mysterious homeland of the Mongol hordes, who for a century and a half had threatened Europe's eastern frontier. These were the same Tartars who were thought by some to have been sent to purge the corrupted Christian West. No wonder these fabulous stories found so receptive an audience, even amongst normally equanimous clerics. Had there not been famine, and earthquakes, and now plague? Had not the pestilence come from the East, from the land of the Tartars itself? Now was not the time to dismiss portents and fatidic rumour. For in a world where such mortality, previously so unimaginable, was suddenly so real, who was to say that these strange things were not now possible?

This quandary was not new: this was an age of recurrent apocalyptic crises. Whilst many ignored the oft-repeated reports of an imminent

Armageddon, the sense that humanity was inexorably moving towards its concluding end-time was universal. In such an atmosphere, any number of events could be read within the context of St John's Revelation and the many prophecies that were its surrogate. These were themselves texts understood with all the rich and imaginative literalism that was a peculiar quality of the medieval mind. Often it only took the mere threat of calamity to excite a hyper-religious response: indeed, such a scare had rippled throughout the Continent only eighty-nine years earlier, in 1260 – the year in which, according to the Calabrian mystic Joachim of Fiore, the last age of man would finally be inaugurated. The collision of this widely believed prophecy with the real and present threat of a Mongol incursion generated considerable alarm. The extremity of penitential behaviour in some places demonstrated just how immediate the disaster was thought to be. In Perugia, a troupe of men was formed, who would gather together and process through the city's streets from church to church, thereby seeking forgiveness from God and from each other in preparation for this end-time. What was unusual was that these penitents – who donned hoods but kept their upper bodies uncovered – carried a flail in their right hand which they used to strike their back over their left shoulder, whipping in time with their chanted lamentations.[56]

Self-flagellation itself was not novel: mortification of the flesh had for centuries been part of the sacramental rite of penance undertaken by monks, in private. This was a public act, however; such open humiliation was normally reserved for criminals. In appropriating and conflating the attributes of the religious order with the execution of corporal punishment, these so-called *flagellanti*, or 'flagellants', created a new ritual all of their own, albeit one that corresponded with an established liturgical form. For these processions were, in a sense, the panicked inversion of the many civic and religious parades that formed the centrepiece of much medieval public ceremony. Yet the flagellant confraternities existed outside the bounds of ecclesiastical jurisdiction and were ungoverned by lay institutions, making the processions all the more problematic for church and city authorities alike, already made nervous by the flagellants' extreme and uncontrolled religiosity. For the church hierarchy, it was not so much the gruesome spectacle that was troubling but the denouement of the flagellants' processions, which comprised a litany of lay confession and reconciliation, a

practice that was certainly heterodox and verged, to some minds, on
the heretical. Nonetheless, the movement soon spread across Italy and
across the Alps; flagellant confraternities were formed in many towns,
all of them adopting the same crypto-religious rule. So popular did
they become that the penitents were sometimes joined, albeit fully
clothed, by civic dignitaries and – despite the misgivings of senior
clerics – by mendicant priests, many of whom identified strongly with
the movement. In the course of 1260–61 processions of flagellants
were seen as far away as Poland. It was a mark of their appeal that
many confraternities survived, especially in northern Italy. From then
on, every time some catastrophe threatened, the flagellants would
re-emerge, to perform their bizarre brand of penance in public
anticipation of the Last Days.

It was all but inevitable, therefore, that the advent of the Great
Death should prompt a widespread revival of the flagellant movement. At first they did not seem to pose a problem: the pope himself
joined a flagellant procession in Avignon in the days immediately
preceding the plague. However, as flagellant confraternities seeded in
Austria, Thuringia and further up the Rhine in the Low Countries,
there was growing concern at the extremity of their mission. Theirs
was a sinister variation on the penitential processions ordered by
bishops all over Europe, one that soon evolved into outright anti-
clericalism. Whilst the bishops' processions were designed to inspire
devotion and reinforce social order, giving a sense of community and
security in turbulent times, the flagellants had the opposite effect,
breeding fear and fomenting unrest. By allowing self-absolution, the
confraternities removed themselves from the reconciling mechanisms
of the church, which the hierarchy was working so hard to maintain.
Clashes with the church authorities only served to increase the flagellants' anti-clericalism. Likewise, many civil authorities were worried
at the flagellants' influence within their communities. Not only did they
whip up a fervour, adding to the anxiety of populations already petrified
by plague, but at their most radical – in attacking the wealthy and the
Jews – they were dangerously subversive. In Strasbourg, as elsewhere
in northern Europe, the penitents were at first refused entry to the
city for fear that their mere presence would provoke violence against
the city's Jews. However, as the plague passed, the confraternities lost
their more extreme edge. Millenarian messages failed to alarm when

the promised Apocalypse had not come to pass – a further reason why Avignon remained unwilling to condemn the flagellants outright, reluctant as they were to stop acts of penitence (acts it had done so much to encourage) even if some of the expressions of contrition were unconventional. It is tempting to suspect that there were more prosaic motives at work too: the pestilence had placed considerable pressure on the papal bureaucracy, which suddenly had thousands of ecclesiastic positions to fill. There was much to do before the papacy turned its attention to these strange cohorts of self-flagellating men.

It took over a month for Bradwardine and FitzRalph to make their way to Avignon. It was a dangerous journey that took the travellers, once safely over the Channel, from the temperate north of France to the Mediterranean south, from the seagulls of Calais to the cicadas of Provence. The last leg was by barge, down the Saône and mighty Rhône, which widened and slowed through the southern dukedoms and counties of France.[57] Just before it reached its delta in the marsh-land of the Camargue, the river made a right turn, giving a first view of Avignon, built up on a rocky outcrop that rose alongside the left bank. Standing proud above the serried roofs of houses and churches was the Palace of the Popes. This was a vast, dominating edifice, severe Gothic, unembellished, windowless except at height and topped by huge projecting battlements. The palace must have transfixed the two archbishops, even though both men had been here before.[58] This was not the city they remembered, however: the curtain walls were being rebuilt, with regular turrets and extravagant crenellations;[59] most obviously, the papal palace itself had doubled in size, all the work of the current pope, Clement VI.[60]

A couple of prominent English visitors were already in Avignon: Thomas Lisle, the absent bishop of Ely, was still loafing around the papal palace, while Thomas de la Mare, the former prior of Tynemouth (and Douglas's host on the night of Neville's Cross), had come to have his election as the new abbot of St Alban's confirmed by the pope.[61] De la Mare had endured a difficult journey to Avignon (a companion monk had to be left in Canterbury, where he died – most likely of plague, while another made it as far as Calais but had to turn back, leaving the archbishop with a much-diminished retinue); his petition was now stuck in the mire of the famously corrupt papal bureaucracy, which was additionally overwhelmed with the avalanche of requests for indulgences, dispensations and appointments that had come to Avignon in the wake of the plague's progress across Europe. Bradwardine, however, was able to jump the queue: he sought one thing alone from Clement VI and his new position gave him immediate access to the pontiff. On 19th July, within days of his arrival, he received the papal blessing, which conferred on him full authority to represent the church's interests in England. Remaining not a moment longer than was necessary, he was soon on his way back home, leaving FitzRalph, de la Mare and Lisle to pursue their various concerns. The new archbishop of Canterbury, now fully fledged, knew that he had much to do.

Neither did the archbishop of Armagh have to wait long before he too had a turn, but his encounter would not go so smoothly. FitzRalph was a popular figure in the curia, well-known from his previous visits when he had won respect for his abilities as both theologian and preacher. He came this time as the emissary of the king of England, so the curial officials found the earliest slot available for him to give a sermon before the pontiff – the ultimate honour for a visiting clergyman. When the day came, sometime in early August,[62] the cardinals – resplendent in purple and red – filed into the cavernous chapel that sat aloft the southern flank of the papal palace.[63] Pope Clement was last to enter, proceeding to the throne placed just before the altar. Midway through the liturgy, FitzRalph rose to speak. This was FitzRalph's moment, when he could put his case in person, over the heads of so many curial officials who made it their business to act as guardians of the pope. He did not waste the opportunity. His text was from St Matthew's Gospel: 'Lord save us: we perish!', the words with which the terrified disciples woke Jesus, who was sleeping through the storm that threatened to sink the boat in which they were crowded.[64] It was clear that the archbishop intended to concentrate on the misfortunes of his people. The English, the archbishop explained, sincerely wished to take advantage of the Jubilee indulgence. Yet, as Edward had wished him to say, the required pilgrimage to Rome was a perilous one. Not wishing to miss an opportunity to show that the English were as much victims of the Continental war as the French, he pointed out that, for an Englishman, travel through France was extremely hazardous. Moreover, if the English were to go on pilgrimage in any numbers, the country would be attacked by the Irish and Scots, who would lay waste to the borderlands, steal cattle and put women and children to the sword. The Anglo-Irish faced additional difficulties: they were devout but poor and thus very few were likely to be able to afford the journey. Even the crossing was now more unreliable than ever, because of the high mortality in coastal areas resulting from the plague. The English, both in England and in Ireland, had borne the brunt of the epidemic, which had so far failed to touch either the native Irish or the Scots. So bad had it been that fully two thirds of the English population had been killed, and the Great Death was still continuing. This nation, now denuded of the larger part of its people, was even less able to defend itself in the face of the hostile nations that threatened it from the north and west.

The archbishop may well have talked up the devotion of the English, even exaggerated what might happen if they were absent from their lands; in his account of English suffering at the hands of the Great Death, however, he played it straight. For he had seen the devastation for himself – both in the colony and in his journey from Bristol to London. FitzRalph's plea cumulated with powerful effect. Yet, impressed as he doubtless was, the pope was aware that if he were to give a plenary indulgence to the entire English nation, absolving them of the requirement of making the pilgrimage to Rome, it would invalidate the whole Jubilee exercise. Besides, the plague was a problem shared by every nation in Europe. Perhaps Clement expressed surprise to FitzRalph that his liege should think that the English were a special case: if the English, why not the Poles, the Flemish or for that matter the French? Indeed, if the journey were so difficult, why had so many important English clerics been able to travel to Avignon in recent months, a journey that was itself equal to half the distance to Rome? Clement may have reflected, with justice, that far from being an innocent request, FitzRalph's petition was little more than a ruse. It did not take much imagination to realize that a good part of the French nobility will have wished to go to Rome in 1350 too, thus leaving Philip VI with even fewer captains on whom to call in the event of an English attack. The pontiff would not be so easily hoodwinked by the English king, a man whose true motives he knew only too well. The Jubilee was not a selective indulgence, nor should it be abused in an English attempt to jockey for advantage in their contentions with the French. It took Clement little time to respond to the petition.

On 18th August, messengers rode out of the palace courtyard, through the city's narrow streets and – once clear of Avignon's gates – at a gallop in the direction of the English Channel. In their knapsacks were letters from the pope – papal bulls – addressed to every archbishop in the British Isles. The order was clear: the prelates should make it widely known that for the Jubilee indulgence to be gained, the Jubilee pilgrimage would have to be made. Yet this was not the sum of it. Also included was an admonition to the archbishops to warn their flocks of the dangers of the 'vain religion' practised by the flagellants – timely advice given that the confraternities had yet to make it over the Channel. In both these messages was a clear indication that Clement was intent on reaffirming both papal authority and religious orthodoxy. It showed, furthermore, that the ecclesiastical establishment was already working hard to restore the *status quo ante*, a signal that as far as they were concerned, nothing of substance had been altered by the coming of the plague.

Archbishop FitzRalph had failed in his first task, yet he still had his original petitions to make, on the primacy of Armagh over Dublin and the miscellaneous financial issues that exercised him. Besides, Avignon had been free of plague for over a year now and although the number of deaths in London had subsided, the epidemic was still making its way through the British Isles. Indeed, there were many regions that had yet to be infected – Scotland and Gaelic Ireland (as Richard had pointed out to the pope) among them. In England, by mid-August, the epidemic had reached as far north as the Ribble and Tees; a quarter of England still lay, therefore, before the advancing pestilence. That neither County Durham, nor north Lancashire, nor some of the more isolated parts of Yorkshire, had yet received the disease, was of little comfort to the communities there. For by now these people had been expecting the epidemic for over a year, awaiting a fate that seemed the more terrible with every word of it that reached them. First there were rumours of a horrific pestilence abroad; then the archbishop's first warning letter was read out in church, just as news came that the plague had arrived on the Dorset coast. Townsmen and villagers will have heard enough through the months that followed

to know what effect the disease was having down south. Their sense
of trepidation can only have been heightened when they were given,
in spring 1349, papal instructions concerning how confessions should
be made once plague had struck.[65] Then, at the end of June, with
the epidemic now in York, there came out of London an ordinance
controlling labour rates and terms, an edict that opened with the
words: 'Since a great part of the population, and especially workers
and employees, has now died in this pestilence'.[66]

Yet here, in the most-northern counties, this proclamation –
expressly framed as a reaction to pestilence – fell on ears that still
awaited news of its definite arrival. Already taut with fright, nerves
must now have been fraying. So it was no surprise that when, on
Wednesday, 15th July, the bishop of Durham's steward began his
summer round of the vast episcopal estate, he was met with terrified
defiance. In the morning he presided over the halmote at Houghton-
le-Spring, a substantial village midway between Durham and the mouth
of the Wear.[67] It was a quick session: no one came forward to take
on new land, for 'fear of the pestilence'. The next day the steward
was at Easington, six miles to the south-east. There he encountered
precisely the same problem: no-one was prepared to take on land on
the usual customary terms, as they 'flatly refused . . . unless they should
still be alive after the pestilence'. Moreover, they refused point blank
'to labour according to the proclamation[68] or on any terms at all'.
Wearily, the steward realized that rather than allow land to lie fallow,
he would have to rent it out because, 'as has become apparent, there is
no other alternative'. It was a concession wrung from him by necessity,
for renting – which broke the feudal bond and implied an equivalence
of tenurial status – was something that conservative feudal lords, of
whom the bishop of Durham was a prime example, were loath to do.
On Friday, 17th July, the steward was at Sedgefield, nine miles to the
south of Easington. On arrival he soon learned that William Kid, 'one
of the lord's serfs', had 'fled by night with his whole family'.[69] William,
because he was a serf, was prohibited from leaving the village without
his lord's permission; this, then, was a serious and punishable offence,
not one committed on a whim. His fellow serfs, unsurprisingly, were
unwilling to take on his land. The bishop's steward had by now given
up explaining that this chaotic state of affairs was a result of the fear
of pestilence, which was evidently the cause of William's flight. The

ensuing halmotes at Stockton and Sadberge, on the road to Darlington, seemed to pass off normally. Nevertheless, the steward can not have been other than shocked by the alarm which had spread around the county, such was the sense of grim expectation – fed by rumour and decree – of the long-awaited Great Death.

Such fear was not misplaced, for the pestilence was, by the day, moving closer. Only fifty miles to the south, it was spreading out of York and the East Riding into the parts around. At some point this summer (it is unclear when) the disease came over the hill into Wharram Percy, down the main street and into one of the houses, carried either by one of the villagers or by a visitor. Perhaps they had been infected in the marketplace at Malton, or even in York itself. In the end it mattered not from where, or from whom, or from how many, the disease was brought in: as everywhere else, the infection of the village – for a while borne unawares – was virtually inevitable. Within weeks of the first deaths much of the village had been struck down, including Walter Heslerton, the unfortunate husband of the lady of the manor, Eustachia Percy. (The whole manor was placed in

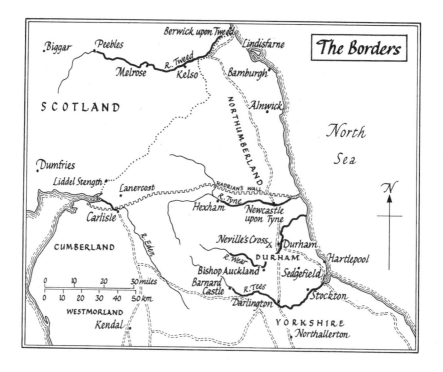

the hands of trustees, as their son was still a minor and Eustachia, who was insane, was incapable of running the estate herself.)

This was good farming country and well-connected to York; yet it is as well to remember that the troubled borderlands were not far away as well. As Wharram Percy's name made clear, the villagers here were vassals of a Northern marcher lord. This was not some theoretical association: Barton-le-Street, only ten miles to Wharram's north-west, had suffered earlier in the century from the Scots' raids. This little village, nestling near the bottom of Ryedale, looked both ways. Not twenty miles to the south was York, from where it most likely received the Great Death, in which almost all its tenants were killed. To the north and west, however, were hills – the beginning of a wilderness that stretched to the Scottish frontier. This was different country: remote, sparsely populated, with poor roads and few towns. Trade was limited; what little existed was mostly in sheep. Not surprisingly, therefore, the pace of the epidemic reduced somewhat, slowed not by the crags and the heather but by isolation and lack of people. These were communities adjusted to hardship – one reason, perhaps, why local accounts of the pestilence are so few.[70] That it was present is certain: further up Ryedale, the abbots of the great Cistercian houses of Rievaulx and Byland both met their end in October – two deaths that cannot be attributed to coincidence. So there *were* deaths, but it seems that in these distant regions, the death toll may have been somewhat lower: if the registers of clerical institutions are anything to go by, the villages of upper Ryedale, the North York Moors and Yorkshire Dales may have lost no more than a quarter of their populations. Perhaps some extremely isolated settlements survived entirely untouched; perhaps the slower speed of spread gave people the warning they needed to avoid making journeys to places already diseased.

That the pace of the epidemic was regulated by frequency of travel and density of population is borne out by the experience of the country around Doncaster. These parts – boggy, wild and oft-bypassed – had, until August, also escaped the plague. For three months this was a disease-free island in a sea of infection: York, Derbyshire and Nottinghamshire had been engulfed since May, north Lincolnshire and the East Riding since June. Eventually it arrived, however. On 8th September, Archbishop Zouche placed an Augustinian canon in the vicarage of Tickhill, a few miles to the south of Doncaster. It was not unknown, but was still unusual, for a canon-monk to take on a parish but the archbishop's hand had been forced, 'by reason of the scarcity of secular [clergy]'[71] who have been taken away from among us by the plague of mortality that hangs over us'.[72] Late in its infection, the supply of priests had now been used up elsewhere. Everywhere uncertainty reigned. When a certain Thomas Allott of Wombwell, twelve miles due west of Doncaster, died, he made bequests 'to my sons and daughters living after this present pestilence'.[73] It was a pathetic testament to the despair which Thomas must have felt, that no one could be sure who, nor how many, would survive.

In south Yorkshire there was one man who we can be sure welcomed the prospect of death: Richard Rolle. A longing for death was a well-developed theme in the writings of this eremitical mystic: 'Jesu, I coveite for to dy / When it es thy paying'.[74] Now, on the last day of September, he gained what he sought, at the Cistercian convent of Hampole, a little community on the road from Doncaster to Wakefield where he had lived for several years. In his own lifetime Rolle had achieved some celebrity, not just for his scriptural commentaries and spiritual manuals – which were numerous – but also among noblewomen, to whom he extended a particular pastoral generosity. There was a whiff of impropriety about Rolle and it was perhaps appropriate that he should end up as spiritual adviser to the nuns of Hampole. The community had suffered from loose discipline for many years, the nuns being censured at one point for wearing fashionable narrow-cut tunics which showed more curves than was perhaps appropriate for those set on a celibate life. They certainly mourned him, these nuns; so too his wider audience – the priests, noblemen and women – who had been attracted to his very individual brand of ecstatic spirituality. Although still relatively young (he was at most forty-four at his death), Rolle had already ensured that there was material enough to sustain the appetite for his work among his growing band of followers. So his passing was not, in that sense at least, premature; it can have come no sooner for Rolle, who had so looked forward to death for much of his life.

In the north-west, the disease had moved from Cheshire into south Lancashire by the end of July,[75] infecting the still inconsequential settlements of Liverpool (which had a population of little more than a thousand) and Manchester. Here there were the usual problems with the carriage of the dead. The villagers of Didsbury had to take their deceased relatives, every one of them, five miles north to Manchester, for there was no consecrated burial ground closer by. Most likely taking advantage of a similar imposition, a certain William of Liverpool persuaded the villagers of Everton to take their dead to his house instead of the churchyard – a service for which he most probably made a charge, albeit at a discount to the church's burial fee. A third of Everton's population (perhaps a half or more of the dead of the village) were brought to William to deal with in this way. Although it is unclear where William disposed of the bodies, we may be sure that it was not where they should have been, for he was hauled up in front of the justices at the next assize to make answer for the scam.

The epidemic had crept over the Ribble by September, establishing itself firmly in the north of Lancashire. Throughout the Fylde peninsula hundreds and thousands died: Lytham, Kirkham, Preston, Garstang, Cockerham, Poulton and Bispham (up the Blackpool promenade) – every parish seems to have been hit.[76] Perhaps a thousand souls perished in Lancaster.[77] Although the pace had undoubtedly slowed, the disease was clearly as lethal as ever; it was also still capable of reaching the least accessible places. The prior of Cartmel, at the foot of the Lake District, died at this time and the threat of infection was clearly serious enough to encourage one John Collesham to seek reconciliation with his abbey of Furness. He had fled because his abbot had refused him permission to make the Jubilee pilgrimage to Rome; that the trip now involved a more perilous journey through plague-ridden countryside perhaps persuaded him it was better to stay put. The confines of the cloister must not have seemed so bad after all.

Over the Pennines and north of the Cleveland Hills, the pestilence made its way across the Tees into County Durham just as it was colonizing land north of the Ribble. The palatinate county of Durham constituted the southern part of the ancient kingdom of Northumbria – the cradle of Northern Christianity, the land of Bede, Jarrow, Lindisfarne and St Cuthbert. There was still something utterly distinct about the north-east, and about Durham in particular. This was the domain of the prince-bishop, whose powers made him a local king. His tenants suffered a lordship that was appropriately oppressive. It was an ecclesiastical hegemony: the bishop had approximately 37,000 acres and 137 villages and that which he did not own was mostly in the hands of Durham Priory. The landscape was varied: brooks rushed down from the high and unpopulated western moorland to the rivers – Tees, Wear and Tyne – that flowed through rolling hills to the eastern plain that lay before the sea. It was in these stark lowlands, between moor and coast, that the vast majority of the palatinate's population lived: small nucleated villages interspersed with farms, inhabited by peasants making what they could of rough pasture and poor land. Life here was not easy – this was hard farming, hard-run. The palatinate was not isolated, however: Hartlepool and Newcastle were notable ports, Darlington was a bustling little town whilst Durham was rich enough to secure a place in the itinerary of most serious Scottish border raids. Even the western valleys saw regular traffic, albeit too often soldiers making their way to the border and back. Egglestone Abbey, sitting at the junction of three trans-Pennine tracks, was at this time still recovering from the depredations of the English 'guests' who had passed through on their way to Neville's Cross.

It seems that Stockton, a small village with a quay and the last crossing point over the Tees before the sea, was one of the first places in Durham to fall victim to the Great Death. It came early enough to affect the end of the harvest, so must have been present by the end of August at least.[78] It is likely that the infection came both from the south, by road, and by the coastal ports as well.[79] The long wait, the news from the south, may have given useful warning to some at least: those villages right on the waterfront seem to have fared far worse than those just a mile or two inland. Jarrow, for instance, on the south bank of the River Tyne, lost 78 per cent of its tenants; perhaps word of the early deaths in Jarrow gave the villagers of Monkton, just two miles away, time to isolate themselves, for there only 21 per cent of the tenants perished.[80] In the townships at the mouth of the Wear, the average death rate was 60 per cent, yet further up the broad river valley the average was closer to 40 per cent.[81] The far lower death toll of the inland villages clearly suggests that many took some positive, preventative action to reduce the risks of infection. However, these survival strategies – if indeed they were strategies – had little overall effect. The average mortality in the priory townships was still over 50 per cent: for every village that was lucky, another was destroyed. At West Thickley, in November, no one appeared before the bishop's steward at the halmote, 'because they are dead'.[82] If anyone had survived, they had already fled. For what could the orphan, the widow and the old man do, in a village near emptied by death? Nothing, it seems, but leave. Wretched survivors, trudging, stooped under the burden of all they could carry, following slow-turning wheels of an ox-drawn cart, treading a miserable and lonely exodus from where they had lived. Some had a place to go: to a surviving relative in a village nearby, or to a town where they might find work. Others, doubtless, had no destination and nothing to do, forced to amble between villages in search of food and a place to rest. Even this, the life of the simple vagrant, would prove too much for one peasant, who was found wandering the countryside, driven mad through grief.

All was not desperation, however. Despite the continued reluctance of some to enter into land, the bishop of Durham's steward found no fewer than 780 new tenants to take on holdings vacated through death, in October and November alone. Coercion certainly played some part in this: on 26th October in Whessoe, a hamlet a couple of miles north of Darlington, the steward tried to commit land to a man called Akres, in the absence of any blood relative living to take the tenement on. Akres refused, however, and so the steward was obliged to back down. Nonetheless, it would be fair to assume that many others had capitulated where Akres had held firm, while some – even in this most oppressive lordship – saw the opportunities to be had amidst this disaster, and took on land of their own volition.

The interminable wait was, at last, at an end: by the close of November, the pestilence had departed from much of the county. The settlements here were so small that once pestilence came, after the many months of dread, it will have lasted but a few weeks. Soon it had moved on, over the Tyne, to the fastness of Northumberland. This was a wild, expansive, ravishing landscape, yet unproductive and further denuded by the plundering Scot. Not surprisingly, very few lived here and those that did were largely in the service of one of the two great marcher lords – Ralph Neville and Henry Percy, both heroes of Neville's Cross. It is little surprise that virtually nothing is known of the Great Death in Northumberland, therefore, as there were not many for it to kill. Whilst the tiny population and lack of anything more than local trade undoubtedly helped slow the pace of the epidemic, the plague did eventually come. Henry Percy drew up his will on 13th September, clearly fearful that the plague was about

to arrive. He would have to wait a little longer yet, for the abbot of
the Premonstratensian abbey at Alnwick, one of the first recorded
victims in the Percy fief, was not taken ill until spring the following
year. Once present, it killed just as it had in the more populated
South: at Belford, not far from the Neville stronghold of Bamburgh,
the cemetery had to be enlarged to accommodate the dead of the six
hamlets around. So it lingered, crawling towards the border, the harsh
winter further slowing it in its tracks. As for Westmorland and
Cumberland, on the west coast, almost nothing is known. The bishop
of Carlisle had ecclesiastical authority here – his flock numbering no
more than were contained by a few large parishes in Suffolk or Surrey.
Although the pope's letter concerning plague confessions was
forwarded to the bishop on 28th April 1349, his register records nothing
for these years; nor does anyone else.[83] It is clear only from later
accounts that the pestilence did, indeed, pass through. It is enough
now, surely, merely to imagine what effect the Great Death had on
this most remote corner of England.

Late on Wednesday, 19th August, Thomas Bradwardine stepped off
the boat onto the quayside at Dover. It was a month to the day since
the archbishop's consecration in Avignon and only two months since
he had left London for Provence. Bradwardine's haste was a measure
of his intent. Now invested with the full authority of first primate of
England, the archbishop made straight for the king and by Friday he
was at the palace at Eltham. No doubt Edward received him with
warmth: Bradwardine had shown himself to be an ambitious candidate
and an energetic appointment, but his loyalty was thus far unques-
tioned. Having discussed the many urgent matters at hand, the new
primate left for London the very next day. During the short journey,
however, he was taken ill. Presumably because the archbishop's palace
at Lambeth was unavailable, Thomas was cared for at the bishop of
Rochester's residence, 'La Place', next door. Four days later, on
Wednesday, 26th August 1349, he died. It was a sudden end to a remarkable career. In a bizarre twist of fate, Bradwardine had escaped the
English epidemic, only to travel to France and promptly die on his
return. William Dene, who records the episode in some detail, does
not state explicitly that the pestilence was to blame. However, it is
likely that Bradwardine contracted plague as he passed through Dijon,

just over three weeks before.[84] Moreover, the speed with which the archbishop was taken ill and the four days he lasted until death all point to plague as the agent of his demise.

News of the archbishop's death reached Edward just as he received reports that the French had abjured the truce. Coming together, these two calamities only served to underscore the extent to which the king was still being forced to rule in response to events beyond his control. As if to emphasize the point, the king was receiving complaints that his Ordinance of Labourers, only sent out on 18th June, was failing to keep a lid on wages. This was no idle bleating on the part of landowners – in Oakham in Rutland, for instance, reapers were receiving 5d. per day in the first week of the harvest, yet in the second week they took home 6½d. – an increase of 30 per cent in just seven days. The cost of harvesting the crops at Brightwell in Oxfordshire was said to be high, as the villeins' works had already been sold and wage-labourers were scarce and therefore dear. At Farnham, where John Runwick had so far held down the cost of bought-in work, 'the plague and . . . scarcity of labour' forced him to offer increased wages.[85] This concatenation of problems had a profound effect on the king, so much so that on 5th September his frustration boiled over. Dashing off a circular to the English bishops, he excoriated his subjects for their iniquity:

> During the pestilences and many evil tribulations with which, by way of warning, a just God now visits the sons of men and lashes the world – showing harshness to his people so that they, in fear and penitence, might call upon his name more humbly – we have been turning the matter over in our mind with intense concentration, and we are amazed and appalled that the few people who still survive have been so ill-fated, so ungrateful towards God and so stiff-necked that they are not humbled by the terrible judgements and lessons of God. For, if their works are any guide, sinfulness and pride are constantly increasing in the people, and charity has grown more than usually cold in them. This seems to presage a much greater calamity (not, I hope, total ruin), and it is to be feared that this will really happen unless God, who has been offended by their guilt, is pacified by the performance of penance for sin and by the prayers of the faithful.
>
> Therefore, . . . we beseech you [to urge] your parishioners and others

with wholesome admonitions, so that, mindful of God's kindness, they
repent their sins and give themselves up to prayer, fasting and the
exercise of virtue, and turn away from evil, so that merciful God might
repel the plague and illness, and confer peace and tranquillity, and
health of body and soul. For we hope that if, by God's grace, the people
drive out this spiritual wickedness from their hearts, the malignancy
of the air and of the other elements will also depart.[86]

Thus ended this most curious rant, which must have been received
with some bewilderment by those that heard it. For the plague was
now absent from much of England; in some parts of the South it had
been gone for months. How could the king threaten a disease that
had already begun to depart? Edward's subtext was the more obvious
for his failure of logic: it was no more than an attempt to frighten the
labourers, suggesting that if they persisted in their effrontery, they
would surely invite a repeat of the divine punishment they had just
endured. Yet Edward's purpose was too transparent: this was none
other than the enraged response of the baronial class, furious at the
insolence of the land-workers who, in their depleted numbers, were
exerting newly found economic power. Both Edward and his fellow
landowners were struggling to react to the consequences of the Great
Death, a catastrophe that had been favourable to many of those that
had survived. That the king's threats proved ineffective only demonstrated that his subjects knew this to be the case.

For not dissimilar reasons, the arrival in London of 120 flagellants
from Flanders around Michaelmas failed to create the millenarian
storm endured by so many Continental cities.[87] Robert of Avesbury,
who might well have seen their spectacle for himself, told how the
men processed around the city twice a day, sometimes in front of St
Paul's, sometimes elsewhere, 'their bodies naked except for a linen
cloth from loins to ankle'.

> Each wore a hood painted with a red cross at front and back and carried
> in his right hand a whip with three thongs. Each thong had a knot in
> it, with something sharp, like a needle, stuck through the middle of
> the knot so that it stuck out on each side, and as they walked one after
> the other they struck themselves with these whips on their naked,
> bloody bodies; four of them singing in their own tongue and the rest

answering in the manner of the Christian litany. Three times in each procession they would all prostrate themselves on the ground, with their arms outstretched in the shape of a cross. Still singing, and beginning with the man at the end, each in turn would step over the others, lashing the man beneath him once with his whip, until all of those lying down had gone through the same ritual. Then each one put on his usual clothes and, always with their hoods on their heads and carrying their whips, they departed to their lodgings. It was said that they performed a similar penance every night.[88]

Bemused Londoners watched but few, if any, joined in. For city folk as for agricultural labourers, warnings of the Apocalypse rang a little empty now. Besides, the men from Flanders probably had little time in which to cause a problem. Winging their way from Avignon were Clement's letters, cautioning the archbishops to beware the flagellants' cult. It seems the English authorities took the pontiff's advice and ordered the ejection of the flagellants from the city.[89] It would be their first and last appearance in London, for on 20th October, following a detailed doctrinal report from the University of Paris, the pope declared the movement heretical and ordered that the flagellants be banned for good. It was a timely decision: these millenarian brethren, who had been foretelling the end-time on and off for nearly a hundred years, faced suppression just as it became clear that the promised Apocalypse had not, in fact, come to pass.

Barbarians

November 1349–1350

There is in every one of us a barbarian tribe, extremely overbearing and intractable.

Themistius[1]

In his Avignon sermon of mid-August 1349, Richard FitzRalph related the tale of the Necromancer of Toledo, who had asked the Devil which country in the Christian world would send most souls to Hell. 'Ireland', the Devil replied, as everyone robbed from each other, never made restitution for their sins and therefore died without true repentance. Returning to the theme on which he had lectured the Anglo-Irish of Drogheda some months before,[2] FitzRalph described to Clement and his court the endemic conflict that so unsettled the island. The English and Irish, he claimed, fought each other out of a traditional and inborn hatred, murder and robbery took place daily and no truce designed to prevent violence ever held. To make matters worse, the Anglo-Irish communities had been ravaged by the pestilence, whereas the native Irish and Scottish people, who were 'of the same tongue', had escaped infection.[3] This assessment of the progress of the disease was correct, or at least had been when the archbishop left Armagh for London in May. Although the epidemic was moving north through England, it was still some way from the border with Scotland; likewise in Ireland, the pestilence had worked its way through the stricken Anglo-Irish communities in their eastern and southern coastal exclaves but had not, as yet, manifested itself among the native Irish of the interior. Yet FitzRalph was not preaching before the papal court to describe the progress of the disease, but was there to plead for the grant of a special plenary indulgence to the English – a people who, he claimed, had been depleted by as much as two thirds as a result of the plague. It served his purpose well to paint a picture of an undiminished, volatile and barely contained Celtic rim, united in a common language, threatening so much damage to the English of both England and Ireland.

Although FitzRalph's description was exaggerated,[4] it cannot have been that different from the one he had given the king when they conferred a few months earlier, at the beginning of June. By then, Edward had most probably heard news of Fulk de la Freigne's death and of the aged Archbishop Bicknor's ill-health, so FitzRalph's warnings can have only added to his concern at the increasingly perilous state of Anglo-Ireland. In addition, Edward was now to be deprived of his energetic archbishop, whom only ten months previously he had charged with negotiating a truce between the contending parties.[5] That attempt had been foiled by the plague and the king must now have feared that the native Irish (like, as he suspected, the peasant English) would use the pestilence to further their own ends.[6] Edward no doubt cast his mind back to his father's sorry reign, when in 1315 there was the calamitous coincidence of the Bruce invasion of Ireland, a Scots incursion in the North and a terrible famine in England, the last of which made it all the more difficult to respond to the Celtic threat. It was clear, therefore, that *laissez-faire* was no longer an option if Anglo-Ireland were to survive: a strong hand was once again required across the Irish Sea. So, on 17th July, Sir Thomas Rokeby was appointed justiciar in Ireland. He was, in several ways, the ideal choice: as sheriff of Yorkshire, Rokeby had been one of the commanders at Neville's Cross and afterwards had been responsible for the escort of the captive King David from the battlefield down to London. His loyalty was unimpeachable, but more importantly, he was an experienced March campaigner. With Scotland king-less and suitably subdued, the North could now be spared this stalwart of its defence. It is noteworthy, therefore, that Sir Thomas did not respond immediately to the king's command. Perhaps the royal messenger failed to make it through to Rokeby's home in north Yorkshire first time;[7] more likely, Sir Thomas – who must have heard the same rumours that were making their way round the villages of County Durham not many miles to the north-east – judged it too risky to travel through the band of plague that now separated the North from the rest of England. This great warrior, whom the Lanercost chronicler claimed 'gave the Scots such a cup that, having sampled it once, they did not wish to taste it again', fought shy of the plague as it made its terrible, inexorable, advance northwards.[8]

In the event, Rokeby's absence mattered little, for within weeks of his appointment pestilence had made its own truce between the pugnacious warlords of Ireland. Thus far the native Irish had ignored the dangers of plague, seeing it instead as an opportunity to prey on the weakened colonists: in Carlow the citizens claimed that the attacks had become so frequent that their town was on the brink of total destruction; so too around Nenagh, a small town in north-west Tipperary that sat right on the boundary between Anglo- and Gaelic Ireland and which had been fought over, like a bone between two dogs, for many years. It had been set ablaze by the native Irish, led by Donnell O'Kennedy,[i] in 1347, only then to be retrieved by Fulk de la Freigne the following year. His death on 17th June 1349 may well have taken place when the Irish tried to recapture the town. Perhaps the pestilence was passed between the two enemies in the mêlée, for it is more than likely that Nenagh, or at the very least the country round about, was in Gaelic Irish hands when, on 10th August, a friar living there died from plague. Nine days later a second friar succumbed. Thus, by the time FitzRalph had begun to insist otherwise to the pope in Avignon, the epidemic had moved at least up to the frontier that separated Anglo- and Gaelic Ireland and may even have crossed it.

As Anglo-Irish Limerick, to the west, had most probably not yet been infected, it is likely that pestilence had come to Nenagh from the east, via colonial Kilkenny and thence across the ancient woods and bogs of north Tipperary, which had long been controlled by Gaelic Irish chieftains.[9] It was late October by the time pestilence had reached the west coast. Limerick, the only remaining western colonial outpost, was also the last English town to be affected, a death being recorded here on 1st November. At around the same time, Matthew Caoch Macnamara,[ii] the lay patron of the Franciscan friary in Ennis (due west of Nenagh and a little to the north-west of Limerick), died. Ennis had only latterly been returned to Gaelic Irish control but further

[i] Anglicized from Dómhnall Ó Ceinnéidigh.
[ii] Anglicized from Mac Con Mara.

north the disease had already reached far into established Gaelic
Irish territory. In Bréifne (roughly Cavan and Leitrim), the plague
took away a prince each from the two predominant families – Richard
O'Reilly,[iii] the king of east Bréifne, and Matthew, son of Cathal
O'Rourke,[iv] whose powerbase was in west Bréifne. Although the
named victims were clan chiefs, the mortality was more widespread,
the annalist going on to make plain that 'great destruction of the
people was inflicted therein'.[10] The epidemic had probably passed
through the drumlins of Bréifne from the east, via Louth and Meath,
where it had killed the bishop earlier in the year.[11] At the same time
it was moving up the Shannon, flowing with the traffic that passed
through Lough Derg and then Lough Ree. The two fronts converged
in eastern Connacht. Thus Moylurg, near Roscommon, was infected
in the closing months of 1349. Even by the standards of medieval
Ireland, these parts were remote, yet still the pestilence did its usual
work: 'great numbers were carried off'.[12] The night before Christmas,
one scribe, Aodh MacEgan,[v] was moved to write this plaint, such was
the terror that the disease inspired:[13]

> I myself am full twenty-one years old, . . . and let everyone who shall
> read this utter a prayer of mercy for my soul; Christmas Eve tonight
> and under the safeguard of the King of Heaven and Earth who is here
> tonight I place myself and may Heaven be the end of my life and may
> He put this great plague past me and past my friends and may we be
> once more in joy and happiness. Amen, Pater Noster.[14]

Conflict, then, around Nenagh or somewhere else, may well have
been the reason why the disease passed from English to Gaelic Ireland.
Yet there were many other means by which the epidemic may have
crossed between the two 'nations'. The Anglo-Irish and native Irish
were not separated by some nicely delineated border but by an unfixed,
undefined frontier-land, which shifted according to the relative
strengths of the barons and princes on either side. Although the
frontier was regularly exposed to great violence (which itself formed
some sort of exchange), it was far from being an anarchic no-man's

[iii] Anglicized from Ó Raghallaigh.
[iv] Anglicized from Ó Ruairc.
[v] Anglicized from Mac Aodhagáin.

land. It was in the interests of both sides to enforce just enough peace to permit cross-frontier traffic, as the wealth of the Irish princes was reliant on a vibrant trading economy. For just as the Gaelic Irish had traded with the Vikings, now they bought and sold from the Anglo-Irish. The fecund Irish isle had much to offer: her many rivers were full of fish, some of which – eels in particular – were sold by native traders. Otters too were hunted in the rivers, and wolves, deer, squirrels and pine martens were caught in the forests that covered perhaps a fifth of the country, their much sought-after pelts being traded abroad. Linen was produced in the north and west expressly for export. The principal trade, however, reflected native Ireland's predominantly pastoral economy. Indeed, the produce of Irish pasture now constituted the larger part of colonial exports: hides from every corner of Gaelic Ireland; coarse wool from the uplands of south-west Munster and highland Leinster; and horses, which Irish princes prided themselves on breeding. All of these products were traded across the frontier and shipped by Anglo-Irish merchants to Bristol and – in far greater quantities – to Flanders. Every bargain between an Anglo-Irish merchant and Gaelic Irish trader presented an opportunity for pestilence to spread from the colony into the territory of the Irish kings.

While many transactions were made in coin, the main means of exchange used by the Gaelic Irish was the cow, a form of wealth that of itself will have aided the spread of plague. For cattle rustling was rife between competing clans and was often the prime object of raids on frontier manors; as the experience of Carlow and Nenagh attests, native Irish raiding continued through the months of plague, making it more than likely that plague passed between the two communities even in those most unstable regions where there was little trade. Moreover, as the raiders often complemented their plunder with acts of murder and rapine, there was a further – very carnal – guarantee of contagion. Even the attempts to prevent incursions, when Anglo-Irish barons treated with their native Irish counterparts, provided opportunities for infection. In 1349, for example, Maurice fitz Thomas FitzGerald, the fourth earl of Kildare, came to an agreement with Murtagh Og O'Connor,[vi] who controlled Offaly. The earl granted him lands for his

---

[vi] Anglicized from Muircheartach Og Ó Conchobair.

'good and praiseworthy service' so long as the relationship remained amicable, for which O'Connor was charged a peppercorn rent of one cow per annum. In less exceptional times there would have been little unusual about such a meeting, yet on this occasion the epidemic may well have spread, silently, from the earl's party to O'Connor's. The many local truces and temporary alliances, of which this was just one, demanded meetings, payments and mutual hospitality. Thus, whether in cross-frontier raiding or in its prevention, there were a multitude of instances in which the one community may have passed the disease, unintentionally and unwittingly, to the other.

Once across the frontier, pestilence travelled with little trouble. Gaelic Irish society was semi-nomadic: for centuries native herders had practised transhumant pasture or 'booleying' – moving cattle into the hills in summer and then down again into the lowland lands in the autumn. Farmers and – in places – their families moved up and down with their cattle, partly in order to defend their property but also because cattle provided (in addition to oats) all the staples of their diet: beef, blood, milk, butter and beef broth. Whilst the location of upland and lowland settlements varied little from year to year, the houses themselves – sometimes no more than a hut of wattle covered with clay and earth – were rarely permanent, even for clan leaders. Although in some places (especially in the west of Ireland and in the more fertile lowlands) there were more-substantial dwellings,[15] since the Anglo-Norman conquest the Gaelic Irish living on the better land had been forced to retreat to the uplands and therefore booleying had become even more widespread than before the English had arrived. Thus, the perpetual seasonal movement of families and small communities ensured that even in the most remote areas, just as in Wales, there was ample opportunity for pestilence to pass from one person to another.

Such remarkable differences between this Gaelic Irish culture and colonial society meant that for all the practical porosity of the frontier – so amply demonstrated by the passage of pestilence from the one 'nation' to the other – the boundary between the two also represented a powerful symbolic limitation. On one side the people were pastoral, clan-based and impermanent; on the other they submitted to feudal power structures, were organized into tidy manorial and urban units, administered through a bureaucracy that had as its model the most sophisticated central government in Europe. Needless to say, both 'nations' and their leaders had some features in common: both professed the same Christian, Catholic faith; both prized deep-rooted (if distinct) literary traditions; both demonstrated a corresponding desire to trade; and in both the majority of the population practised subsistence agriculture. Yet such similarities were shared by almost all the peoples of Western Europe; these two cultures were so discrepant as to make them almost irreconcilable.

As both nations cleaved to very different (and very mixed) identities, the way they perceived the frontier was also characteristic. For the native Irish, the frontier-land was substantially similar to the loose borders that separated the many different Irish clans, although it was increasingly viewed as the limit of their freedom, beyond which lay land held – unjustly – under foreign occupation. In this sense the frontier did much to engender an embryonic sense of nationhood within the Irish as a whole. The same was true of some colonists who, feeling increasingly separate from their mother country, came to regard their proximity to the frontier and their involvement in frontier warfare as central to their unique identity; the frontier had already become the anvil on which a distinctive Anglo-Irish culture was hammered into being. For the English more generally, it was in the very nature of the colonial enterprise that the frontier came to represent so much more. There was a confusion at the heart of all this, for Ireland was at once a land of plenty but also, as one knight commented some years later, 'a strange, wild place consisting of tall forests, great stretches of water, bogs and uninhabitable regions'.[16] Another noble traveller, whilst entranced by the beauty of the native Irish people, was shocked not only by their bare feet and legs but by the way they showed 'all their shameful parts, the women as well as the men'.[17] Thus, for the English the frontier formed not just the extent of the colony and of royal administration too, but the limit of civilization itself.

There was nothing new in English prejudice: it had existed at the time of the conquest and even before; indeed, it had been used to justify the first Anglo-Norman expedition to Ireland and the subsequent establishment of a colony. When Prince John, the fourth son of Henry II, made his first visit to the island in his appointed capacity as king of Ireland in 1185, the nineteen-year-old prince, with his rowdy

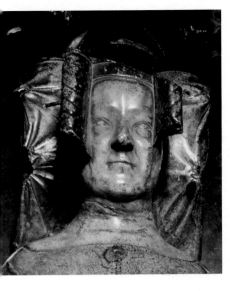

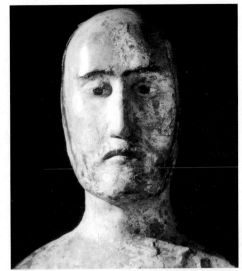

(*Above*) Philippa of Hainault, faithful consort of Edward III (*above right*), the consummate warrior king. They lost one daughter, Princess Joan, in the Great Death and two others – Mary and Margaret – died during the second epidemic.

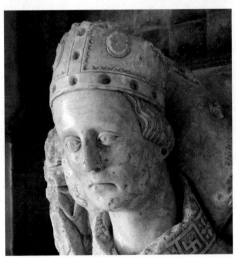

William Edington, bishop and administrator, was responsible in large part for the recovery of royal finances after the Great Death and the ambitious attempt to control wages.

Hapless David II of Scotland, captured at Neville's Cross, was incarcerated in England while his realm was ravaged by plague. After he returned in 1357, he ruled to impressive effect.

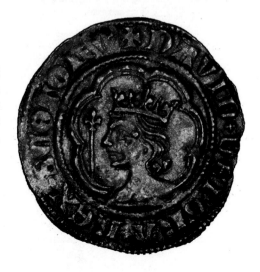

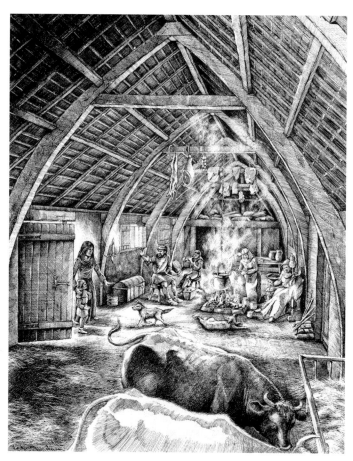

Although many peasant homes, like this recreation of a Northern 'cruck' house at Wharram Percy, were kept scrupulously clean, such close living quickened the spread of pestilence.

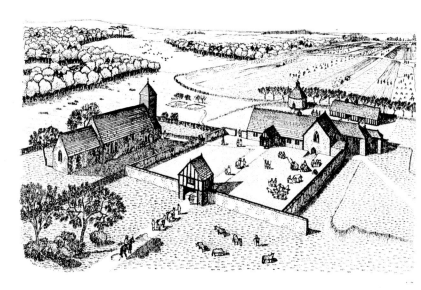

Rural communities were dominated by the manor house and church, as at Faccombe Netherton in Hampshire. The land of the manor was divided into strips and farmed in rotation.

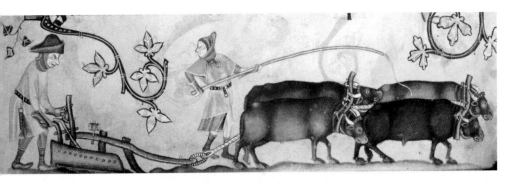

The lives of peasants, both men and women, were hard and changed only with the seasons. The Black Death elevated some and impoverished others but for most the monotony and graft continued.

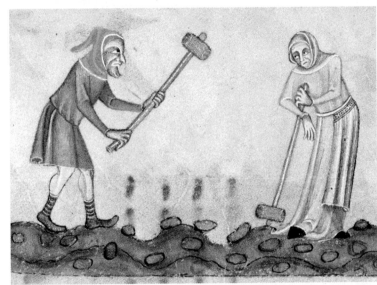

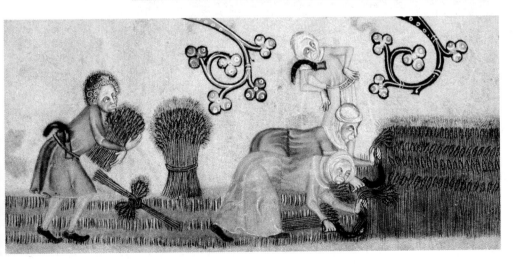

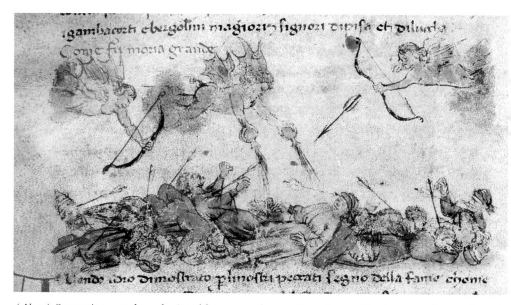

(*Above*) Scourging angels as depicted by an apothecary from Lucca. Pestilence whipped through Europe, carried along the trade routes that crossed the Continent. Widely believed to have been caused by corrupt air, the disease was rapid and indiscriminate, killing humble and mighty alike. (*Below*) The mortality was unprecedented everywhere: cemeteries, like this one in Tournai, were soon filled with the dead.

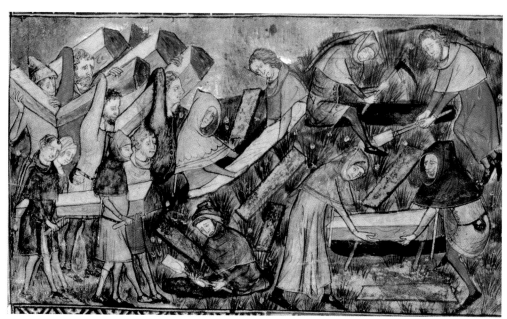

In London, mass graves were dug to the west, at Smithfield, and to the east, by the Tower (*right*). While some bodies were interred alone, most were laid in trenches.

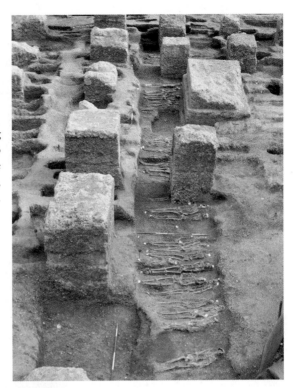

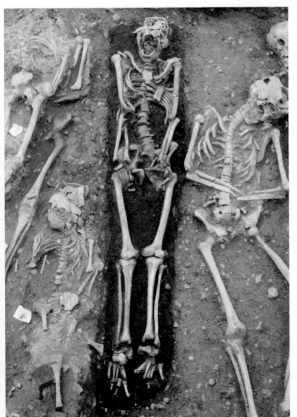

The more wealthy were afforded a coffin, charcoal-lined in the case of this central skeleton. Most, like the victim on the right, were dropped into place, one on top of another, as is clear from the bodies on the left, while the corpses of children were used to fill in the gaps.

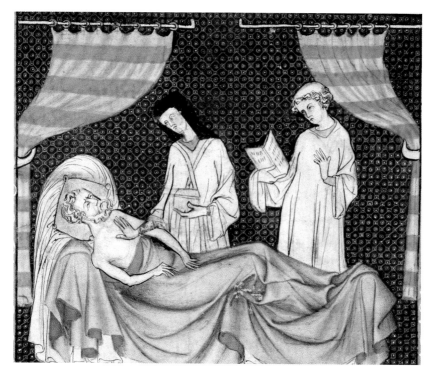

The 'good death': time to pray, a final confession, and priestly anointing. Yet many were denied this last ritual when pestilence took hold, as either death came too quickly or the local priest had been struck down.

William Wykeham's New College at Oxford was just one of several similar foundations intended to address the shortage of well-trained priests created by pestilence.

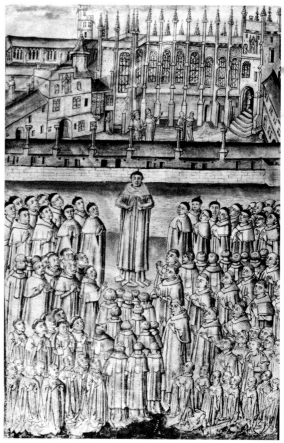

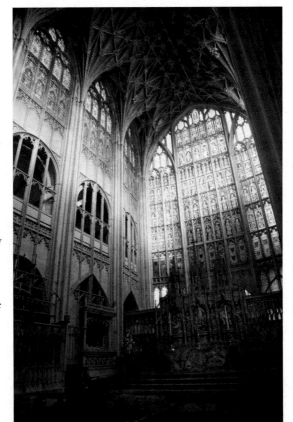

(*Right*) Work on the choir of Gloucester Cathedral was temporarily disrupted by plague. Here a new style (later called the Perpendicular) had already begun. The quality of the very best work of English artisans – like the east window at Gloucester and (*below*) the innovative priory church at Edington – was little affected by the mortality.

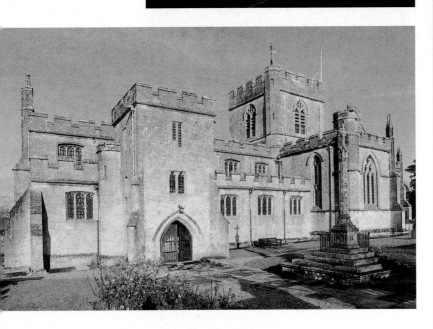

(*Right*) Legislation designed to prevent the display of new-found wealth banned many from wearing fine clothes and jewellery, such as this delicate silk and silver gilt chaplet, from a hoard buried in Germany at the time of the plague.

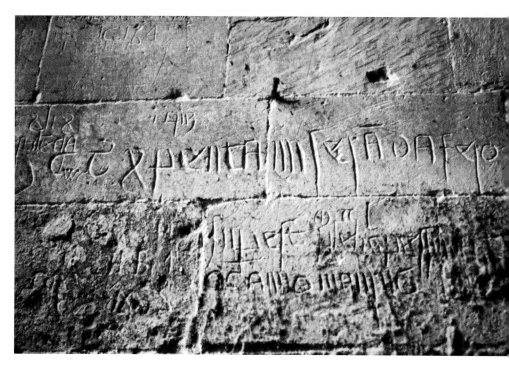

'A pitiable plague departed… leaving a wretched people to witness another plague, and in the end a mighty wind, Maurus, thunders throughout the world'

Wracked by repeated misfortune, the villagers of Ashwell etched their painful record into the stone of the tower of their church.

companions, tugged at the beards of the Irish chieftains who greeted him at Waterford.[vii] Insulted, these Irishmen later told the king of Connacht, Rory O'Connor,[viii] that John had behaved like an ill-mannered child. It was too generous a description, for this delinquent never did learn to behave as he should. When in August 1210, John – then king of England as well as Ireland – received the submission of Cathal Crovderg O'Connor[ix] (Rory's much younger brother and successor as king of Connacht), he laughed at the brave warrior when he saw him riding bareback, as was the Irish custom.

Although King John achieved a greater mastery over Ireland than any other medieval English king, it was not long before the royal chuckle began to ring a little hollow, for the Gaelic Irish kings came increasingly to act together in their rejection of English rule. In this sense, the presence of the English had done more than anything to give the Irish clans, who already enjoyed some sort of common identity, a common cause as well. Indeed, it was to the eternal shame of the Irish kings that it had been one of their own – Dermot MacMurrough[x] – who had first invited the English to Ireland, in a tragically misguided attempt to secure the High Kingship for himself; instead, Henry II supplanted the role for himself. At least now there was a single enemy on which all of them could focus; fittingly, Dermot's successor as king of Leinster, Art MacMurrough,[xi] was now foremost in that campaign.

Not that this meant that the Irish were in any way united. The Irish princes never eschewed their internecine rivalries: they persisted in the cattle raiding that so destabilized the pastoral economy and the horrendous violence that brought such ruination. One early fourteenth-century Gaelic poet bewailed this self-destruction: "tis Eire herself which has ruined this isle of ours; we find the land too tempting an object of attack.' However, that the Irish continued in equal measure to be divided amongst themselves and despised by the English helped (paradoxically) to preserve what was left of their territory. The colonists

---

[vii] John had been made king of Ireland in 1179.
[viii] King of Connacht 1156–86, High King of Ireland 1166–86; anglicized from Ruaidrí Ó Conchobair.
[ix] King of Connacht 1202–24; anglicized from Cathal Crobderg Ó Conchobair.
[x] Dermot MacMurrough, king of Leinster 1126–71; anglicized from Diarmait Mac Murchadha.
[xi] King of Leinster 1347–61.

had little interest in the bogs and mountains that lay beyond their cultivated manors, nor did they want much to do with what they perceived to be the wild barbarians who lived there. Moreover, they had always found it easier to fight and treat with the Irish piecemeal, separated as they were into so many clans, rather than launch the kind of wholesale invasion that may well have finished the native kingdoms off. This policy ensured that the Irish never managed to rally round a single leader but at the same time condemned the colonists to cohabiting with their indigenous neighbours. The result was perpetual instability, especially where the two sides ran up against each other, at the frontier. Ultimately, this volatile relationship favoured the Gaelic Irish, who were free to wage guerrilla war on the poorly defended colony, thereby reducing that portion of Ireland under the dominion of the English crown to the shrunken and dishevelled state that Edward III contemplated now.

It was this pathetic situation that greeted Sir Thomas Rokeby when at last he arrived in Dublin to take up the justiciarship on 20th December 1349. In addition to the depredations that followed the Irish raids, the hard-pressed Anglo-Irish colony was also trying to recover from the after-effects of plague. Rokeby had travelled through English counties half-emptied by pestilence; the country around Dublin had suffered in kind – at Colemanstown, a township in the manor of Newcastle Lyons a few miles from Dublin, only three tenants remained out of the sixteen that had lived there before the plague. Rokeby would soon discover that such a grievous loss of population and income obtained in every other part of the colony. As if this were not enough, the native Irish around Dublin, who had presumably shaken off the plague some months before, were raiding with renewed ferocity.[18] Elsewhere on the island the colonists were faring rather better, as much of Gaelic Ireland – from Thomond (roughly Clare) to south Ulster – was now in thrall to the same plague that had all but burnt out in the colony. Wherever the Gaelic Irish were stricken, there came a respite in cross-border fighting. Rokeby used the hiatus well. He moved first to clear out the Augean stables that the colonial administration had become, setting up an enquiry and placing the treasurer under arrest. Then, heeding the pleas for help from Carlow, Rokeby ventured out against the Leinster Irish, who – having endured the full term of the pestilence – were now safe to attack. Sir Thomas subdued their fighting bands and made the chieftains personally responsible for the maintenance of peace.

Far away, on the other side of the island, the pestilence maintained its westward march, unhindered by the wet Irish winter, even to the most distant hills of Connacht, where among many others it took William O'Dowd,[xii] the bishop of Killala, and Cathal O'Flaherty,[xiii] whose family dominated wild Connemara. The epidemic was now conquering territory never touched by the English nor even subjected to nominal Norman rule. Whilst nothing is known of the plague's progress in north Ulster or Kerry, we can assume with confidence that pestilence soon penetrated these places too – rapid and lethal, just as in the colony, just as in England. Among the survivors was Aodh MacEgan, whose Christmas prayer had been answered. On the anniversary of that desperate plea, he inscribed the same page again:

> A year ago this night since I wrote these lines on the margin below and may I by God's will reach the anniversary of this night. Many changes. Amen and Pater Noster.[19]

Many changes indeed. Yet although he was freed from the threat of plague, Aodh was still apprehensive about the future. The reason could well have been the English. For just as the plague receded in Gaelic Ireland, Rokeby's troops advanced against the native Irish, showing a determination that had not been seen – at least in the west of Ireland – for many decades. By the winter of 1350, when Aodh penned his thankful lines, Rokeby had done with Leinster and was now campaigning in south Thomond. On his appointment, this redoubtable marcher knight had been warned by Edward that Ireland was 'not in good plight or good peace'.[20] That Rokeby showed such willingness to reverse this state of affairs was for Ireland certainly something of a change. It cannot have been a welcome one for the native Irish, who had just suffered a mortality far greater than even they could inflict on themselves, or hope to mete out on their oppressor enemy. Satan, FitzRalph had alleged, was even-handed in his judgement of the peoples of Ireland: the distribution of misfortune and disease throughout the island had been correspondingly fair.

★   ★   ★

[xii] Anglicized from Ó Dubdha.
[xiii] Anglicized from Ó Flaithbheartaigh.

Edward III's interest in Ireland rose and fell in inverse proportion to his preoccupation with France, so it was fortunate that the post that Sir Thomas Rokeby was ordered to fill became vacant before events on the Continent drew the king's attention in that direction once again.[21] In the last week of August 1349, word reached Westminster that Philip VI had appointed a captain-general in the Saintonge,[22] with specific orders to raise an army and recapture territory held by the English to the north of Bordeaux. Edward's response was immediate: on Friday, 28th August, he appointed a panel of lawyers to investigate this breach of the truce, which had been signed only three months earlier and was supposed to have been valid for a full year. He did not need advice as to where the cause of the problem lay, however: it was in Gascony, where skirmishing had persisted despite the several promises made by Bishop Bateman at Guînes in May. Suitably attired in the fig-leaf of English legal rights, Edward sent the earl of Lancaster to Bordeaux in order to secure the duchy's frontier and force the French back into a truce.

In truth, Edward cannot have been surprised that the peace had unravelled. Not only had he anticipated a conflict concerning his secret treaty made with the Flemish in the autumn of the previous year[23] but his ever-efficient government had continued to collect taxes in preparation for the resumption of war, despite the dual obstacles of mass mortality and epidemic disease.[24] Writs were sent out on 16th July 1349 for the tax commissioners to renew their visits, even though pestilence was still raging in the Midlands, peaking in Staffordshire and spreading through the North. The writs contained a novel feature: the taxmen were ordered, in addition to their normal duties, to seek out and fine those contravening the new Ordinance of Labourers; all the money they received was to be sent back to the Exchequer with the usual revenues from taxation. Thus were the 'excesses' of common labourers to be taken away and put to use in furtherance of the king's foreign affairs.

It was a measure of the resilience of royal administration that it was able to effect the wishes of the king and council with such assurance and agility, maintaining a service to the crown despite the losses it had suffered through the months of plague. The Chancery lost three of its twelve senior officials, the Exchequer two of its senior clerks, while both the King's Bench and the Common Pleas lost attorneys and recording clerks.[25] These numbers were not great but, given that the corps of senior officials numbered only a few dozen, they were significant.[xiv] Fortunately, however, there were clearly enough clerks to fill the shoes of those who had died. (Indeed, Edington brought the veteran administrator William of Cusance out of retirement in July 1349 to run the wardrobe; he resigned, when things had settled down, after six months in the post.) In the provinces, however, royal officials had only limited clerical back-up, yet Westminster still expected county accounts to be presented as normal. So when the sheriff of Devon failed to render his account on the due date he was fined, a penalty he successfully disputed by explaining that he had been grievously ill (not, we must assume, from the plague) and had had no one to send in his place as his under-sheriff and all his other officials were dead from plague. The family of Robert Wymond, a tax collector in London, was even less fortunate, for no sooner had Robert dropped dead than the officials in Westminster ordered his property be seized as surety for debts that he still owed the crown. This was in May 1349, whilst plague was at its peak in the capital.[26] So although the plague may have created bureaucratic delay, it very rarely brought about administrative neglect. The royal accounts of the Tower of London give an eloquent example of this. The 1349 ledger begins in one hand, which then ceases, but despite the death that this almost certainly indicates, another hand resumes the entries to conclude the year.[27] Thus, regardless of the demise of so many local officials, the loss of senior clerks at Westminster, the death of not one but two chancellors, the continuing mortality and the fearful disease itself, the royal bureaucracy carried on: the Chancery remained open and the Exchequer kept to its customary terms, even extending through the summer months in order to help clear the backlog that had built up as a result of the plague.

Philip VI's administration, by contrast, had – in similar circumstances – been brought to its knees, to the point where for a while French government ceased to function. Why not so in England? Some credit is due to Edward, whose efforts in building a bureaucracy that could be relied upon to govern in his absence had endowed his government with remarkable resilience. Thus Westminster Hall was able to

[xiv] Among the dead was Thomas Clopton, the Keeper of the King's Wardrobe, who died in July only a few months after he had taken receipt of the goods of le Laurence from Richard Large. See Ch. 8, p. 178.

continue working through the epidemic, with the king in hiding from the disease. Edward's subjects had their own demands of the institutions of government as well, however, and these did not go away. Indeed, quite the opposite: Westminster Hall had to remain open through the plague months precisely because of the huge quantity of petitions, charters, accounts, tax returns and other business that was brought through its doors, much of it generated as a result of the plague. That Westminster could respond was in part a function of the nature of medieval English government, which – while sophisticated in comparison with other European powers – was by modern standards extremely limited. With so small a staff and so little complication, there was less that could go wrong in a time of crisis. Yet this was no ordinary crisis, for not only did the mortality kill crown officials but the epidemic spread fear and threatened panic, something from which Edward's clerks were not immune. So, while pestilence swirled all around, the king's officials showed great individual courage, just as his administration had demonstrated considerable corporate strength.

The experience cannot have been other than formative: this bureaucratic body had now proved that it had life and fortitude all of its own. Such new confidence may well have been the reason why the king's ministers felt able to take on new competencies – such as the control of wages and the terms of labour – which, if successfully discharged, would mark the greatest single encroachment of government on everyday life since the repressive innovations of William I. Yet this was not part of some great political design, nor evidence of a long-term trend that only we, today, may discern. Rather, it was the response of tested individuals within a strengthened bureaucracy to the specific circumstances that prevailed as a result of the plague.

Unlike his administrators, the king had been conspicuous in his absence throughout the crisis – just like other great magnates, he hid away from the epidemic. Edward's duty was not to lead the nation through this, or any other, natural catastrophe; nor was it to attend to the welfare of his people: the monarch's purpose was the proper ordering and defence of his realm, whose boundaries it was his right to define. It was in a return to this role that Edward re-emerged from seclusion in the summer of 1349. Having addressed himself to the breakdown in the truce across the Channel, he turned his attention to Canterbury, whose archbishop had died but two days before:[28]

Thomas Bradwardine, the third to hold the English primacy within a year, had been in office for only thirty-eight days. Now the king was faced with finding yet another replacement. The Canterbury monks proceeded to their election on 20th September. By now well-tamed, they chose correctly once again: it was to be Simon Islip, Keeper of the Privy Seal – another member of Edward's cadre of loyal administrators.[29] (Although the pestilence had long since departed, Bradwardine's belated death had made everyone nervous again, so Islip was enthroned in private, in order to keep the risk of infection to a minimum – much to the chagrin of the priory monks, for whom the installation of an archbishop was traditionally an excuse for celebration.)

The autumn of 1349 was otherwise relatively uneventful for Edward. Indeed, he found time to go to Hereford – a rare journey, as he seldom ventured beyond Oxfordshire. The king was bidden to the city at the invitation of Bishop Trillek to celebrate the translation of the bones of St Thomas Cantilupe to a new shrine in the cathedral. On 25th October there was to be a great service, which Trillek hoped might mark the beginning of a recovery among his traumatized flock: in his mandate to the senior clergy of the diocese ordering them to attend, he recalled the time that the bones of another St Thomas – Thomas Becket – were moved to a new shrine, 'after which all things prospered'.[30] How they must have hoped and prayed that this miracle would be repeated, for these priests and their parishioners had just experienced something of the torments of Hell.

The return journey to Hereford allowed Edward to survey the changes the Great Death had wrought on his realm: the crowdless roads, the uncultivated fields, the half-emptied villages, the newly enlarged churchyards, the unoccupied houses, abandoned mills and silent forges, all showing the early signs of dilapidation and decay. It surely had a profound effect on him; on his return to Westminster his impressions were certified by the large number of petitions his officials had received, complaining that many places would be unable to meet the demands of royal tax collectors, in large part because of the difficulty of finding and securing labour, at least at a reasonable rate. An inventive approach was devised, which might address both problems at the same time. On 21st November a new ordinance was sent out, proclaiming that the fines being raised by prosecutions brought under the original Ordinance of Labourers should be set against the current tenth and fifteenth. This was technically reverse hypothecation – putting the excess in wages towards a reduction in the burden of taxation. It was another innovation to bear the mark of Treasurer Edington's remarkable mind upon it.

Edward's primary concern, however, was not the relief of the nation but the ability of his Exchequer to gather in the tax that he had been promised by parliament before the pestilence had struck. So long as he was without a truce with France, Edward needed cash in his Treasury coffers so that he had the resources to be able to repulse any attack on his Continental possessions. News from Avignon that Richard FitzRalph had failed in his attempt to win a plenary Jubilee indulgence from the pope only served to compound his concern. He had hoped by this plan to prevent a mass pilgrimage to Rome which might deprive him of good soldiers and capable captains. Now that his ruse had been dashed, Edward sent out a decree on 1st December forbidding anyone to leave England, excepting those such as 'well-known merchants' for whom travel was necessary. The king was clearly on edge. He had good right to be. The threat would be realized even sooner than he had thought, though not in the form that he had feared.

The royal family and court were at Havering for Christmas, yet on Christmas Eve their celebrations were interrupted by the arrival of some shocking news: Aimeric de Pavia, the mercenary commander charged with defending Calais, had struck a deal with Geoffrey de Chargny, who had already caused so much trouble to the garrison, to allow entrance of a French force in return for a very considerable bribe.[31] The betrayal was scheduled for the morning of New Year's Day, only a week away, but the unreliable Italian had since got cold feet and had sent this message to Edward telling him of what was in the offing.[32] Appalled at the prospect of losing what he had won with such effort only two years before, Edward immediately cobbled together a force from his household soldiers and set out for the coast, accompanied by those few nobles, the Prince of Wales and Sir Walter Manny among them, who had been his guests at Havering for Christmas.

In not more than a week they were across the Channel and – after slipping anonymously into Calais harbour – hidden within the fortress town itself. Early on the appointed morning, Geoffrey's French force marched over the causeway that crossed the marshes which separated

Calais from the surrounding country and gained entry, as previously arranged, through the town gate, utterly unaware that there was an English force within. Just as the first group of French soldiers had made its way under the portcullis the drawbridge was quickly raised: Edward's trap had been sprung. The English – led by the redoubtable Manny – pounced on the intruders and then rode out from the town to set about the main force, sending de Chargny's soldiers across the marshes in flight.

With Calais saved, Edward relieved Aimeric de Pavia of his duties and sent him on a pilgrimage to Rome, where multitudes from around Europe were converging for the Jubilee. Eager that Aimeric should speak openly, often and well about what had happened, he sent the mercenary off with his pockets full of gold, the same that had been given him first as an enticement by the French, which Edward – all of a sudden full of magnanimity – now permitted him to keep as a reward. It was, of course, none other than a recycled bribe, whose necessity betrayed the pretension of Edward's claims and the base reality of his trespass in France.

Edward took his noble French prisoners from Calais back to London, where they joined the band of knights and princes that the English had captured during the several successes of recent years, among them Sir William Douglas of Liddesdale and David Bruce, king of Scotland. For these two men the Calais escapade only heaped misfortune upon their long run of bad luck. The king and his lieutenant had just passed their fourth Christmas in England; now it looked as though they would have to see through several more. It was Robert the Bruce who had wrung the famous victory of Bannockburn out of Edward II; it must have been to Edward III's considerable satisfaction, therefore, that he now held the fate of this younger Bruce in his hands.

More than the victory of honour he had secured, David's captivity brought with it the promise of peace in the Borders and an opportunity to re-establish English influence in Scotland itself. None of this could be achieved, however, by following a plan that involved Edward's old client in his wars with Scotland, Edward Balliol. Balliol was now ageing and unpopular, and had shown himself to be unequal to the challenge.[33] Edward was increasingly of the view that he now had most to gain by dealing directly with David himself, even though this would represent an about-turn on the policy to which he had adhered, albeit inconsistently, for the best part of twenty years. For despite the captivity of the Scots' king and the subsequent expeditions of Neville, Percy and Balliol into Scotland, the Scots were once again asserting themselves forcefully in their lowlands, the same where the Northern barons had been fighting only a matter of months before. It was apparent, therefore, that if Edward were able to come to an agreement with the Scots, whereby they would be bound to keep the peace, honour English claims in Scotland and ensure the payment of the ransom, then all would gain something from their king's release.

The draft terms of such an agreement were drawn up in 1348. They had as their basis the recognition of David as vassal-king of Edward III. For Edward this was a cosmetic concession; for the Scots it was an extraordinarily onerous demand, as its acceptance would mark the end of the independence of the Scottish crown and signal their final submission to the claims of overlordship first made by Edward I in 1291 – claims that had been in large part responsible for the appalling carnage that had filled the near sixty years that had since passed. Negotiations between the two kings' parties were further slowed by Balliol, who was proving hostile to any deal that compromised his claim to the Scottish throne. It was in an attempt to get the pretender to relent that Edward sent a memorandum to Ralph Neville in 1349, asking him to apply pressure to Balliol 'because [he] will not agree to good ways of establishing peace such as would seem reasonable to one side and the other'.[34] Yet Neville would find it hard to fulfil his mission, for Balliol had been forced by his Scottish opponents to retreat into Galloway – separated from Neville's castle at Bamburgh by more than a hundred miles of border country.[35] This may have been well-known territory to Neville but it was a region made extremely dangerous of late, not only by the activities of the lord of Douglas but – by the close of the year – by the presence of plague.

The Great Death had been creeping towards the border through the autumn of 1349 and probably seeped through during the winter. Although trade had been outlawed because of the war, the Scots were completely unprotected from the disease. The boundary between the two countries, although formally agreed in 1328, was respected by neither side:[36] the English had never ceased in their attempts to capture and secure land north of this boundary and in response the Scots had continued to fight the attempted occupation as well as making regular – albeit passing – incursions of their own into the northern English counties. In reality, therefore, the demarcated border meant very little; this was instead a broad frontier that stretched from Lanark and Lothian to Cumberland and Northumberland, encompassing all the country in between except the western extremity of Galloway, which remained not only fervently Scottish but the last Gaelic-speaking region south of the Clyde. Inherently there was a lack of stable lordship in this region, which allowed criminal gangs on both sides of the border to operate with impunity. One common practice was to kidnap someone from over the border for ransom, which would in turn be paid for in cattle stolen in some other cross-border raid. With pestilence all around, every one of these *bagarres* presented an opportunity for the disease to make its way over the border and into the villages which the Scots bandits used as their base.

The March was certainly a lawless place, even by the standards of the medieval North, beset by brigandage and the pillaging raids inflicted by both nations' armies. Yet for all its dilapidation, the March retained many of the features of the developed agricultural economy that had prospered when times had been more benign. Until its capture by the English in 1333, Berwick had been the wealthiest town in Scotland, boasting long-established trading links with Flanders, France and the Baltic ports. The town's market had since lost much of its Scottish hinterland but it still continued to attract goods from both sides of the border, in large part because the bridge here was the most heavily used crossing over the Tweed. Further up that river, at Norham, Coldstream and – a few miles into Scottish territory – at Sprouston, there were more bridges, linking the roads that ran on both sides of the Tweed valley from Berwick to Kelso. Here was the first of the great Border abbeys which, with Jedburgh, Dryburgh, Melrose and Peebles, controlled huge tracts of border pasture and farmland. The vast production of these abbeys was traded not only in Scotland but in England and abroad; Melrose, for instance, had a flock, rather later in the century, of 15,000 sheep and was widely famed for the wool it produced.[37] Even on the western border, which was in every sense more remote, fords and tracks allowed passage from Cumberland into Annandale and Nithsdale, the same that David had used to cross the frontier on his last campaign in October 1346. Thus, despite the bans imposed by royal governments and the best efforts of local thugs, cross-border trade persisted, now carrying with it a lethal fellow traveller unseen.

By its nature, very little of this illicit cross-border traffic – both in goods and in violence – was a matter of record. The official account of how pestilence crossed into Scotland was left, therefore, to English chroniclers, who took great delight in the humiliation of the Scots. In an episode several of them repeated with sardonic relish, Scots troops (most probably those of William, lord of Douglas) descended from Selkirk Forest upon the English of Teviotdale in the joyful certainty that God had favoured them 'by the foul death of the English'.[38] As the native Irish had already found, however, the pestilence showed no such favour. So here, in the rolling Borders, the disease was passed from the English frontiersmen to Scots farmers, traders and warriors, all of whom returned home to their families and villages, unwittingly spreading the disease around. Once established in the Borders, there was nothing to impede the passage of pestilence throughout Scotland: from Selkirk a road ran via Peebles and Biggar through upper Clydesdale, where it joined the road from Crawford that ran to Glasgow and Dumbarton. There was a main road from Biggar to Edinburgh too, just as there were main roads to Edinburgh from Berwick, via Haddington, and from Roxburgh, by Kelso.[39]

It is possible that even before plague-carrying travellers arrived in Edinburgh by road, pestilence had already taken hold, via its long-established trading links with the Low Countries and with Bruges in particular. Scots merchants had possessed exclusive trading rights in Bruges since the last century, one that had grown as trade with Scotland's nearest neighbour was disrupted by war; since Berwick's fall, the sea route diverted to the next nearest significant burgh – Edinburgh. As the Great Death had arrived in Bruges in July 1349 and was present there until October, it is entirely likely that it had been transported to Edinburgh by the autumn – by which point the English epidemic had still not reached the border – and was manifesting itself by Christmas.

Edinburgh and the other large Scottish burghs had been founded along English administrative lines but had been built with the Continental pattern in mind. Although the urban populations were very small, the houses were tall and tightly packed, with narrow frontages crowding the streets; unique to Scotland, however, were the long 'backlands' that ran out behind. Only the church and the very wealthy built in stone; everywhere else buildings were made of the same materials used out in the villages – timber frames filled with wattle and daub, thatched with heather or straw. In Scotland as elsewhere towns provided the best place for the plague epidemic to expand and then explode into the surrounding countryside. It was only a matter of time, therefore, before the epidemic made its way out of Edinburgh northwards, crossing the Forth with the ferrymen of Queensferry into Fife and across the narrow bridge at Stirling, from where the road ran on to Perth. With Dundee and Aberdeen, Perth was one of three great burghs that lay in a line to the north-east of Edinburgh, a string of ports and market centres for the predominantly English-speaking people who lived in the eastern lowlands that ran, roughly, from Stirling to the valley of the river Spey. Well-travelled roads connected these burghs, along which travelled consignments of hides, cereals, manufactured goods, wool and fish, just as they did between the many towns of England and colonial Ireland.[40]

Here also there is very little to prove that plague passed through; it should not be doubted, however, that it came to every one. St Andrew's cathedral, only a short journey from Dundee, lost twenty-four (a third at least) of its canons, while in Aberdeen a chaplain named John Fordun left an account of the epidemic that could only have come from someone who had seen the Great Death first hand:[41]

In 1350 there was a great pestilence and mortality of men in Scotland, and this pestilence also raged for many years before and after this in various parts of the world, indeed, throughout the whole globe. So great a pestilence has never been heard of from the beginning of the world to the present day, or recorded in books. For this plague vented its spite so thoroughly that fully a third of the human race was killed. At God's command, moreover, the damage was done by an extraordinary and novel form of death. Those who fell sick of a kind of gross swelling of the flesh lasted for barely two days. This sickness befell people everywhere, but especially the middling and lower classes, rarely the great. It generated such horror that children did not dare to visit their dying parents, or parents their children, but fled for fear of contagion as if from leprosy or a serpent.[42]

The pestilence spread out from the burghs into its hinterland, just as in England, just as it would be expected to do. Perceton, for example, the farmstead near Irvine, most probably received the disease from the flourishing little burgh of Glasgow, just over twenty miles to the north-east. Perceton was in many ways typical of the hybrid manors, or 'touns', that had been established in lowland Scotland over the previous 200 years, whose *modus operandi* made the transmission of plague through these parts nothing but certain. Set within a rectangular site, enclosed by a moat and palisade to give protection against both English and local bandits, there was a simple manor house, barns and a corn-drying kiln (which hinted at the added difficulty of cereal agriculture in these northern climes). Touns like Perceton possessed many of the features of the English manor (a court, a mill, and the vestiges of military service) but the binds between the lord (or 'thane') and peasant were, in relevant ways, different. As in England serfdom had largely disappeared but the rigid system of labour services that persisted in so much of England and colonial Ireland was not widespread. Instead, both the more-substantial peasant landholders ('husbandmen') and those with minimal holdings (cottars) held land on a short lease, paid for out of a cash rent generated in part by the sale of surplus crops (including oats, flax, barley and rye) in local markets.[43]

Nonetheless, the relationship between thane and bondman was still essentially feudal, one that had enhanced – as in England – the beneficial effect that successive good harvests and low levels of epidemic disease had had on fertility. As a result, Scotland's population, in common with those of most other countries in Europe, had boomed over the previous two centuries. In tandem, more and more marginal land was being farmed, so that in places agriculture extended into the barely fertile uplands, at an unusual height in excess of 300 metres above sea level. Thus, on the eve of the Great Death, there were something approaching a million mouths to feed in Scotland, a number that was sustained only because more of the country was under cultivation than ever before, or since. All these people, all this food, all this trade: the pestilence will have had no difficulty in spreading through the lowland touns of Scotland, killing at least a third – probably more – as it went.

Lowland Scotland only constituted half of the country's territory, the rest forming the Highland region, which enjoyed somewhat different economic and political traditions. Largely Gaelic-speaking, the society of the kin-based clans that dominated the Highlands bore closer resemblance to their Gaelic cousins across the Irish Sea than they did to the mostly anglicized Lowland Scots. It would be a mistake, however, to paint these two regions – Lowland and Highland – as entirely separate and different, for they were not. Although the Scots of the south and Lowland east had long ago switched from speaking Gaelic to English, their customs – in law, kin-based landholding, military service and much else – all showed that they shared with the Highlanders a common Celtic inheritance. Just as Lowland society, regulated by modified Anglo-Norman feudal structures, retained many traces of far older Scottish customs, Highland society was not immune from the innovations that the immigrants had introduced. Lowland burghs, for instance, had become more and more important to the Highland economy, as it was in their markets that Highlanders were able to sell their predominantly pastoral products – milk, meat, wool, hides and bone; in return they purchased manufactured goods and small luxuries, some imported from abroad. So whilst Glasgow communicated with Perceton and other manors to the south, it also dealt with the Highlands that lay to the north and north-west. There could be no stronger symbol of these links than the new stone bridge that had been built to cross the Clyde in 1339, enabling traffic to pass between the lowlands around Renfrew and the hills and sea lochs of Bute and the Cowal peninsula to the north. The growing unity between Lowland and Highland Scotland was accompanied and advanced by the interlinking of their respective noble chiefs, both noble castes, for instance, having immigrant blood. Thus, any separation between these two parts of Scotland was in many senses less real than apparent.

To the extent that any divisions remained between Highland and Lowland society, however, they will have done almost nothing to prevent the passage of the Great Death from the burghs and Lowland fields to the islands and Highland hills. For as Lowland cultivation pushed into the foothills of the Highlands it was all the more likely that the epidemic would pass from lowland agriculturalists to upland pastoralists. There was every reason, therefore, to suppose that the Great Death moved into the Highlands both through local mixing between people in the fields and villages of the Highland foothills and through political contacts and normal trade.

That the Great Death was as active in the Highlands of Scotland as it was elsewhere in the British Isles can be assumed with some confidence, therefore. Indeed, the fact that the Great Death passed between the Anglo-Irish and the Gaelic Irish, and once established then spread quickly around, makes it all the more likely that the same should be true for the Gaelic Scots, whose settlements and farming practices were akin to those of the Gaelic Irish and who, moreover, enjoyed a far more open relationship with their Lowland neighbours than the native Irish ever achieved with the Anglo-Irish colonists. The mountains of Scotland posed their own challenges but even here there is strong parallel evidence to suggest their infection by plague. Norway, which received the disease about a year before Scotland, had a similar Highland population living in comparable terrain.[44] There, fortunately for the historian, the records are better: they show that the epidemic passed through the sharp-sided valleys at almost the speed that it achieved in the more densely populated flatlands of France and England.[45] Finally, an Icelandic annal clearly states that the 'pestilence visited the Shetland Islands, the Orkney Islands, the Hebrides and the Faroe Islands'.[46] At the time Shetland and Orkney were both Norwegian possessions but the Hebrides were in the hands of John MacDonald, lord of the Isles (Uist) and William, earl of Ross (Lewis and Skye). If the disease was able to move quickly through the Gaelic Irish, penetrate into deepest Norway and make the jump not only to the Northern Isles but to the Scottish Hebrides, there can be little doubt that the Great Death spread to the extremities of Scotland, completing its terrible journey across the full extent of the British Isles.[47] Throughout Scotland, as elsewhere, every barrier that might be imagined to impede the movement of people and the progress of disease, be it physical or political, ultimately had no effect. Thus, as it travelled from the toe of England to the tip of Scotland, covering the distance in a little over two years, the Great Death provided the greatest single proof of the ever-increasing extent to which the lives of medieval people, for all their manifold differences, both defied containment and were, in subtle ways, interlinked.

12

Resurgam

1350–1351

Fortune gan flateren thenne tho fewe þat were alyue[i]
William Langland, *Piers Plowman*[1]

Edward's celebratory banquet at Calais was hardly at an end before
messengers had set sail for England, carrying the happy news. The
heroic defence of Calais had been a personal triumph. Many, however,
still had deep reservations about the king's Continental policy, especially that class of taxpayer represented in the Commons. The Calais
adventure was a perfect rejoinder to the doubters. As required, the
dutiful new archbishop of Canterbury, Simon Islip, immediately wrote
to the bishop of London, Ralph Stratford, commanding him to 'advance
the general rejoicing'.[2] Not afraid to associate the defence of Calais
with what he claimed was another sign of divine favour – the end of
plague – Islip prompted Stratford to 'bring the king's victory and the
remembrance of the pestilence to your people's notice'. Penitential
psalms should be sung and the usual processions begun, so that his
flock may sincerely contemplate 'the past and present gifts of God'.
For not only had the nation survived 'the amazing pestilence which
lately attacked these parts' but now 'our magnificent king' had subdued
'certain enemies . . . wonderfully to his authority, conquering the great
host by his military skill and putting it to flight'.[3] It is doubtful that
Londoners were as excited as the archbishop intended them to be:
after all, it had not even been a year since Ralph Stratford had stood
with Sir Walter Manny by the side of the new burial pit at West Smithfield, readying it through consecration for the many thousands of

[i] Fortune then began flattering those few that were alive.

bodies that were being carted from the city's gates every day. The warrior-knight might now be a hero of Calais; Londoners were more concerned, however, with the task of putting their lives, and their city, in order again.

King Edward had lost but one child to the pestilence; most of his subjects had lost much, much more. Little Thomas Worlingworth, the son of one of London's leading goldsmiths,[4] first lost his family and then his adoptive parents: his mother and father had died within a couple of days of each other at the beginning of May 1349 and the orphan, who was no older than nine, had been left in the custody of John and Joanna Bret, who were most likely old friends of the Worling-worths. No doubt they were fond of the boy, and he of them. Within weeks, however, John Bret died and was buried at West Smithfield, leaving a bequest for the new chapel that Sir Walter Manny planned to build there. Thomas, already orphaned once, was now without his adoptive father. He still had Joanna, however; but within eighteen months she too had died, although the pestilence – having long since left London – was not to blame. So John Hiltoft, another goldsmith, took over the boy's legal wardship and it is likely that he took him in.[5]

Although the Great Death had brought Thomas tremendous loss, it had also given him an enormous and early fortune. He was just one among many individuals who found themselves, all of a sudden, in possession of new wealth. Many had never expected to have been left so much, so soon. The estate of William Greyland (who had worked tirelessly, settling the wills of his friends and relations before succumbing to the plague himself) passed, together with a number of shops and tenements belonging to William's sister Johanna Colchester, to a certain Richard Sterre. Thus, as a result of these coinciding deaths and in the absence of any other heirs, Richard was the adventitious beneficiary of a significant portfolio of property.

The Great Death was indeed a giant lottery. Some were spared, others were killed. Families and estates vanished for ever, while a fortunate number came into an inheritance. Many were impoverished: the vast majority owned very little, and family and community were the intangible assets that sustained lives; when these vanished, the poor had nothing to support them. Some, however, especially those who already had means, were able to make use of the many opportunities for profit thrown up by so many deaths. Thomas Harewold, for instance, moved quickly in 1349 to buy up the shops of a widow whose husband, a rich mercer, had died. Harewold's fellow grocer, William Thorney, acquired a new shop in St Antonin's parish immediately after the death of a vintner but he, like many, had no time to enjoy the benefit of his new asset as he fell victim to the plague within a matter of weeks. Yet wherever there was death, there was opportunity, and so a certain John Weston, who had began his city career as a roper, now changed his allegiance to the grocers because of the openings created by the many vacancies made by the Great Death. Thomas Worlingworth had been an unwilling participant in this black roulette; men like Harewold, Thorney and Weston had played actively and with enthusiasm.

The religious foundations of London were also the beneficiaries of this massive transfer of capital and cash. Many suddenly found themselves, in the space of a few months, with decades' worth of bequests. The friars made the greatest gains in this gruesome windfall. As plague receded, benefactions had poured in – not just on the execution of the wills of the dead but from those thankful to be alive. The brothers put the money to work as soon as they could: the Crutched Friars[6] near Tower Hill started construction of an expensive new chapel in 1350. In the same year the Carmelite (or Whitefriars) of Fleet Street began rebuilding their church with funds given by the earl of Devon, the mayor and commonalty of the city, and numerous less exalted London citizens whose names no longer survive. On the other side of the city the Augustinian (or Austin Friars) were at a similar game, pressing on with the completion of a new nave to their church (paid for in part by a bequest from Humphrey de Bohun), which would soon stand high among the tenements crammed close by.[7] None of this compared with the riches amassed by the Franciscan or Grey Friars, however. This first and largest of the mendicant orders had been bequeathed so much property during the epidemic that it had become one of the largest landlords in the city. The king was so concerned at this that on 15th October 1349 he ordered the mayor to prevent the Franciscans from developing any more land for profit, as they 'ought to live by begging according to their rule',[8] at least until the crown had established whether they had legal title over everything they now claimed as their own.[9]

Believing that the city government, London's civic policeman, was looking the other way, a far smaller landowner used the pestilence to make a speculation of a different kind. Certainly no one noticed the modest building project under way in Watling Street, where builders continued to work through the pestilential months of 1349. It was an impressive house, at least more impressive than that which had been there before: for it was not only far higher than the previous building but also had many more windows. The property's owner clearly hoped that, amidst all the pestilential confusion, no one would notice his many contraventions of the city's tight planning regulations, which gave neighbours considerable rights of objection to new developments. Perhaps the neighbours here had died and there was no one to care that the new house both overlooked the rear of the next door building and blocked the light from its yard. In the great scheme of things it was a minor infraction. Yet this small construction project in Watling Street showed something that was true of Londoners through the ages: whatever was thrown at them, many still kept their eye fixed on the main chance. It was this, rather than any action by the city authorities, that had kept the city going.

Not that this should diminish the achievement of the mayor, John Lovekin, and his aldermen during the terrible months of plague. The maintenance of civic administration in London was testament to the constancy of its institutions and the persistence of its officials, despite the extraordinary volume of business officials were required to work through. It was a personal achievement too for Lovekin, who had assumed the mayoralty just as pestilence appeared and had guided the commonalty through the vicissitudes of the plague year. He must have been thankful to have survived. The son of a wealthy fishmonger, Lovekin had grown up in the Surrey town of Kingston, on the southern bank of the Thames. He had built an impressive fortune upon his inheritance, owning one of the large river-front houses, not far from Sir John Pulteney's house at Coldharbour. Yet he had never forgotten where he had come from and had further endowed a chapel dedicated to St Mary Magdalene in Kingston that his father had built. Just before the plague he had commissioned the great mason William Ramsey, who had recently remodelled the cloisters of St Paul's, to design a new building for the site. Although Ramsey had perished in the epidemic, Lovekin at once set about completing the project, realizing a little jewel that its creator would never get to see; it is one of the few remaining examples of Ramsey's work, with its neat corner turrets and uncomplicated elevations, innovative and complete.

Although the pestilence had now departed London, Lovekin's successor, Walter Turke, had to contend with new problems that even his predecessor did not have to face. Half-emptied but now free of plague, it was no surprise that the streets of the metropolis drew people in from the countryside around. Inevitably this created problems of its own. So many newcomers, vying between each other and with surviving Londoners, made a sure recipe for dispute. Besides those looking for honest work, some of whom were prepared to sleep rough, there were doubtless many who were interested only in crime, not least in the many houses standing empty which seemed to invite burglary. Whilst these were not new problems in themselves, the sheer scale of the immigration posed a fresh challenge to the city's sheriffs. So concerned had they been that they had approached their counterparts in Westminster to ask that they be granted indemnity in any police action that they took. The crown had been more than happy to grant this, and on 29th December 1349 had sent a writ to the Guildhall giving them all the powers they could want. Noting the 'many evildoers and disturbers of the peace who have come armed there . . . , and others of whom there is notorious suspicion or found wandering by night . . . , as well as others who have broken the peace there, and in the present great concourse of aliens and denizens to the city and suburbs', the writ stated that 'now that the pestilence is stayed, it is very necessary for them to cause the king's peace to be inviolably kept . . .'.[10] This was London as it had always been: bustling, dangerous, chaotic, full of promise and the object of dreams. It was hardly a city overwhelmed by grief.

Numbered among the dead of London were near on half its 'free' citizens – the electorate and commercial mainstays of the city. In 1350, as soon as the many inheritances had been settled, the city clerks drew up a new register of the freemen in each ward. Although many of the names were familiar, the faces were different: the influx of immigrants and the huge turnover within existing families of freemen had given a refreshed, more youthful, complexion to the capital's citizen body. A similar process was going on in towns across England. In Canterbury 136 new burgesses were added to the city roll between 1349 and 1351

– so great a number that it was felt that not all were sufficiently versed in the city's regulations. So, on 20th September 1351, the city ordinances were read out aloud in the burghmoot for the benefit of the many new freemen who were not aware of all their provisions. There were 109 admissions to the freedom of Norwich between 29th September 1349 and 2nd January 1350. For every new freeman who had made it onto the city rolls, there may have been ten or more immigrants not rich enough to purchase the freedom of the city. These figures suggest a very considerable degree of urban immigration. Even this, though, was not sufficient to repopulate these towns and cities completely. In Norwich four of the city's fifty-one churches were abandoned, for want of parishioners.

Civic life was quick to revive. Some of the new citizens of Norwich were doubtless involved in the foundation of the new Tailors' Guild in 1350; in Lincoln the Guild of Corpus Christi came into being in the same year. The latter's foundation deed tells us much about the impatience felt by so many ambitious townsmen – many of them immigrants – who, seeing the opportunities that the mortality had made for them, were all the more frustrated by the restrictions that were imposed by the old ruling order. The guild, the statutes explain, had been founded by 'folks of common and middling rank'. Neither the mayor nor the bailiffs would be allowed to be members, unless they be of 'humble, good and honest conversation' and abide by the same rules of election and conduct as everyone else. Further, 'no one shall have any claim to office in this gild on account of the honour and dignity of his personal rank.'[11]

The rapid replacement of burgesses was testament to the resilience of provincial municipal administration. This was not an isolated act of civic will, however, but a sure reflection of the robust commerce that many towns continued to enjoy. The signs are not dramatic but they are definite nonetheless. There was, for instance, clearly still life in the Wiltshire cloth industry, which centred on the new town of Salisbury,[12] while in Yarmouth there may have been an absolute fall in demand for herring, but not in terms relative to the number of merchants now vying for business.[13] Further up the east coast at Grimsby, a prosecution for wool-smuggling in 1350 demonstrated that the custom was at least worth evading, a sure sign of revived demand.[14] In Coventry the turnaround was more definite still. The fall in the value of rents in the immediate aftermath of the pestilence, no doubt a response to the glut of property on the market and the poor sentiment among buyers, was already corrected by the summer of 1350. In that August, St Mary's Guild, which had become the trustee for so many dead merchants' estates, was able to rent some shops in Gosford Street on a full-repairing lease at a good rate. Clearly Coventry had already bounced back.

The loss of population in Cambridge, however, had a severe short-term effect. Not long after the plague had receded, the vicar of the church of All Saints in the Jewry was granted a stipend by the diocesan officials because 'parishioners have in the meantime suffered for so long from the pestilence, which is well-known to be taking hold in this year, so that the oblations of those coming to the said church are by no means sufficient for the necessities [of living].'[15] Yet within months of the plague's exit from the university town, there was once again activity all around; indeed, it was almost as if the passing of the pestilence had reinvigorated the still young university. Edmund Gonville continued with his collegiate foundation, while Bishop Bateman, relieved temporarily in early 1350 from his diplomatic responsibilities, embarked on a project all of his own – the foundation of Trinity Hall.[16] In the same year King's Hall, which had suffered grievously during the pestilence, expanded along what is now Trinity Street and the following year Pembroke Hall (which had been founded just two years before the plague, in 1347) acquired a hostel for accommodation on its current site. It was not just the university that was building: in 1350 the Franciscans set about enlarging their church, which catered for both townsmen and the academic community.[17] Thus was Cambridge growing again by the time the first new year after the plague had passed. Whatever damage the disease had done, it had been temporary.

Oxford, on the other hand, was suffering terribly from the depredations inflicted by the pestilence, which had heaped misery onto what was already a declining town. If the Crutched Friars had been sensible, they would have seen this to have been the case; their foundation, made in the aftermath of plague, proved to be short lived. They needed only to have looked over the road at the house of another small mendicant order, the Trinitarian Friars, which was served by a sole brother at the time. In 1351 the king repossessed the land. On the other side of Merton College was St Edward's, which had not had a vicar since 1349; it probably lay empty from that date, never to be used again.[18] Unlike in Norwich, these empty churches gave a true indication of a town in decay. Moreover, the continued depression in rents showed that recovery would be a long time coming. The chantry established in the will of the wealthy burgess Nicholas Garland, dedicated to St Thomas the Martyr in the church of St Mary Magdalene in St Giles's Street, just beyond the North Gate, ran into trouble almost as soon as his testament had been granted probate. The property he had endowed the chantry with had lost so much of its value that it was not sufficient to cover the cost of the chantry priests. So a fraternity was quickly established, with the modest entrance fee of 6s. 8d., so that additional sums could be raised towards the cost of the foundation. It was a pretty picture in how the pestilence had changed the circumstances of Oxford townsmen, even those who were dead, for now Garland was forced to share his chantry with less-estimable burghers, the prayers for his soul thereby reduced because of a post-mortem fall in the worth of the assets he had left. It remained to those still alive to do all they could to bring about a recovery. Thus, on 20th April 1350, the burgesses lifted all charges and tolls they had previously imposed on merchants, not only because of the pestilence but because of the earlier collapse in trade.

Oxford was not alone in the doldrums. The collapse in rents in Winchester, for instance, showed no sign of reversing,[19] while Dunwich – long ago reduced by the invading sea to little more than an impoverished fishing harbour, pleaded with the king in 1351 to have its feudal levy reduced. Yet both these places, like Oxford, were – to a greater and lesser extent – all suffering before the pestilence came their way; the mortality only served to accentuate their decline. Without exception, those towns which had a vibrant economy before the Great Death recovered quickly from its effects. In this way, pestilence did little to alter the fate of a town but merely accelerated a trend already in place.

Buoyed by their victory in Calais, the returning troops were greeted by miserable scenes at home. The January landscape was not bare as it should have been, but unkempt. Much of the crop planted as usual in the autumn of 1348 and spring of 1349 had not been harvested and so lay collapsed, rotting in the fields. Acres of dead thistles showed where not one but two ploughings had been missed. As William Dene reported, the county was 'spoiled and wasted and stripped of all its possessions. The shortage of labourers and of workers in every kind of craft and occupation was then so acute that more than a third of the land throughout the whole kingdom remained uncultivated.' The little villages and hamlets of the Weald, which had turned out to cheer many of these men on their return from the triumph of Crécy and capture of Calais, had been half emptied. Houses were left cold by death, 'buildings and walls were crumbling' through desertion.[20] It was not just the reduction in cultivation that was evident: at Chartham, near Canterbury, the river fishery, which had previously been rented out for 22s. per year,[ii] was now standing disused for want of fishermen (little wonder that Dene complained there was 'a shortage of fish').[21] At Meopham, just beyond Rochester, the brewers had reduced their output by 40 per cent, whilst at Tudeley, near Tonbridge on the western side of the county, the two forges belonging to Thomas Harry were lying idle on account of the Great Death.

The devastation of the countryside and the dilapidation of villages, according to the refrain of almost every observer – whether they be monastic chronicler, royal escheator or local manor clerk – was a result of the mortality caused by pestilence. It is important to make plain, first of all, that the death rates among different parts of the population had differed. Among the magnates there were very few losses: the deaths of Sir Robert Bourchier, Thomas Wake and the marcher lord Hugh Despenser were rare exceptions.[22] Such light mortality among the fifty or so great lords undoubtedly reflected a low overall death-rate among the wider noble class, which has been calculated, with some accuracy, to have been 27 per cent.[23] It is a similar estimate to the death rate among the English bishops who suffered only three losses (which can safely be attributed to pestilence) during the plague years – a figure that equates to a mortality rate of no more than 20 per cent.[24] There were no deaths among the Welsh bishops and none recorded for Scotland, although it is possible that the death rate among bishops in Ireland might have been slightly higher than among their counterparts in England (perhaps because their ministry was more personal than was that of many of the grand magnate bishops of

---

[ii] i.e. £1.10.

England), approaching a death rate of a third.[25] The bishops' registers indicated a higher mortality rate still among the English clergy,
of between 40 and 45 per cent, a figure that is often matched (where
it is known) by the rate of death among the men and women in religious houses. The relatively low mortality among the elite of nobles
and bishops says little, therefore, about the virulence of the epidemic
but more about the ability of these favoured groups to move out of
harm's way, or alternatively seek safe seclusion until the pestilence
had passed, as did Humphrey de Bohun and also the king.[26] For the
vast majority of people, who had no option but to stay within their
town or village, empirical and anecdotal evidence points to
a death rate of around 50 per cent, sometimes less but very often
considerably more.

The first economic consequence of this enormous mortality was
a fall in prices. There may be some truth to Henry Knighton's view
that the collapse was first triggered by 'the fear of death . . . , for
there were very few who cared for wealth and possessions'. However,
sentiment alone was not enough to keep prices down after the
plague had gone, for the laws of supply and demand applied now
as much as they had done before. The crop planted in 1348 was sown
for double the population left to consume it after the harvest in
1349; as Knighton had it, 'in the year of the plague . . . there was
such an abundance of grain that almost no one cared for it.'[27] This
was enough to cause prices to tumble, so much so that it was not
even worth harvesting some of the crop.[28] It would be reasonable
to expect there to have been some upward correction over the course
of the following season, 1349–50, as less land was sown by a smaller
labour force for fewer mouths: prices should, therefore, have returned
to their usual level. Yet still prices remained stubbornly low, held
down by the surplus still remaining from the previous year and –
through remitted rents – a reduction in the capital cost of cultivation. Thus, in Somerset the cost of wheat in 1350 was still down by
about a half its pre-plague level, while that for oats and barley fell
by nearly three quarters.

Even this might be to underestimate the spectacular reduction in
prices that immediately followed the Great Death. Although the population was now around 50 per cent of its former size, the number of
coins in circulation remained as it had been before the pestilence. This

changed relationship was equivalent to a massive increase in the money supply, leading to rapid inflation. While this was not sufficient to counteract the collapse in prices, it did make that fall appear less dramatic than it had actually been. The real drop in commodity and livestock prices had, therefore, probably been even more precipitous than the figures given in the manorial accounts suggest.

Wages, on the other hand, went up, as manorial accounts and the complaints of employers made abundantly clear. In Somerset, a reaper cost 6½d. per acre in 1350, whereas before the Great Death he will have charged only 3d. At Pré, in south Hertfordshire, a labourer could earn 4d. for threshing a quarter of wheat in 1350, double what he could have earned in the early 1340s. At Teddington in Middlesex, meanwhile, carters and ploughmen saw their annual wage rise from 4s. 6d. and 6s. respectively, to a common rate of 11s.[iii] The carpenters and tilers employed by the reeve John Runwick at Farnham in Surrey to build stabling for all the animals received as heriots charged between 6d. and 10d. per day, instead of the 3d. they had been paid before the pestilence came. In short, labourers everywhere were demanding and receiving higher pay.

The new scarcity of labour certainly accounted for a good part of the widespread rise in wages; it was also true, however, that inflation was at work here too. All things being equal, the fall in prices should have produced a corresponding rise in the buying power of labourers (their 'real' wage), dampening a good part of the demand for higher wages. However, wages increased as prices declined, and despite the (inconsistent) implementation of the Ordinance of Labourers, pay remained high. Inflation was to blame: given that some workers were in a better negotiating position than others, it is unlikely that this near-universal rise in wages would have occurred had the money supply contracted in line with a much-reduced population. Instead, there was more coin in circulation relative to the number of people handling it and its value, therefore, fell. Labourers were right to ask for more money for the same work, as money was now worth less. To employers, however, the effect was to make the rise in wages appear greater than it actually was in real terms. All of this was

[iii] i.e. from approx. £0.23 and £0.30 to £0.55, equating to a rise of 144 and 83 per cent respectively.

perfectly clear to contemporaries, even if they explained the problem without the benefit of modern economic terms: 'the threshers, labourers and workmen were so well-supplied with cash', said William Dene, 'that they did not need to worry about paying the full price for . . . foods.'[29]

This was not the sum of landowners' problems, however, for the mortality among tenants had caused an immediate and dramatic fall in rents. The extent of this collapse was made plain by the inquests held by the king's receiver (or 'escheator') into the value of the estate recently owned by Margaret, late dowager countess of Kent and sister of Thomas Wake of Liddel, whose lands she had inherited – albeit for four months only – after his death.[30] On 12th January the jury at York reported (just as they had done only a few months before) that rents were drastically reduced because of the death of tenants.[31] In Lincolnshire, eight days later, the jury from the countess's manor of Greetham told how the commuted payments from the villein tenants had fallen by a third, whilst rents from free farmers had dropped by more than a half.[32] Jury after jury testified as to the fall in income across the late countess's estates: in Northamptonshire revenues were greatly reduced on account of the plague, while a Cambridgeshire jury recounted a litany of mini-disasters, from ruined houses to a mill now worth less than a sixth of its pre-plague value of £2, which 'because of the pestilence . . . could not be let at a higher rate'.[33] Here rents had dropped by 69 per cent[34] and feudal revenues from the manor court had fallen from 13s. 4d. to 3s. 4d. as a result of 'the death of tenants there' – a decrease of 75 per cent.[iv] These were the plain financial results of half-emptied villages, unharvested fields, idle mills and untended cattle – not that these astounding losses were unique to agricultural estates: the lead mine at Ashford in the Water, by Bakewell in Derbyshire, for instance, was worth only a twentieth of its previous value in 1351 because of the dearth of labour for hire.[35]

While landowners had enjoyed a one-off bonanza from the many heriots received on account of the mortality, and from the rush of entry-fines and marriage-fines that followed, these were rarely sufficient to offset the loss in rents, the reduction in available customary labour, fewer feudal dues, the reduced income from the proceeds of

[iv] i.e. from £0.67 to £0.17.

local justice, the reduced income from market sales and the dramatic rise in the cost of employing labour to work on the demesne. Across the kingdom, landowners had experienced an unprecedented fall in their revenues and destruction of their capital, all within the space of a couple of years. In short, lords were experiencing a classic profit squeeze, made more acute by the distorting effect of inflation.

Landowners attempted a variety of strategies to restore the profitability of their estates. Lords were powerless to do anything about the fall in prices and largely impotent in the face of greater wage demands; they could, however, do something about the revenues of feudal landholding. The first imperative was to keep tenants in their manors, paying some sort of rent. The Prince of Wales's official reduced the rents of his tenants at Drakelow, Cheshire,[v] by a third, as they had 'threatened to leave . . . unless they were granted such a remission . . .'. The remission was 'to last until the world improves and the tenements come to be worth more'.[36] Other feudal impositions were likewise often reduced: at Lessingham the steward reduced the marriage fee payable by a butcher's widow by 75 per cent, citing the demands of the times in the official manor record, while the earl of Oxford[37] was forced to remit labour services on his manor of Aldham near Hadleigh in Suffolk, in order to ensure that his tenants stayed put – a humiliation the earl's pompous steward tried to disguise in the record 'as a special favour'.[38] The abbot of Eynsham, Nicholas Upton, renegotiated the labour services of Walter Dolle and the other villein tenants of Woodeaton, so that instead of Walter rendering over 160 days' labour a year to the abbot,[39] he would instead work for twenty-six days and pay a cash rent of 13s. 4d.[vi] Clearly both sides were happy with this deal: the tenants of Woodeaton did not leave the village, which they had threatened to do unless a new agreement were struck.

Some landlords responded to declining revenues with more-radical action than the temporary remission of rents, feudal charges or labour services. In the Oxfordshire village of Upper Heyford in 1350, the lord still had twenty-three empty villein houses and over 600 acres of customary land standing uncultivated, so the following year he offered small parcels of the vacant land on five-year cash leases to the tenants

[v] Now part of Rudheath.
[vi] Approximately £0.67.

who still remained. Elsewhere landowners decided to lease their demesne, like the manor of Hampstead, belonging to the abbot of Westminster, who let the whole of the demesne in 1350 to an enterprising farmer named Richard Hanningham, for a term of five years at a cost of £10 per annum. Where leases were already in place, the terms were often renegotiated, as at Ormsby, in Lincolnshire, where the lease on one parcel of land, which had previously been renewed every year, was now let for life.

There were those lords who came to an accommodation with their villein tenants, or simply leased their land out; there were others, however, who went the other way and fought hard to preserve the landholding structure that had existed before the Great Death and with it the terms under which land had previously been let and cultivated. The steward of the bishop of Winchester's manor of Downton, just south of Salisbury in Wiltshire, compelled villeins to come forward and pay the entry fee to fill three of the twelve properties still vacant by 1350. At Wargrave in Berkshire, on the south bank of the Thames, the bishop's officials went so far as to turn the clock back in order to safeguard manorial income. The villeins here had for a long time had their *opera* commuted to a fixed rent but now that wages had risen and workers were so scarce, it suited the steward to demand that these services were once again performed, as their value in labour was now worth more than in cash.[vii] The tenants cannot have been happy, as they were now forced to return to bonded labour when they had been used to working as they pleased.

Yet even on those estates where feudal power was most uncompromising, lords recognized that if they were to extract any income from their ravaged manors, they would have to find some accommodation with those tenants who remained. Thus the bishop of Durham's (notoriously oppressive) officials adopted a nuanced approach, discriminating between those villages that were truly needy and those that were not, reflecting in turn variations in plague mortality and the degree of previous poverty. So when in April 1350 the tenants of Heighington, Ricknall, Middridge and Killerby argued for a reduction in their rent to 12d., they were refused, the record tersely noting that 'the steward does not agree'.[40] Yet later in the year the bondmen

---

[vii] Approximately £2.17. It would be eighty-three days' labour, assuming a post-plague wage of 6d. per day (approximately £0.03).

of Easington pleaded poverty and were remitted every penny of their rent. Where the bishop's steward continued to show no latitude, however, was in the flight of bondmen from their village: when Thomas Carleton left Sedgefield without permission in the autumn of 1350, the charges attached to his tenement were put upon his brother and another surety until they had brought him back. It was a harsh penalty for these two remaining men to bear.

Thus, lords' responses to their reduced incomes differed manor by manor, estate from estate. The Prince of Wales attempted to retain his tenants by inducement; the bishop of Durham achieved the same by force. Some, like the bishop of Winchester, might rescind commuted *opera* to get the cheap labour they required; others, such as the abbot of Westminster, simply leased out their demesne. As was becoming clear, the world left by pestilence would be fashioned by the need of each lord and each peasant to find an accommodation with one another, so that both might retrieve something from the misery and devastation they had been left.

Not content with berating labouring peasants, William Dene was as ready to direct his fulminations at his brother clergy. 'Priests', he claimed, 'making light of the sacrifice of a contrite spirit, took themselves to where they might receive a stipend greater than the value of their benefices. As a result, many benefices remained unserved by parish priests, whom neither prelates nor ordinaries were powerful enough to bridle. Thus spiritual dangers sprouted daily among the clergy and laity.'[41] It was an impression that firmly lodged itself in the collective memory of the Great Death. Two decades after Dene delivered his tirade, William Langland was to write much the same thing:[42]

> Persones and parsche prestis pleyned to þe bischop
> That here parsches were pore sithe þis pestelence tyme,
> To haue a licence and a leue in Londoun to dwelle
> And synge þer for symonye while seluer is so swete.[viii]

[viii] Parsons and parish priests complained to the bishop / That their parishes were poor since the pestilence, / Requesting a licence to live in London / And sing there for simony while silver is so sweet.

Another twenty years on, in the 1390s, Henry Knighton explained that the pestilence had caused 'such a shortage of priests everywhere that many churches were bereft of the divine office: of masses, matins, and vespers, of sacraments and observances', so that the cost of retaining a chaplain had more than doubled, while the much-reduced ranks of prospective ordinands were largely made up of widowers whose literacy was limited and grasp of theology non-existent.[43]

Although Langland and Knighton were writing decades after the Great Death, the problems they identified were clearly recognized at the time. There had been an effort to control clerical wages as early as the summer of 1349, when at least five of the English bishops had enrolled the provisions of the Ordinance of Labourers into their regis-ters and several had sent out supplementary instructions demanding that stipendiary (or wage-earning) clergy take no greater wages than they had been used to before the pestilence.[44] However, unlike the lay lords, the bishops had one advantage that the barons did not possess: they could 'create' priests, whereas the barons could not conjure up new workers, much as they would have wished. There was a limit, however, to how much new ordinations could help solve the shortage. Not only had there been as many deaths among trainees as among ordained priests but it was also difficult to accelerate the training of ordinands without compromising the proficiency of the resulting clergymen. If followed by the book, the journey to priesthood was a long and involved process, an accretive education that only half of all entrants would eventually complete. Faced with a sudden shortage of priests, the first option open to the bishops was to allow exceptional candidates to proceed to ordination earlier than was normally allowed by canon law, something that required the permission of the pope. Thus, in the autumn of 1349 Simon Islip petitioned the pope to allow each of the bishops in his province to ordain twenty men under the age of twenty-one, a request that was supplemented by individual petitions from some of the English bishops, asking variously that they be able to hold more ordinations than was normally permitted and even to ordain men of illegitimate birth, something long proscribed by the church.[45]

In theory, there were already sufficient priests to take over from those who had died. For while there had been approximately 10,000 beneficed clergy in England on the eve of the Great Death, there were probably four times that number who worked for a wage, rather than living off the tithes and other revenues of the parish as did beneficed clergy. So even if half of all priests had been taken by the plague, there were still as many as 20,000 stipendiary clerics to fill the shoes of the 5,000 parish priests who had died. In reality, however, this was inconceivable, as a great number of the stipendiary clergy were not deemed to be suitable to take on a benefice of their own: many had only a rudimentary education and, in any case, benefices were often reserved for the sons of the well-to-do, who in some instances might own the advowson (the right to appoint the rector) of the church where the son would eventually be installed. Although some wage-earning priests enjoyed some status – working as vicars (standing in for absent rectors) or as royal clerks – most stipendiary clergy were seen as little more than skilled wage-labourers who, at best, could expect to sing masses for the dead or work as auxiliaries to parish priests. It is no surprise, therefore, that William Dene criticized wage-earning priests in practically the same breath as he complained about peasant labourers: for Dene, as for his contemporaries, they were much the same class of worker.

The mortality changed the balance of these two classes of priest. Whilst very few stipendiary clergy would even have been considered for one of the many benefices that remained empty, they were nonetheless able to demand higher wages for their work. Indeed, the wages were in some cases so attractive that those clergymen who struggled on in a poor benefice were tempted to resign their position and sing masses instead. In the diocese of Hereford about half the vacancies in 1350 related to priests resigning their cures or moving to another parish, whilst in Lincoln there were an extraordinary 166 resignations during 1350. While the number of beneficed clergymen moving to wage-earning jobs was probably quite small, their actions were felt all the more for the real shortage in priests that the bishops felt they could promote to parishes.

Those priests demanding higher wages posed a simpler challenge. Employers could either increase pay or cut services. Archbishop Zouche bowed to the market and accepted in 1350 that he must pay more to get more chaplains, offering stipendiaries 6 marks each per annum.[ix] This may well have been the decent thing to do, as it is more than

[ix] i.e. £4.00.

likely (as Thomas was to claim) that some priests were driven to extreme poverty. Indeed, poverty may lie behind the tale of William, a priest of Waltham in Essex, who was convicted in 1350 of holding up a woman for her purse – for which the locals gave him the nickname 'William the One-day Priest'. With stories like this doing the rounds, it is easy to understand why some patrons were so reluctant to compromise and place an untested stipendiary priest in charge of one of their parishes. It was probably for this reason that Zouche (who seems to have been comparatively forward-looking in dealing with these problems) on a few occasions appointed a decent deacon to take care of a parish, as at Birstall in Nottinghamshire, where the archbishop collated Deacon John Rillington to the vicarage on 8th January 1350, in the belief that a good deacon was better than a bad priest, even though they were unable to say Mass for their parishioners or hear their confessions.[46]

The majority of William de la Zouche's colleagues resorted to outrage, however. Not that their admonitory instructions stemmed the complaints sent to the bishops about the conduct of their clergy, many of them probably from those same noble employers who were lobbying the king to do something about what they saw as peasant labourers' excessive demands.[47] By the time the Easter of 1350 passed, Archbishop Islip had become convinced that admonition was not enough. After a provincial council, attended by most of his bishops, he published a new constitution to apply to the whole province of Canterbury, dealing with the several ills that he claimed were afflicting the clergy.[48] 'Priests of the present day', Islip stated:

not realising that divine intervention spared them from danger in the past pestilence not for their own merits but so that they could perform the ministry committed to them by God's people and the public benefit, and not ashamed that their insatiable avarice is despicably and perniciously taken as an example by other workers among the laity, now take no heed to the cure of souls . . . but rather leave [their cures] completely abandoned . . . not content with the payment of adequate wages but demand excessive salaries so that they can revive old extravagances, and thus for the bare priestly name and precious little work they claim greater profits for themselves than those who have the cure of souls.

The result of this 'excessive affluence' was that many in the clergy
were being sucked down into 'the whirlpool of voluptuousness', a
moral degradation easily seen in 'the trimmings of their garments,
their fancy hairstyles, their haunting of taverns and gambling dens,
and their disgusting pursuit of carnal lust'. To a degree, these were
perennial complaints, and Islip's response was in large part to be
expected. He ordered his bishops to enforce residency and to ensure
that 'the best and most suitable chaplains' should be appointed to
parishes.[49] However, this much was out of the ordinary: given that
'simple priests can scarcely be satisfied with salaries twice as big',
priests' wages were to be regulated according to a set scale. Every
bishop was to report back to their primate by 8th September, giving
details of offenders against the constitution and the progress that had
been made in tackling excesses. When John Gynewell failed to respond,
Islip shot back a letter, accusing him of scornful and contemptuous
disobedience. But the bishop had his reasons. Archbishop Zouche,
whose archdiocese marched with Lincoln, was offering higher rates
of pay; if Gynewell did not do likewise he could never hope to attract
the clerics he needed to fill the many parishes still without a priest.

For all its fury, Archbishop Islip's ordinance seemed to have no effect
on the numbers of chantries or colleges of chantry priests. A considerable number of new foundations had been added since the wills of
the wealthy were put into effect. Among the new larger foundations
were the College of Clifton and three new chantries in Newark parish
church (both in Nottinghamshire), in Norfolk the College of Thompson
and in Suffolk the College of Raveningham. Nor did any rise in wages
necessarily affect existing institutions: the huge College of Cotterstock
in Northamptonshire, for instance, continued on regardless. Yet for
smaller endowments, where the revenues barely covered the cost of
the required number of chaplains (as with Nicholas Garland's chantry
in Oxford), there were often problems, leaving these moderately
wealthy benefactors in the same boat as those poor villagers who,
lacking a parish priest and therefore the sacraments, might fairly blame
the pestilence for endangering their chances of salvation.

It was not a complaint, however, that most could make by the
close of 1350, as by then the concerted efforts of the bishops had
ensured that most parishes were being served once again by a priest.
Although it is probable that some were less well-educated than their

predecessors, and many came from less distinguished families, there was no reason at all to say that the quality of their piety was any different from those who had gone before. It was, by almost every measure, a remarkable collective achievement by the English church, one driven primarily by a desire to prevent those same spiritual dangers that worried William Dene so sore.

For all the upheaval in the church, the appetite of the pious to make the Jubilee pilgrimage to Rome was undiminished. Only a few names survive but they alone provide a vignette of English society with which Chaucer would have been content. There was a monk from Robertsbridge in Sussex named John Crump, as well as the Midlands mason John Palterton and his assistant, Thomas Woffeld, both of whom left donations before they departed towards their 'new work' in the cloisters at Westminster Abbey, whose completion would have to await their return. A certain John de Sutton also went to Rome, possibly the same aged knight who had just opened a college of priests at Sutton in Holderness.[x] The prominent London merchant Andrew Aubrey asked permission to take leave of the kingdom with his eldest son, a chaplain, a servant and the huge sum of £40 for expenses. There was even a Cistercian brother from St Mary's Abbey in Dublin willing to make the journey. These were the privileged few, however, for after the pope's refusal of a plenary indulgence for all Englishmen, the king had issued a general ban on foreign travel in order that the kingdom was not weakened in the face of the continuing threat from France – an injunction that he repeated on 28th January and again on 23rd June. Despite the odd exemption, therefore, many of those who wished to go to Rome were prevented from doing so, for which reason the mayor and aldermen of London petitioned the pope that a Dominican friar named John Worthin should be allowed to give absolution in the city on the pope's behalf. 'May your Holiness', the councillors intoned, 'deign to know that, by permission of the most High, a dreadful mortality has so cut off our merchants, that our citizens who, as it were, usually dispense their services in all realms, are no longer able in person to visit your most Holy See, even though they should be involved in cases which are reserved for your Court, without a ruinous expense, while the present wars are going on.'[50]

[x] See Ch.10 pp. 226–7.

Edward's prohibition was a sensible precaution, for despite all the travails endured by the French people, their king still threatened war. Edward might well have wondered at the lunacy of Philip's position, for no matter what the provocation endured by Philip VI at the hands of Anglo-Gascon adventurers during the summer of 1349, his premature termination of the truce had been a rash decision. Philip could be forgiven for not being in his right mind: the epidemic had only lately claimed his queen, Joan of Burgundy, as well as Bonne of Luxembourg, the wife of his son and heir, John, duke of Normandy. His court had been utterly dislocated by the pestilence and royal administration had all but collapsed. Although the French offensive in Gascony during the following autumn had been a measured success, the English response, unleashed by the earl of Lancaster, had been wounding. So Edward's luck, once again, carried him through: paralysed by recrimination and indecision, the French council of war had no other option than to sue for peace, and thus a truce was signed – after the usual theatrical preludes – by Bishop Bateman on 13th June 1350, to last until August the following year. It was ignored, as usual, by the adventurers who fought on both sides: one of the English messengers sent to take the news of the peace to Bordeaux was lynched even before he made it to his destination. Pestilence, it seems, had done nothing to reduce the rancour between these two old foes.

Even before the ink had dried on the new truce, however, men were being arrayed along the south coast for the first time since the plague had passed. They were charged with guarding the shore against the Castilian navy, which had been harassing Channel shipping despite the fact that the Spanish had put their signature to the treaty at Guînes. The disruption to trade was serious, causing a doubling in the retail price of Gascon wine in London. The Spanish antics were all the more irritating given that it had only been two years since plague had scuppered a marriage alliance between the two nations. With the French now held at bay by a new truce, Edward was able to deal with this menace once and for all. So the king ordered ships to be requisitioned and then went down to Sandwich himself in order to lead the attack. Their opportunity came when, on 29th August, the Castilian fleet was spotted cruising close off the south coast, near Winchelsea. The English unfurled their sails and set their boats on a direct course with their enemy.

The English were in good spirits. Edward stood at the bow of his own ship, dapperly dressed in a black velvet jacket and a black beaver-skin hat – an outfit, Jean Froissart claimed, that greatly suited him. He had musicians aboard, who played dance tunes as they approached. Then, as they got close, the king ordered the band away and served a cup of wine to his comrades. Fortified, he directed his squadron straight into the middle of the Castilian fleet. Medieval naval battle was not sophisticated – like a maritime escalade repulsed in turn much as a garrison would defend their town. Each boat was kitted out with two 'castles', constructed in wood, one at the bow and another at the stern. As soon as they crashed into each other, the ships were locked together with grappling irons and then, under the cover of much arrow-fire, the English attempted to scale the Spanish castles using ropes and ladders, avoiding where they could the rocks and boulders hurled down on them by their enemy. The English suffered many losses and the Prince of Wales's boat sank, although only after he had managed to board another. By nightfall, however, Edward's sailors had got the better of the Spanish and the king was able to return triumphant to his wife, who had watched the whole encounter from the cliff-top at Winchelsea. Her relief was certainly great, for not only had her husband and first-born son survived the battle, but so too had her ten-year-old son, John of Gaunt, who had gone as his older brother's esquire. The king and two princes had hardly returned to dry land before momentous news arrived from France. Edward's nemesis, King Philip VI, was dead.[xi]

Whilst waiting at Sandwich for the Castilian navy to come into view, Edward had received the troubling news that, during the sessions of the justices of the peace there had been a riot at Eynsham, in Oxford-shire. By the royal account, a crowd had assembled and had assaulted Thomas Langley, one of the local gentlemen and a justice of the peace, forcing him to run into the abbey to seek safety, barricading himself inside the abbot's chamber. The mob, knowing he was within, threatened to burn the building down if he did not surrender the indictments submitted to him and all those offenders who were in the justices' custody awaiting trial; more than likely, a good number of

---

[xi] He died on 22nd August 1350, at the abbey of Coulombs, forty miles west of Paris. The news will have taken about a week to arrive on the south coast of England.

those accused had committed offences under the Ordinance of Labourers. The king was certainly infuriated: he ordered that the rioters of Eynsham be brought to 'speedy punishment'.[51]

Although there was a history of raucous behaviour in Eynsham, the villagers would not have been alone in protesting against the new cap on wages.[xii] In November 1349 the cordwainers of London complained that their servants threatened to strike unless they received higher wages, and the corporation had them thrown into Newgate gaol until they gave that idea up. The following month the bishop of Bath and Wells, Ralph Shrewsbury, had been besieged by an angry crowd wielding bows and arrows, iron bars and stones, inside the church at Yeovil, where he had been celebrating a Mass in thanksgiving for the end of plague. The problem here was most probably the recent re-proclamation of the ordinance, which Shrewsbury may have even have made himself. At nightfall the mob had dispersed so the bishop was able to make it to the rectory but in the morning the thugs came looking for him again and he was forced to shutter the doors until a troop of his retainers arrived to rescue him. The offenders, sixty in all, were ordered to public penance – a remarkably lenient punishment given the distress they must have caused and the injury they had done to Shrewsbury's attendants. Perhaps the bishop had some sympathy for the outrage shown by the townsmen, for as he continued his journey round the diocese the problems with which they were having to contend were plain for him to see.

The Ordinance of Labourers not only provoked hostility, it was unequal to the task of controlling wage rates. Despite the fact that the royal decree had been repeated on a further two occasions since its issue in June 1349,[xiii] and the keepers of the peace had been instructed to enforce the statute,[xiv] inflation and the competition for wage-labour ensured that most lords and most labourers preferred to run the risk of contravening the ordinance, especially those clauses relating to wages. Whilst employers greatly resented what Knighton called the 'workmen's arrogant and greedy demands', they were unwilling to threaten their supply of labour by suing for redress.[52] Besides, the

---

[xii] See Ch. 7, p. 154.
[xiii] 21st November and 8th December 1349.
[xiv] On 20th February 1350.

ordinance was loosely drawn, stating only that labourers should receive 'salaries which were usually paid in the country where they were working in [1346] or in some other appropriate year five or six years ago'.[53] So open to interpretation was this clause that in London the mayor's council issued its own, more detailed, ordinance, which stipulated wage rates precisely and, moreover, fixed the prices of a whole range of items, from a pair of sleeves to a tun of Cretan wine.[xv]

There were prosecutions, however: the breach-of-contract clause was useful to a whole range of employers, not all of them lords. In Thornbury it was used as the basis for private suits of trespass between prominent villagers. Thus in spring 1350 William Hatheway claimed that the wealthy villein, Thomas Picher, had taken a servant from him; Thomas was acquitted. Thomas Fader, another well-to-do villein, was accused of luring William Parker's servant away; in this instance the accused was found guilty. The ordinance also provided a means by which lords might compel the indolent or the criminal to work, like the four men of Wigan who were accused of being vagabonds and vagrants by night and would not work by day; shockingly, one of the gang was a chaplain. It was a priest, however, who came to the rescue of Richard Digg, a common labourer of Preston St Mary in Suffolk, who had been bound over by the constables to work in the village. Father Thomas remonstrated with the constables about what he perceived to be this gross injustice and as a result Richard returned to his old ways, only working when he wished. It was obstreperous behaviour such as Richard Digg's that William Dene found so objectionable: 'no workman or labourer was prepared to take orders from anyone, whether equal, inferior or superior, but all those who served did so with ill-will and a malicious spirit.' With an apocalyptic flourish, Dene concluded that 'it is therefore much to be feared that Gog and Magog have returned from hell to encourage such things and to cherish those who have been corrupted.'[54]

An opportunity to address the deficiencies of the ordinance came in the New Year of 1351, when parliament was called. The Lords and Commons had not met together since 1348, not since the Great Death:

[xv] The first articles of the London ordinance dealt with the building trades, reflecting the particular demand for masons, carpenters, plasterers and tilers that had been created by the current construction boom in the city and on the king's projects at Westminster and, latterly, at Windsor.

the scheduled parliament of 1349 had been first postponed and then cancelled, and Edward had not shown any urgency to summon the assembly again, not least while he did not have to. It was the longest period without parliament since Edward had succeeded to the throne (and would remain the greatest hiatus during his fifty-year reign). Parliament could not, however, be prorogued indefinitely, for although the triennial grant still had a year to run, the wool custom had expired.[xvi] It was, in the event, a momentous assembly, for the legislation passed in 1351 represented the most significant package of statute law since 1340. The influence of pestilence was clear from the petitions submitted prior to the opening session on 9th January. The magnates were pressing, once again, their demand that their children born abroad should be legitimized in terms of inheritance, something that was clearly all the more important given the deaths of male heirs during the epidemic; the great merry-go-round of priests in the wake of the mortality, much of which was thought (wrongly) to be directed from Avignon, led to a petition on the limitation of the pope to make direct appointments to English ecclesiastical positions; in these difficult times for urban trade, the towns wanted legislation on the prevention of forestalling (cornering) markets and the control of river traffic; and all this was in addition to the petitions submitted by both rural landlords and urban employers asking that the Ordinance of Labourers, granted eighteen months previously at the height of the epidemic, should be beefed up and given a statutory basis.

The king and his ministers listened carefully to these requests from the Lords and Commons; they may even have encouraged some themselves. Edward's assent duly came: an act was passed legitimizing children of nobles born abroad; a statute was granted depriving the papacy of all its rights to appoint clerics in England over the head of the king, something that Edward no doubt felt justified in doing given Clement VI's refusal to offer an alternative indulgence to the Jubilee pilgrimage to Rome; the towns were given what they wanted on forestalling and river traffic; and finally – the *pièce de résistance* – a statute of labourers was enacted.

The statute opened with an explicit recognition that employees had

---

[xvi] Granted in 1347, it was due to expire in September 1351 and thus required parliamentary renewal.

'no regard to the said ordinance [of labourers] but rather to their own ease and exceptional greed ... for which the Commons pray for remedy'.[55] The remedy they received was comprehensive: as well as reiterating the clauses requiring labourers to work and to keep to their contracts (whose terms were also controlled), specific rates of pay were set down as the maximum allowable – weeding was to be paid at no more than 1*d*. per day; mowing 5*d*. per acre or per day; reapers of corn no more than 2*d*. per day, or less if that were the case in 1346 or before. A master carpenter was limited to 3*d*. per day but a normal carpenter only 2*d*. Tilers and masons were to receive 3*d*. and their mates 1½*d*. Craftsmen – shoemakers, tanners, saddlers, goldsmiths and the like – were again prohibited from taking more for their products than in 1346, a control not simply on prices but on what these men could earn for their labour.

The statute also specified a mechanism for enforcement, the absence of which had been another fault of the original ordinance. All labourers were to swear an oath before specially appointed justices of labourers, or their lords or their officials, that they would abide by the statute. Those breaking this oath were to be punished in the stocks or required to go before the justices, where they would have to pay back any excess wage and fined for their misdemeanour. There were some important exceptions, which indicated the special pleading of a number of powerful interests. The statute was not extended to the Welsh, for instance, as they provided a large seasonal labour force which would move down from the hills and across the border at harvest-time, thereby falling foul of the clause on length of contract. These few concessions notwithstanding, the statute was nothing less than a full-scale attempt to regulate wages nationwide and to criminalize those who wished to exert their lately improved bargaining power. In scope, it was without exception the most ambitious piece of legislation yet put before parliament and approved by the king.

The government lost no time in enforcing the new statute. On 15th March 1351, just two weeks after parliament had been prorogued,[xvii] joint commissions of peace and labourers were appointed throughout England.[xviii] Soon presentments were being made by juries across

[xvii] 1st March, 1351.

[xviii] In relying once again on the justices of the peace, it was clear that the administration wished to use the existing judicial infrastructure.

England and, shortly after, judgements made by the travelling justices. In Essex four labourers were accused of refusing to work for more than double the rate ordained by the statute. Hugo Plomer was indicted at Market Overton in Rutland on 29th June for selling church candles at what was deemed to be an excessive price. Fines collected around Hitchin in 1351 show that men were arraigned from small settlements (2s. from tiny Meppershall) as well as large villages (36s. 9d. from Pirton). The towns provided considerable returns: £5 from Ware and £10 from St Albans alone. In total, Hertfordshire yielded the remarkable sum of £122 6s. 3d. to the Treasury in 1351.

Whether enforcement of the statute was having any deterrent effect it is difficult to tell, for even where a reduction in wages is recorded, it may be suspected that clerks made false entries so that their lords avoided prosecution for paying too much;[56] indeed, it is likely that wages were often made up by the addition of food allowances, which were easier to wash through the accounts. What is clear is that the law was sufficiently enforced to cause, like the ordinance before it, some considerable anger. In Tottenham, in 1351, the justices had to flee their session and the offenders due to go before the bench were sprung from their gaol by sympathizers. In the same year five men appeared before the Devon bench, chaired by Hugh Courtenay, the earl of Devon, to answer charges that they had broken into a house and taken the legal documents relating to the enforcement of the statute that were being kept there, which doubtless recorded the indictment of one of the thieves. However, there was no repeat of the kind of violence witnessed at Eynsham or Yeovil and it seems that objectors increasingly focused their efforts towards evasion, in whatever form that might take.

Greater use was being made of the statute in its first year than landowners had ever achieved with the ordinance that preceded it. By that measure, the new law was a success. It was certainly a radical innovation: for the first time central government had stipulated wage levels for labourers and had nationalized those price controls that previously had been the preserve of local lords and urban councils. This was not half of the administration's plans, however. Having dealt with wages, the treasurer Edington turned his attention to prices. It was widely known that when coin was short, prices fell, so Edington did the opposite: he increased the amount of coin in circulation in an effort to push prices up. There were new, larger-denomination coins,

like the half-groat and groat (4*d*.), which could be used in small transactions that otherwise might involve two or four pennies. It was an
old trick of moneyers wishing to inflate prices, for not only did it
make higher-priced transactions easier but it had the psychological
effect of further devaluing the common penny. Coupled with the
controls placed on wages, it was hoped that the recoinage would help
to restore manorial profits nationwide.

Meanwhile, measures were put in place to stimulate trade. Much
to the chagrin of many townsmen, freedom of all foreign merchants
to trade within England was reaffirmed.[57] Although the defeat of the
Castilian fleet off Winchelsea in 1350 did little to make the Channel
any safer for merchant shipping, a commercial treaty with Castile the
following year – coupled with the continuation of the truce with
France – ensured that exports could recover: 35,000 sacks of wool were
shipped in 1350–51, almost as much as had been exported ten years
earlier. The propagation of trade by the crown was not, of course, a
philanthropic exercise: the excise on wine was increased, the farm of
customs was relet,[58] the tax on cloth was reintroduced,[xix] and the wool
merchants were tapped for yet more loans. This was a co-ordinated
policy on the part of Edward's royal administration, intended both to
reassure worried landowners and urban producers and to protect
the crown's crucial customs and tax revenues. Not only was this an
astute political move, but it was the best that Edington and his
colleagues could do to shore up royal income. Whether the measures
had any effect in doing anything to counter the macroeconomic effects
of the mortality remained to be seen; nonetheless, in terms of both
its novelty and its ambition, this was by any measure an impressive
demonstration of administrative competence.

After the fracas in Yeovil, Bishop Shrewsbury celebrated Christmas
and in the New Year resumed his peregrination of the diocese of
Bath and Wells. By early February he was at Keynsham Abbey, an
Augustinian house midway between Bristol and Bath which had lost
its abbot during the pestilence.[xx] On St Valentine's Day, 1350, he made
his report; he was not enamoured by the canons, nor enraptured by

---

[xix] The aulnage, or assize of cloth.
[xx] See Ch. 3, p. 60.

what he had seen. The gates were not supervised properly; the public were allowed to wander around as they wished; there was no proper control over the costs of the kitchen; the canons were eating and drinking outside the monastery; and (despite the rising cost of wages) the abbey was employing far too many servants for the amount of work that had to be done. All these defects were to be corrected, and the canons were also told that they were not to keep dogs, especially sporting dogs. The new regime must have come as something of a shock to the canons, who had got used to living in this house of ease.

Shrewsbury's experience was not unique. There were miscellaneous reports of the collapse of religious order in houses across England, such as in Lenton in Nottinghamshire, where the prior sought the sheriff's assistance in arresting three of his monks who had apostatized and were wandering round the countryside without their habits. In Malmesbury, Wiltshire, the townsmen discovered that one of the brothers of the ancient abbey there had sired a daughter 'of a handmaid' during the plague year. Reports such as these, however, can be found in almost every year of the fourteenth century. Although they were not as frequent as later 'reformers' liked to make out, there had always been abuses in English monasteries, an unsurprising fact given the tens of thousands of religious that there were at this time. As Bishop Shrewsbury's ordinance showed well, there were mechanisms in place to deal with the corruption of the spiritual life, a process that was not stopped by the advent of plague. Nor should we imagine that the number of cases of poor behaviour among the religious hugely increased as a result of the pestilence: no contemporary chronicler suggests that this was the case.

There was a recognition, however, that the mortality presented new challenges to the monasteries. The order of St Augustine, which had the largest number of religious houses in England, convened a chapter in 1350 at Northampton. The assembly was routine but had been delayed by the pestilence and, as was to be expected, it was the effects of that mortality that dominated the agenda. A report was presented to the assembled abbots and priors that the priory of Ivychurch, on the road out of Salisbury, had lost its prior and twelve canons, leaving only a solitary canon – James Groundwell. With no alternative, James had been made prior. Although he was said to be of good character, this was a position that he had probably never aspired to hold, even though there were no brothers left over which to rule. Forced to take on the single-handed management of the abbey and its estate, poor brother James had allowed the religious life of the monastery, which was now a *de facto* hermitage, to collapse. The chapter ordered that canons from other, more fortunate, monasteries should be sent to revivify Ivychurch and all other houses in a similar condition. The instruction worked, for by April there were already enough new canons to have an election for a new prior, and brother James – who must have been very relieved – was able to resign the responsibilities he had never sought. Even in a large monastery, like the Cistercian priory of Meaux in east Yorkshire, the deaths of so many brothers had a deleterious effect on the management of the monks' estates. A monk of Meaux wearily commented that because 'the abbot, prior, cellarer, bursar and other experienced men and officials had died, the survivors made misguided grants of the goods and possessions of the monastery'. This monk's main concern, however, had been the death of 'the majority of our tenants'.[59] It was this mortality, and its financial consequences, that was to pose the most serious and widespread challenge to the monks and nuns of England.

The pincer action of decreasing prices and increased costs had as serious an effect on ecclesiastical landlords as on their secular counterparts. Many monasteries, especially those which were having problems before the Great Death, were soon starting to show the effects of the squeeze. The new abbot of Ramsey, Richard de Shenington, found upon his accession that the house was 2,500 marks in debt – a quite astounding sum.[xxi] Much of this debt had been incurred before the Great Death but the impact of the pestilence had made the situation far worse, so in 1350 the abbey was forced into the fire-sale of one of its smaller possessions, the village of Weston-cum-Brington, in which all the bondmen had in any case died.[xxii] A little under twenty miles towards Cambridge from Ramsey, the epidemic seems to have been the death knell for the small house of Minoresses of Waterbeach: the nuns were impoverished but had long resisted merging with the house at Denny, nearby, but in 1350 the king told the few who stubbornly

---

[xxi] £1,666.67.

[xxii] Now Old Weston, near Brington, both in Cambridgeshire (formerly Huntingdonshire).

remained that they had to repopulate their house or be forced to move. They moved, and the buildings were soon desolate.

Bishop Trillek of Hereford had previously been asked to intervene to help settle the dispute between Denny and Waterbeach but he had declined: he had enough of his own challenges to meet. The least of these, but requiring attention nonetheless, was at the abbey of St Peter in Gloucester, where Abbot Staunton was having problems with the monks. The whole choir was half demolished and work had not yet resumed on the new roof, a tricky project further complicated by the need to find a new master mason, as here too William Ramsey had been overseeing the works. The reduction in the abbey's revenue forced Staunton to replace the monks' clothing and food allowance, providing them with their vestments and victuals direct, but these luxuriant monks did not like this and complained to the bishop. They were not to wait long to be rid of their tight abbot, as Staunton died the following year. Because of his austerity measures, however, and the rise in pilgrims occasioned by the Great Death, the abbot's final account shows he had been able to right St Peter's finances in that short time, leaving a surplus of 1,000 marks.[xxiii] There were many who struggled to recover, however,[60] and Bishop Trillek worked assiduously with each abbey to try to rebuild their fortunes, for the simple reason that – as Archbishop Zouche explained in a similar case within his own diocese – 'unless help is provided very quickly in the form of generous financial support, divine worship will be lessened . . . and the exercise of hospitality and other pious works cease altogether.'[61]

The energy with which prelates, laymen and religious set about the restoration of monastic fortunes is deeply impressive. It would be a mistake to overstate their task: the clergy in their entirety were still wealthy enough to be able to pay a tax of a tenth of the value of their movable goods, amounting to £15,000, in 1351, which was only 17 per cent down on their previously assessed value.[xxiv] It was clear, however, that the shock of the plague had focused minds, and those who felt responsible had determined that struggling houses should not be allowed to go under. For although they were not proliferating as they had done two centuries before, monasteries and other religious houses were still greatly valued by the public. Indeed, people

[xxiii] £666.67.
[xxiv] i.e. £18,000.

were now flocking to the cathedral shrines – most of which were monastic foundations – in unprecedented numbers, their piety heightened by the horrors they had survived.

The spirit of renewal was all-pervading. Thomas de la Mare, the new abbot of St Alban's, lost little time on his return from Avignon in convening a chapter-general for all English Benedictine houses.[xxv] As a result of this assembly, de la Mare introduced new ordinances for the order in 1351. While aimed at reform, the revised laws were practical and humane. Brethren were to attend every service, in its entirety; they were not to sing 'without point or sense, like smiths beating iron on an anvil', but with great expression, although appropriate cuts were permitted to ensure that services did not go on too long; novices were to endure a strict regime so that they might get used to the rigours of monastic life; monks were to abstain from idle conversation, but serial offenders were to be more harshly punished than the occasional miscreant; the heads of houses were to remain in their monasteries as much as possible; and – perhaps in recognition of the panic caused by the plague – sub-priors were to visit the sick of the monastery every day. Most importantly, monks were to live and lead by example – to abhor fraudulent or unlawful contracts, to refrain from false claims while selling, to oppress no one or make unjust exactions, and to avoid temptations of the flesh – women, food and drink. These were rules aimed simply at improving the religious life. Although the provisions which removed some of the hurdles to profession – such as the memorizing of saints' stories by heart – might seem to be part of the effort to counteract the fall-off in recruitment, within the context of all the other ordinances it is clear that de la Mare's intention was simply to focus on true spirituality and not on rote and unfelt oration.

The same mixed pattern of crisis, stasis and renewal could be seen in hospitals, most of which were also fraternal foundations. Two hospitals in London display these contrasting fortunes well. The circumstances of the hospital of St James in Westminster went from bad to worse – the plague had killed all the brothers save Walter de Weston, who, on account of the fact that he was the sole remaining brother, had been made master in 1348. However, after two years of

---

[xxv] All of them, that is, except Canterbury, which refused (as it usually did) to attend.

mismanagement, culminating in a double burglary in 1350, when goods and legal records were stolen by none other than a fellow priest, the hapless Walter was charged with allowing the house to fall into dilapidation and removed. This was not a problem encountered by the Augustinian hospital of St Mary Spital which – like the London friaries – benefited from a flood of donations during the plague year. With the money they made a number of investments, buying land, tenements and shops in Shoreditch and Hackney – so significant a series of acquisitions that the hospital set up a trust to make the purchases in order that they might avoid legislation that had been passed in order to prevent the alienation of property to religious houses in just this way.[xxvi]

Not that laws like these were a problem for the hospital of St Katherine by the Tower, which had for two centuries enjoyed the patronage of successive queens. Queen Philippa was very partial to this house, and had supported the rebuilding of the hospital church before the Great Death to designs by William Ramsey. Although the great mason had not seen his plans fully realized, the queen was determined that St Katherine's should reach completion so, in 1351, she secured a new charter for the hospital from her husband the king, which set out a constitution for the hospital and bestowed the residue of previous endowments on the house so that they could afford to finish the work. However, even in its unfinished state and with its architect dead, St Katherine's was having an influence on a new generation of masons. The corner turrets on the choir were being repeated by the mason who built to Ramsey's designs for John Lovekin's chapel in Kingston, while the mason responsible for the new church of the Austin Friars in Broadgate drew directly from the way that Ramsey had arranged the windows, roof and bays at St Katherine's. The completion of this church of St Katherine, therefore, represented renewal in more ways than the simple fact of a new building.

The length and breadth of the land, very obvious changes were taking place. The population of every settlement, every family, had been cut – on average – in half. Prices had dropped. Land was more plentiful and labour was more scarce, so surviving villeins argued for better

[xxvi] The Statute of Mortmain, 1279.

terms and surviving workers could demand higher wages. Some manors were faring better than others; one monastery was in trouble while a neighbouring friary might be spending the receipts from a deluge of donations.

Yet there were other, more subtle, repercussions of the mortality. The wrecking of so many families, for instance, was having various effects. The proliferation of orphans, many of them by dint of succession young tenants in their own right but not legally able to enter their land, meant that an unusually large number of tenements were being farmed by guardians; where an orphan lacked even an uncle or cousin, they were made the shared responsibility of villagers. Where not even an orphan survived to take on land, new tenants were taking up vacancies. In the Winchester manors, for example, the proportion of hereditary land bequeathed to sons fell from 38 per cent in 1348–9 to 25 per cent in 1349–50. Conversely, land taken on by un-related villagers increased, from just 16 per cent of land transfers in 1348–9 to 44 per cent in 1349– 50, an increase in a year from less than a sixth of all transferred land going to unrelated parties to nearly a half.[xxvii] These dry statistics describe a profound shift in landholding: the hereditary link between the villein family and a plot of land was being ever more rapidly eroded, as land was passing out of the family as never before.

The surfeit of vacant land presented many opportunities. There were some who had not previously had tenements of their own and were now able – through some little cash inheritance, the rise in wages or a fall in entry fines – to be able to become a tenant for the first time. However, those who benefited most tended to be the wealthier peasants and those who possessed the spirit of enterprise, just as had been the case after the previous calamity, the Great Famine of 1315– 18. Stephen May, a villein of Codicote in Hertfordshire, was an extra-ordinary example. In 1351 the lord of Codicote, the abbot of St Alban's, granted Stephen all the lands of the lately deceased Robert and J. atte Strete, all the lands of the lately deceased Reginald Alleyn, and all the lands of the lately deceased Edward atte Hache, for a term of eight and a half years at 20s. per annum, with 'all the service and customs belonging to the said lands'. Thus Stephen took on the land that had

[xxvii] See Ch.7, p. 161.

once been farmed by four other tenants, in addition to that land he had previously possessed. (Stephen was allowed to demolish only one of the houses, however, and would, therefore, have had to maintain all of the rest – a clause in the agreement that showed, together with the length of the term, that the abbot expected at some time in the future to be able to let the tenements separately once again.) Similarly, John Runwick, the reeve of Farnham, took on five acres that had been owned by his neighbour, at a cost of 18*d*.[xxviii] This new obligation, together with the strain of working through the torrid months of plague and the exhausting few years that followed, was a heavy burden, so John resigned his responsibilities as reeve. He had worked with great energy through this time: it is no wonder he now wanted a quieter existence.

There were many, however, who could neither afford nor manage to take on any more land, even when it was passed to them in inheritance. Some refused their right, some fled, a few were compelled to take up the land nonetheless; many had seen no improvement as a result of the pestilential mortality of 1348 and 1349. Almost every village in every part of the land saw something of the remarkable range of changes in fortune that followed the years of plague. A return visit to some of the villages already encountered serves well to illustrate the point.

The Deverill villages of west Wiltshire were re-forming themselves in the wake of plague. John Peter, the patriarch of a family living in Monkton Deverill, survived the pestilence, although he and his wife Agnes had probably lost two sons during that time. John was well into his seventies, however, and when John died a natural death in 1350, Agnes – who cannot have been young herself – had to take on the responsibility for the family's small brewing business, without, of course, the help of her sons. John's death marked the end of a successful village dynasty. The man had worked hard: to his dying day he continued to pay for the commutation of autumn works that had first been remitted thirty-one years earlier in 1319 and since then he had been able to save enough money to be able to help each of his surviving children – girls as well as boys – to take on property of their own. Yet as far as the Peter name was concerned, it was all for

[xxviii] i.e. £0.08.

naught, as after Agnes's death none bore it in Monkton again. Yet the demise of one family created openings for another. Peter Boket, the labourer from Monkton, was able to take on eight acres in his own right in 1350, for which he paid 20s.[xxix] – a significant sum for a labourer who had previously had no land. Perhaps it was a plot previously occupied by one of John Peter's sons, or by John Peter himself. For Peter Boket the shock of the mortality was surely tempered in time by the excitement of the new opportunities that were now on offer.

By the time the ploughs cut their first furrow at Thornbury, on the shore of the Severn, in the spring of 1350, the pestilence had been gone for over a year. Those intervening months had seen an unprecedented number of land transfers and a slew of advantageous marriages, yet the changes continued long after the many new couples and landowners had made their new homes. John Fish, the villein tenant who had gained both a wife and land out of the plague, was nominated by the earl's bailiff to take on some land left vacant by the plague. (The unfortunate man found that whilst he had been led to believe that the land came with tools, most of them had been stolen by Robert in the Hale, who had clearly helped himself to them while the tenement was unoccupied. Robert was one of the wealthiest villeins in the manor; this behaviour explains, perhaps, one reason why.) By 1351, however, there seems to have been a tentative upturn in the demand for land, at least to a point where compulsion was no longer required. That year William Hyndewele and William Suotor voluntarily entered land that had been vacant for two full years. Having been out of cultivation for so long, the tenement had degenerated into a terrible state, so the terms the two men secured were particularly good: the entry fine was a token gift of two capons and all subsequent rents were to be rendered not in services, as previously, but in cash.

Yet despite the progress of some who had previously had very little, the windfall created by the mortality tended to land in the laps of those who already had most – and they were keen to protect what more they had gained. Thus, when the Statute of Labourers came to be enforced in Thornbury, it was no surprise to find that the jury consisted entirely of prominent villein tenants, men like the nefarious

[xxix] i.e. £1.00.

Robert in the Hale who had possessed, by the standards of villein peasants, significant wealth before the Great Death. One of Hale's fellows on the jury bench was the same Thomas Fader who had, the previous year, been successfully sued for enticing a servant away from another tenant. Unlike Fader's dispute, the cases brought before the jury in 1351 were not spats between wealthy peasants but simple prosecutions of lowly wage-earners, all of whom pleaded guilty. The case of Robert White is instructive. Robert had held no land before the plague and had subsisted from labouring and a little brewing. The 6s. 8d. he gave to marry Cecilia Adams in the summer of 1349 was probably the sum of his life savings: it was certainly a large amount for a landless worker. With the marriage came a cottage and the six acres her father had held. It was not much, but it was a foot on the ladder. Like so many others, Robert had tried to do a little bit better for himself and put up the price at which he had offered his labour. Yet the bigger tenants in the village soon put a stop to Robert's modest advance and had him arraigned because 'he did not come to work taking a reasonable wage by the statute'.[62] This was not the work of some oppressive noble lord but the action of a peasant elite, keen to protect their own margins by holding down the cost of the labour on which they depended.

Robert White, at least, could console himself that he had gained something from the pestilence. Others were less fortunate. It would be little surprise if Matilda Wilcox felt that her survival had been a mixed blessing, for she had buried two husbands within six months. There were many, however, whose situation was worse still – those who, through the deaths of those who supported them, were forced into impoverishment or, worse still, destitution. The Cheese family, burgesses of Thornbury manor, managed to get by before the Great Death, but young Eleanor Cheese appears as a debtor to the church-wardens in the summer of 1350 and the following year was fined for picking the loose ears of corn dropped during the harvest in the fields; even then she was judged to be so poor that the fine was allowed to drop. There were enough of these unfortunate folk who had only just managed to avoid privation before the plague but had since been pushed to the point of ruin.

There was, therefore, a significant and rapid change of fortune in the lives of many survivors – some up, some down; a very great number, however, carried on the daily struggle to feed and clothe themselves just as they had done before. For these people, almost all of whom had suffered the loss of family and friends, the mortality had made little difference to the way they lived their lives, other than to laden them with a new burden – the great grief that the pestilence had brought.

The impoverishment of Eleanor Cheese, advancement of John Cole, prosecution of Robert White, and all the other goings-on in Thornbury were of little interest to the manor's lord, Ralph Stafford. The redoubtable soldier had been in England since he had gained control of the manor in 1347, although that was due to a lack of anything to do on the Continent rather than any devotion to his estates. Ever at Edward's service, Stafford spent the years at home acting as the king's fixer. In 1350 he accompanied Sir William Douglas north of the border to treat with the Scots, and agreed a marriage between his daughter Beatrice and the son of the earl of Desmond.[xxx] Desmond had been in London for the duration of the plague waiting to plead his innocence before Edward against the charges of brigandage levied by the king's ministers in Dublin. Finally, in November 1349, Edward granted him a pardon. The Stafford marriage would ease the necessary rehabilitation of the erstwhile bandit earl. In recognition of his efforts, Edward elevated Ralph Stafford to an earldom, in 1351. Yet there were none of the usual estates that came with so grand a title – only an annuity, albeit 1,000 marks a year.[xxxi] This gift was an indication of the remarkable solidity of the English nobility in the aftermath of the plague. Grant of lands had, in the past, almost always followed the prior attainder of some errant lord's estates, and were thus as much a sign of contention as they were a mark of favour: that the king had no lands to grant was a sign of concord in the realm, and his favour had to be shown in cash. Moreover, Stafford's annuity was testament to the remarkable survival of the English nobility during these years of plague: for unlike in Thornbury and virtually every other village in the country, there had been no failed lines of heredity among the magnates and consequently there was no new land to be distributed around. Thus, while the position, continuity even, of so many peasant

[xxx] The son being Maurice fitz Maurice FitzGerald.
[xxxi] i.e. £666.67.

families was affected by pestilence, the English noble estate retained its shape and structure. This, and the survival of all its principal person- alities, did much to ensure that the changes wrought by plague, both subtle and overt, were contained within the existing systems of feudal control.

Like any community, noble society was forever beset by bickering and dispute, suppurating jealousies and hereditary injustices. It was the mark of a good monarch that contention was managed carefully. Success in battle and the booty that came with it naturally made this task all the more easy. Edward, therefore, should take much credit for the happy state of his nobility during these mid-century years. He had many failings but his ability to gather together the great men of England, both noble and ecclesiastical, in unstinting loyalty to the crown was a most definite quality. By the standards of what was expected of a king, he had also acquitted himself well in the after- math of this Great Death.

As he was not engaged on campaigning, Edward was afforded during this period greater leisure than he had enjoyed for many years. He diverted himself just as one would expect this noble-king might. St Stephen's was substantially complete, inside and out, by the close of 1351, thereby bringing to fruition Edward I's foundation. Now Edward felt able to embark on a project of his own. Once again he was to follow in his grandfather's footsteps. When he had been Prince of Wales, Edward I survived a storm on the return leg of a crusade and had founded a Cistercian monastery at Vale Royal, in Cheshire, in pious thanks. Edward III determined to do the same, ostensibly in commemoration of his victory at Winchelsea and the many moments of salvation from the wrath of the sea. Yet, there was, perhaps, an ulterior motive. For Edward chose to place his new foundation by East Smithfield cemetery in London, the same purchased by John Corey, most probably on his behalf, at the beginning of the pestilence. Could this new monastery, almost abutting Queen Philippa's new hospital church of St Katherine next door, be a thankful offering for Edward's salvation, and the survival of all but one of his family, through the past months of plague?

Yet perhaps this is too generous an interpretation. The edge of a large city was an odd place to put a Cistercian monastery, whose monks preferred the seclusion of a distant and hidden valley. The

Tower of London was hardly an aid to contemplation, yet here it dominated the view. An explanation may be found in the peak months of the London plague, when Edward had banned the digging of a new cemetery by the walls of the Tower. Perhaps he was concerned about the health of the castle, perhaps he was keen to stop a threat to the revenues of his own cemetery nearby. Just maybe, the abbey was instituted partly in propitiation for that act – a long-planned idea transplanted to the location of private guilt. Whatever the reason, the abbey, named St Mary Graces, could not hide its anachronism so close to the many new friary churches emerging from within the city walls.[63] If nothing else, it was a sign of Edward's romantic conservatism, an attribute he shared with his fellow nobles. It was certainly further evidence of the respect in which he held his grandfather, who had become for Edward an imagined and idolized surrogate father, after whom he was named but whom he had never known. It just may have been, however, the achievement of a man not usually given to reflection, acting on a rare instance of self-reproach.

13

Reorder and Reaction

1351–1360

Deep in deepest Connacht, somewhere between Lough Corrib and Lough Ree, the poets and harpists, jesters and bards of Ireland came together at Christmas, 1351, in the house of William O'Kelly,[i] the princely patron of Hy Many.[ii] The gathering was celebrated by one of those present in the poem 'The Poets of Ireland to One House'; it may well have been that Aodh MacEgan, the plaintive scribe who thanked God for his survival at Christmas the previous year, was among their number. How he will have marvelled at this famous scene, which the annalist would later declare caused all who went there to be 'well pleased'![I] For whatever the reasons O'Kelly brought these men together, this must surely have been first and foremost a celebration of the Gaelic nation, its fortitude in the face of the English occupation, and its survival from the recent horrors of plague.

The pestilence, and a brief visit from the new English justiciar Sir Thomas Rokeby, had brought native Irish attacks on colonial possessions to a temporary halt, but as soon as Rokeby had returned to Dublin, and the epidemic had abated, the raiding started over again, heaping yet more misery upon the stricken colonial outposts in the west. Some of the most vulnerable western manors, like Rinndown on the west bank of Lough Ree, were abandoned during these years. A report from the diocese of Cashel, in the mid-south, claimed that 'lands and rents had been all but totally destroyed by the king's enemies and by the mortality of their tenants in the last plague'. The towns on the south coast were suffering terribly. The townsmen of Cork pleaded in 1351 that the mortality had been so great that many houses

[i] Anglicized from Uilliam Ó Ceallaigh.
[ii] Anglicized from Uí Mhaine.

still stood empty,[iii] while the small settlements on either side of Youghal – Inchiquin and Kinsalebeg – were now totally laid to waste, after the pestilence had finished what had been started by many years of Gaelic Irish attacks.

The colonial manors further east, meanwhile – spared the worst of native Irish assaults – retrieved what they could from the wreckage left by the mortality. As in England, rents were remitted and land was let: anything to keep people on the land working the fields.[2] Yet in many places there were still no takers, so, where lords had too few servants to cultivate the land themselves, it lay abandoned, just as it did in the wilder west.

That even a partial recovery on colonial estates was possible was thanks in large part to the efforts of Justiciar Rokeby, who had brought the Leinster Irish under control and instilled a semblance of order in the colonial administration. Those functions of royal rule that had been suspended during the plague were, in time, resuscitated, and royal coffers – for once – were beginning to fill.[iv] Yet, this recovery in revenues was only temporary, for without the one-off receipts of death and inheritance, the diminished state of the crown manors was soon laid bare. Moreover, the proceeds from customs, reflecting a widespread depression in the colony, fell by a third and did not recover. Thus by 1352 Irish Treasury officials recorded crown revenues of around £1,570 per annum, only half what they had been before the Great Death and a quarter of the amount remitted at the turn of the century. Although there was a slight (and short-lived) recovery in later years, royal revenues never returned to their pre-plague level.[v] This was as much a reflection on the continuing decline in trade as it was in a fall in agricultural income, for the combined effect of a slowing of exports

[iii] See Ch. 4, p. 88.

[iv] The justiciar's court in Dublin resumed its sessions in January 1351 and held no fewer than sixty-seven sessions that year, in order to clear the backlog of cases that had piled up over the previous twenty-four months of adjournment, which meant in turn that there was a surge in the proceeds of justice. Moreover, the extraordinary number of entry fines and heriots resulting from the mortality produced a rare increase in revenues from the crown estate. Taken together, by the end of the 1349–50 financial year royal officials were able to show a return that exceeded the pre-plague norm.

[v] It should be remembered that because of inflation, even reaching parity with pre-plague income was equal to a loss of real income.

to Spain, persistent attacks by the Gaelic-Irish, and the depopulation and degradation of the colony all meant that both exports and imports maintained their pre-plague decline.

Rokeby saw these problems immediately and knew that substantial reform of both the colony and its administration was required. The Irish parliament of 1350 had made a start, passing legislation against absentee landlords, and the enquiry that Rokeby had instigated into the management of the Exchequer culminated in a reforming royal ordinance of March 1351. The following autumn, he convened a great council to discuss the many challenges that the Anglo-Irish faced, one of which – the successful division of the colony by belligerent Gaelic Irish into two parts – was borne out by the need to hold two separate sessions, one in Dublin and another in Kilkenny. The product was a set of twenty-five ordinances which, it was intended, would form the foundation upon which the Anglo-Irish colony could be rebuilt. As well as the standard proclamation of the freedoms of the church and the primacy of Magna Carta, the ordinances repeated the recent royal decrees on the operation of the administration in Ireland and introduced the Westminster Statute of Labourers passed earlier that year. There was an attempt to stop the pollution of English practice by Irish custom, by limiting marriage alliances, private truces and the use of Irish law. However, the ordinances conversely ordered marcher lords to adopt the Irish praxis of 'kin-liability', which made the local lord responsible for the arrest of felons and incarceration before trial. In England, this responsibility had for centuries fallen to travelling crown justices and latterly local magistrates. However, as none of this apparatus operated properly in Ireland, it was conceded that, for practicality's sake, the Anglo-Irish would have to adopt the less regimented traditions of local justice that were current in the native community.

This revealing compromise pointed to the larger challenge facing the colonists: that, for all Sir Thomas Rokeby's energy, the colony could not afford to consolidate and re-extend itself without an accommodation with the native Irish nation. This implicit acceptance that the Gaelic Irish could not be overcome under current circumstances was itself a departure, albeit an unsurprising one. Quite simply, the incentive to conquer was no longer there, as for the king and for increasing numbers of landowners Ireland had become a loss-making enterprise, a fact that the additional problems caused by pestilence only served to underline.

Granted parole in late 1350 to lobby the Scots for the peace treaty agreed between kings Edward and David, it was not long before Sir William Douglas returned to the Tower bearing bad news: the border country had been laid waste by Balliol's invasions and the plague had wrecked what the marauders had not touched. Moreover, Robert Stewart had rejected David's deal. The king and Sir William tried again in early 1352, personally pleading with the regent to agree to Edward's offer; but Stewart had little difficulty in persuading his peers to refuse the proposed treaty, pointing out that its acceptance meant that their years of suffering would have been for naught. These Scots were not prepared to pay £40,000 only to forgo their independence. So the king and his warrior companion were soon back in the Tower.

Driven near mad by imprisonment, Sir William forsook his loyalty to David and came to a private arrangement with the English king; yet he was murdered by his cousin almost as soon as he returned to Liddesdale. Thus deprived of his lieutenant, King David grew increasingly desperate. By 1354 he had agreed new terms for a treaty, which ceded yet more sovereignty to England and increased the ransom to £60,000. The Scots consented to the terms, at Berwick, on 13th July 1354. Yet, with French encouragement, they soon went back on what they had agreed and David, who had been waiting at Newcastle to be handed over once the first instalment of the ransom had been paid, was returned south to Odiham Castle, in Hampshire. He had been sixty miles from freedom.

Even if Edward had gained nothing tangible out of King David's incarceration, his absence from Scotland at least helped to promote peace on the border. This was a help, as Edward was once again focused on France, where his position was increasingly fragile. Distraction raids conducted by Walter Manny, the duke of Lancaster and John Beauchamp through the spring and summer of 1351 had been repulsed and Bateman, brought once again to Guînes, was forced by the French – who for the first time in years enjoyed a sliver of advantage – to agree to yet another, highly unsatisfactory, holding truce. Yet in early January 1352 a renegade English captain captured Guînes itself in flagrant violation of the temporary peace, bringing the two nations closer to full-scale war than at any time since the Great Death had passed.

Edward received the news of this unexpected prize from a furious French embassy, which came hot foot over the Channel to remonstrate with him. The king was in Westminster, preparing for the 1352 session of parliament, which was about to begin. The French protest added a further complication to what everyone knew would be a tricky session. Even though no campaign was imminent, the king planned to ask parliament for a new grant of taxation, in order that he could keep his options open on the Continent and meet a French challenge, should it arise. The Commons were extremely wary of agreeing to precautionary grants, however, and in any case were in no mood for a return to conflict: the triumph of Crécy, which had for several years sustained the English lust for war, was now obscured from their collective memory by the all-consuming horrors of the Great Death. Manorial incomes were depressed, making the payment of tax more onerous; to make matters worse, the clergy were refusing to pay the second instalment of the £18,000 subsidy they had granted the king the previous year, over the crown's appropriation of vacant benefices for royal clerks. Conscious that an accommodation was necessary with all these groups if any hope of a new taxation was to be realized, Edward's ministers quietly encouraged the submission of petitions in advance of parliament on those issues where the king was happy to concede legislation. Thus when the time came Edward would make great show of the royal indulgence of his subjects, lay and clerical, hoping that in turn they would reciprocate in cash.

In the event, the crown got what it bargained for, but only because of the serendipitous arrival of the furious French ambassadors. Nonetheless, the king was forced to pay dearly in statute for his three-year tenth and fifteenth: there were reforms on the vexed issue of feudal military funding and service, new regulations concerning weights and measures, and for the nobility a significant (if largely symbolic) statute on treasons, which formally limited the arbitrary powers of the crown. The clergy too received the statute protection they had sought and duly agreed to complete the payment of the subsidy as they had said they would.

Finally, parliament addressed the enduring problems caused by the

Great Death: the instances in which villeins could claim their liberty were curtailed, while all the profits from actions brought under the Statute of Labourers were to be deducted from the assessments for the new tenth and fifteenth, just as they had been in 1349. However, unlike the former rebate, in which deductions were made in the districts in which the penalties had been levied, parliament agreed that the receipts of the justices would be used to offset the tax owed by those places in greatest need of relief. This was not what the Commons had wanted (members had hoped that by bringing prosecutions under the Statute of Labourers they might directly reduce the tax bill for their own area); the crown, however, was insistent that its distributive scheme should go ahead, even though the disbursement of monies collected by the justices to the towns and hundreds claiming distress required an extraordinarily complicated bureaucratic procedure to be put in place. The crown's reasons were simple, and had very little to do with charity. Petitions were still arriving at Westminster from towns and districts in distress, pleading that their assessment for taxation, unaltered since 1332, should be reduced; most cited the pestilence as the chief cause of their impoverished state. To accede to these pleas would not only reduce the income from taxation but would set an unfortunate precedent. So Edward's ministers reasoned that, if they were to direct labourers' fines and 'excess' wages towards the most devastated areas, then they could more easily refuse their requests for relief. Thus the new rebate embodied the intriguing notion that the ill-gotten wages of wilful workers in one area might be used to allay the hardship of taxpayers – great and small – in another, thereby righting some general imbalance brought about by the plague. This was not just a clever bureaucratic fiddle, which went some way to assuage the concerns of hard-pressed taxpayers at no cost to the Exchequer: it was none other than the first 'redistributive' measure introduced by the English state.

In their novelty and manner of implementation, the measures of 1352 further extended the ambition and reach of Edward's administration of his realm. The genius behind this was that of the treasurer, William Edington. It was clearly he who had devised the rebate scheme and it was the ingenious bishop who saw the advantages of regulating weights and measures, which would help reduce customs fraud. This in itself was crucial to Edington's strategy for maximising the proceeds of indirect taxation, which he correctly saw as the only means by which his monarch could be made financially independent. At the very most, the tenth and fifteenth only yielded £37,000 per year, which was insufficient to fund large-scale foreign campaigns: the campaign of 1346–7, which included Crécy and the siege of Calais, had cost well over £200,000. As Edward's many defaults meant that he was unlikely to be able to continue to fund the war from loans, Edington set about clawing as much as he could from indirect taxation, which (usefully) did not require parliamentary consent. Having taken the collection of customs in house after the collapse of the Chiriton tax-farming company, Edington reformed the entire system for taxing wool exports, establishing legal points of sale to foreign merchants in important inland English towns. The so-called wool 'staple' was approved in October 1353 and within a year had already borne fruit: receipts had increased by 265 per cent, from £42,800 in 1352–3 to £113,400 in 1353–4. Although a boom in wool exports was to make this an exceptionally good year, receipts from customs were maintained far above the figure achieved before Edington's reforms were put in place. Furthermore, the rebate helped to ensure that the triennial grant, despite the continuing problems left by the mortality, achieved 96 per cent of its assessed value in the year of its grant (1352) and in each of the following two years. This was not the sum of it, for Edington ensured that proper accounting and budgeting were introduced in all the departments of the royal administration, so that tax revenues, once collected, were properly spent. Taken together, these measures ensured that even if Edward had not been able to afford to go to war in 1352, within three years he was in a position to campaign on the Continent without recourse to credit. Despite the Great Death, the English king – unlike his bankrupt French enemy – was now richer than he had ever been.

In the first three years of the operation of the staple in England, only foreign merchants were permitted to export wool from England. Although this was deeply unpopular with domestic merchants, it brought much-needed foreign currency into the country and attracted foreign trade, as merchants bought not only wool but increasingly sought out finished cloth. As a result, exports of cloth (which had been growing before the Great Death) continued to expand, so that by the end of the 1350s the number of cloths shipped from English ports was ten times the number exported on the eve of the plague.

The chief beneficiaries of this boom were the cloth-producing towns. Coventry, which was almost certainly larger by the end of the 1350s than immediately before the plague, was by 1355 busily constructing new walls – that surest sign of urban prosperity and prestige. Despite the proximity of competing Coventry, Leicester had probably recovered its population by 1354, when the town clerk recorded as many local taxpayers as there had been in 1336. That half the list comprised new names – many of them from the villages nearby – showed clearly how that recovery had been achieved. Immigration fed the resurgence of all these growing towns, some of which were so hungry for new citizens that they were prepared to permit mercantile freedoms to women, who had previously been excluded from civil privileges. In Colchester – another cloth town – the extraordinary number of new burgesses included one or two women: a small number but significant nonetheless.[3] The new guild of the Blessed Virgin Mary in Hull, established in 1357, had among its founder members a few single women, and it is clear that they intended that there should be even more: one of the purposes of the guild was to provide loans to poor members, both men and women, who wished to set up their own businesses in the town.

Ambitious young men and women were attracted to flourishing towns that offered good opportunities; those places which were already in decline, or were encountering problems as a consequence of the plague, failed to attract the new immigrants that they needed to replenish their populations. Winchester was in decline long before the Great Death, a trend that its subsequent depopulation only confirmed. Norwich produced cheap worsted – the wrong kind of cloth for export; it failed to recover as did Coventry and shops made vacant in the pestilence were still empty in 1357, by which time they were falling into disrepair. Yarmouth's fortunes were done no favours by its leading townsmen, who sought the protection of the crown rather than trying to adapt to a shrunken market. The Statute of Herrings (1357) for which they lobbied backfired when what few traders remained went elsewhere, so Yarmouth's 'protections' had to be suspended the following year.

The attempt to rig the herring market in Yarmouth was enough to cause ructions in the town, as up and coming burgesses became increasingly angry at the actions of the old merchant monopolists, whose business the disastrous statute had been intended to protect. Similar disputes were repeated in many towns, as established merchant elites sought to shore up their position in the face of ambitious and forceful rivals. In Beverley in 1356 500 townsmen broke into the guild-hall and disrupted the election of new members to the council, in an unsuccessful attempt to break the oligarchy that the richest merchants of the town had recently formed to run the town. The merchant princes of London achieved a similar coup in the capital, although their reaction was directed against foreign competition, not fellow townsmen, and was rather more short lived. In 1351 the new mayor, Andrew Aubrey, suspended normal ward elections and restricted seats on the common council to representatives of the larger guilds. Their intention was to force the crown to back down on its promotion and protection of foreign merchants, but when it became clear that the king would continue to uphold the rights of the Flemings and Hansards, any residual support for the new regime ebbed away and, once Aubrey's term had come to an end, ward elections soon returned, conducted just as they had been since ancient times.

Contention and competition were the stuff of medieval civic life and disputes of this kind were common enough. However, the coincidence of so many urban disturbances in these years points to the destabilizing effect of the Great Death, which catalysed tension into dissent. The mortality had opened the door not only to incomers and ambitious survivors, but to the young inheritors now coming of age. Thomas Worlingworth, the London orphan whose first adoptive parents had also died, was only released from the wardship of John Hiltoft in 1358. Thomas walked away from the London court of wards in control of a significant estate, one which few men, let alone one who was barely twenty, might ever expect. There were many like Thomas in the towns of England after the plague: not with his wealth, maybe, but adoles-cent orphans with adult means. They were part of a fresh generation of townsmen – immigrants, aspirants and inheritors – who had been promoted more rapidly through the agency of plague. Their presence not only changed the age structure of towns but altered their internal economic dynamic too. Money was in the hands of new people, and new types of people. It is not difficult to see, therefore, why tension quickly built between this refreshed urban class and the established civic elites, especially in those towns where there was an entrenched mercantile party keen to protect its position and wealth.

However, where the main obstruction to urban ambition was a franchise holder, such as a monastery or great lord, townsmen were more likely to come together against this outside power than indulge in fractious dispute. Arguments with feudal overlords were often as old as the towns themselves; it is all the more striking, therefore, that so many found their resolution during these post-plague years. In York an ancient dispute between the citizens and St Mary's Abbey over the jurisdiction of the suburb of Bootham was resolved in 1354 by an agreement brokered by Archbishop Thoresby, which passed all rights to the common council of the city. In Coventry too the townsmen at last achieved success, for in 1355 they assumed administration of that half of the city previously governed by the prior, as well as that half in the possession of the king's mother. That these franchise holders were willing to consent to the townsmen's demands reflected a shift in the balance of urban power, away from the feudal authorities of old and towards an ever more assertive and self-confident commercial urban class. It was a process begun long before the Great Death but one which pestilence had nonetheless accelerated.

The continued decline of Oxford was arrested to some extent by the rapid recovery of the university, which was soon thronging with students, who returned to the university in no fewer numbers than before the pestilence drove them away. Among them was a young John Wyclif, who arrived at Oxford in the months following the end of the pestilence, just as one of his future opponents, Uthred Boldon, became warden of Durham College. Uthred's greatest pupil, Adam Easton, came to Oxford from Norwich cathedral priory in the mid-1350s to begin his doctorate in theology and his contemporary and friend, Thomas Brinton, also from the priory in Norwich, was at Gloucester College at much the same time. Each of these men would come to have a significant influence on the late fourteenth-century church, and they all rubbed shoulders at Oxford in these post-plague years.

Before going up to Oxford, Thomas Brinton had spent a couple of years at Cambridge, which prospered after the Great Death. Unlike Oxford, which maintained a broadly stable academic population throughout these years, Cambridge grew, as was evident from the several new colleges that were established during the 1350s. Edmund Gonville's foundation was the first of these, for although he had died in the summer of 1351, William Bateman – who only the previous year had established his own college of Trinity Hall nearby – brought the college to completion. To these two new foundations was added a third in 1352, when the townsmen of Cambridge, incorporated in the fraternity of Corpus Christi, won the support of Henry Grosmont (whom the king had recently elevated from the earldom to the dukedom of Lancaster) in setting up a college; their endowment was made possible, no doubt, as a result of the many bequests made by the guild members who had perished in the Great Death. (Those that survived them were certainly ambitious: this was the only college to be established by townsmen in either university.) The influence of the pestilence could be found in more colleges than just Corpus Christi, however: it is probable that Bishop Bateman's intention that Trinity Hall should specifically propagate learning in canon law was prompted by the deaths of so many learned clerks during the pestilence, while Lady Elizabeth's new statutes for her earlier foundation of Clare Hall, which she granted in 1359, expressly stated that the college was instituted for the furtherance of knowledge to be applied to divine worship and the good of the state which, 'in consequence of a great number of men having been taken away by the fangs of pestilence, is now beginning lamentably to fail'.[4] It was with a similar regard for clerical education that Archbishop Simon Islip founded Canterbury Hall in Oxford, in 1361, and William Wykeham established the New College of St Mary in 1379.

These new colleges were sure evidence not only that Oxford and Cambridge were thriving but that their purpose had to some extent been reoriented as a consequence of the mortality. This is not to claim that the pestilence had much effect on the academic standing of either university, both of which forfeited so few of their leading scholars during the plague. For in truth, the English universities, and Oxford in particular, had lost their former lustre some time ago: several great minds died during the decade before the Great Death, while other luminaries had moved away.[5] Besides, Oxford had long before given up its two most famous stars, the Franciscans John Duns Scotus and William Ockham, over to the Continent. It was a doubly unfortunate loss, for Duns Scotus and Ockham both brought about a radical

reorientation of Catholic philosophy, away from the great systems of
Bonaventure and Thomas Aquinas, which had combined God and His
creation in one inextricable whole, towards a critical examination of
the intrinsic qualities of Godhead and its relationship with human
thought and action. This was, by its nature, a fissiparous academic
tendency, one which, coinciding with the war with France that so frustrated regular scholarly exchange with Paris, resulted in the English
universities following a more independent intellectual drift. Thus, even
when peace with France meant that cross-Channel exchanges could
resume, the universities continued along the rather insular course that
they had followed in the years before the Great Death. For as their
focus moved to the unglamorous but necessary task of improving
the education of the clergy, it was unsurprising that the schools should
concentrate on a more practical, applied style of scholarship, rather
than on the theoretical disputes to which they had made so significant
a contribution earlier in the century.

The death of William of Ockham in 1347 had removed one of the
final obstacles to the reconciliation of the papacy with Ockham's
Franciscan order, who had been at odds for half a century over the
ownership of church property.[vi] While Ockham's death certainly made
peace with the papacy possible, it is not too fanciful to think that the
horrors of the pestilence helped to make the *rapprochement* actual.
Wishing to make best use of this newfound amity, and well aware of
the demand for friars to help with parish work after the deaths of so
many priests, the Franciscans pushed the papacy to look again at the
restrictions on friars that had prevented their involvement in parish
life.

It is doubtful whether this rather arcane discussion would have
had any impact in the British Isles had it not been for the fact that
the pope asked Richard FitzRalph, amongst others, to look at the
matter on his behalf. FitzRalph was still in Avignon at this point, having
unsuccessfully lobbied the pope in 1349 to grant the English a plenary
Jubilee indulgence, and was now arguing his case for the primacy of
his archdiocese over all Ireland. Edward III had withdrawn his support
for the archbishop as soon as he had failed in his first objective: the

---

[vi] Since the publication of the bull *Super cathedram* in 1300 by Boniface VIII.

king's priority was to secure order in Ireland and the absence of the archbishop of Armagh, arguing the toss over his privileges in Avignon, did nothing to further this end.[vii] Angry at FitzRalph's failure to return to his see, Edward recalled him from the papal city, an order that the wilful archbishop chose to ignore.[viii] Surrounded by the lavender, cypresses and olive groves of Provence, FitzRalph could have been forgiven for preferring the pleasures of Avignon to strife-ridden and rain-sodden Armagh. Yet it was the intellectual challenge posed by the pope that kept him there, not the comforts of the papal court, as this was an issue on which FitzRalph had recently developed a keen interest. For the archbishop had seen for himself some of the sharp practice employed by the friars in Ireland during the pestilence.[ix] Whilst in plague-stricken Drogheda, the brother of a dead man had come to the bishop, complaining that the friars, who had been named as executors of the dead man's will, had refused to give over some property that had been bequeathed to him. When the archbishop summoned the friars to explain themselves, they impudently told him that he had been appointed their conservator in order to protect them, not pass judgement on their actions. This snub infuriated the prelate and spurred him to reflect on the privileges enjoyed by the mendicant orders. The seclusion enforced on him by plague, and his subsequent long wait for decisions in Avignon, had afforded him much time to do precisely this. Now FitzRalph was able to give his answer, before the

[vii] FitzRalph probably devoted his sermon of 6th December 1349 to this issue. He will not have heard yet from Westminster that the king had withdrawn his support for his claims. In fact Edward had already appointed John of St Paul, who had lately filled the vacancy left on the death of Archbishop Bicknor in Dublin, as Primate of Ireland.

[viii] On 18th February 1350. Edward also wrote to two papal bureaucrats who were investigating the primatial issue, lobbying them to come to a conclusion that favoured Dublin and not Armagh.

[ix] The origin of FitzRalph's animus against the friars, with whom he had had good relations before the late 1340s, may lie with Hugh, archbishop of Damascus, who was also an Augustinian friar. In 1345 Hugh had gone round John Grandison's Exeter diocese, improperly usurping the bishop's authority and allegedly living a scandalous life. In 1348 he had then been sent to be Zouche's suffragan, most likely to get him as far from Grandison as was possible. This was just at the point that FitzRalph was on probation with Grandison, whom he admired greatly. No doubt Grandison told FitzRalph about the affair and the two had discussed the friars' more general contempt for the rights of the secular clergy.

pope. On 5th July 1351 the archbishop preached a sermon before the papal court that denied the presumed pastoral rights of the mendicants in the strongest possible terms: they should not hear confession, nor should they be able to bury the dead, and their ability to preach should be circumscribed. With that, FitzRalph returned to lobbying the pope for his rights in Ireland, and when this proved to be unsuccessful made his return there.

The archbishop arrived back in his diocese by late summer, 1351. He immediately got to work on dealing with the problems that had been left by the Great Death. As in England, there was a serious shortage of priests: before he had died, Alexander Bicknor had been given permission to ordain forty illegitimate men and twenty potential ordinands who were still underage so that he could try to make up numbers. Vacancies had caused the usual abuses: John de Briane was allowed to receive the revenue from five English posts as well as a canonry, prebend and deanery of St Patrick's Cathedral in Dublin while he was at university. On seeing the effect that the degeneration of the Anglo-Irish clergy had had on the pastoral care of the people, FitzRalph called two provincial synods, the first in 1352 and again in 1355, specifically to address the problems he had found. His constant concern was that the church should lead by example and place itself at the centre of community life. With this in mind, he upbraided his bishops and clergy for indulging in drunkenness and fornication rather than tending to the needs of their flocks.

Yet FitzRalph found his attempts to build an ecclesial utopia constantly frustrated by the friars, who had grown in influence in the wake of the Great Death. In 1350, in the archbishop's absence, they had been given unfettered rights to preach, hear confessions and bury the dead. FitzRalph thought them to be especially pernicious in Drogheda, where they had grown rich from bequests made by wealthy merchants and the fees earned by offering (increasingly popular) private confessions. There was now a two-tier Christianity in the town: it was precisely this fragmentation of the communal church that FitzRalph most feared. Clearly conscious of the recent flood of bequests that had followed the Great Death, FitzRalph attacked the merchants of Drogheda in no uncertain terms. In life, he claimed, they fiddled their books to avoid paying tithes, and only gave away their riches once they had died, and then often only to the friars. Such false charity, he proclaimed, was no aid to salvation. However, for the archbishop the merchants were merely the conduit of evil, not its source: that claim to infamy belonged to the friars, whose hunger for donations and endowments lured parishioners away from their parish priests and thus undermined the unity and purpose of the church. Duly exercised, the archbishop set to work on a vast treatise, *De Pauperie Salvatoris*, which not only repudiated the friars' privileges but denied the whole validity of the mendicant orders.

Archbishop FitzRalph was not alone in his distaste for the mendicants. The closed orders despised them (John of Reading, a Benedictine, claimed of them that 'superfluous finery was everywhere: in their chambers, at table, in riding – all contrary to the requirements of their order and prompted by the devil')[6] and many bishops agreed with FitzRalph that the friars encroached upon their spiritual domain. However, the malice directed at the friars from other clergy had done nothing to diminish their appeal; if anything, establishment opposition only reinforced their standing among the laity. Mendicants of all stripes – Franciscan, Dominican, Austin and Carmelite – encouraged donations both from the rich, who had traditionally funded monastic foundations, and from people of fewer means – from the widow to the urban tradesman made good. This lack of exclusivity was a powerful fundraising tool, for in offering the most humble an opportunity to be remembered before God in death, it lent an extra badge of piety to those rich people who gave the friars the bulk of their bequests. The result was that the friars emerged from the Great Death stronger in numbers and funds than many of their secular and religious counterparts. Their relative strength contrasted with the weakness of the secular clergy in the immediate aftermath of the plague, for which reason some bishops were willing to use the mendicants to supplement their pastoral efforts. Bishop Trillek of Hereford commissioned friars to help the stretched Herefordshire clergy in the years after the Great Death, and it is little surprise, therefore, that the new house of Carmelites established in Ludlow in 1350 was already ordaining new brethren by the end of 1352. For a similar reason Bishop Hatfield licensed Carmelite friars to give sermons in the diocese of Durham in 1353, 'that there should be more preaching that the souls of the people might be fed'.[7]

Whatever FitzRalph's feared there was little danger of the mendicants usurping the traditional role of the secular clergy in administering to 'the people': that task was simply too big. The prelates had to ensure that the parish clergy were present in their villages, were well-disciplined and dutiful in caring for the needs of their parishioners. This last challenge was particularly pressing, for the pestilence had forced the bishops to concentrate on the problems of allocating clergy and providing the sacraments, which inevitably eclipsed the careful assessment of the quality of clerical preaching and teaching, which was the usual stuff of episcopal visitations. To help with this, the archbishop of York, John Thoresby, devised in 1357 a Latin manual for parish priests, to help them instruct their parishioners in the rudiments of the faith.[8] In common with FitzRalph, Thoresby enjoined the clergy to lead by example and to ensure that the parish church remained at the heart of community life. Manuals like this had long been used: many had been based, as was this one, on Archbishop Simon Peckham's seminal instructions of 1281. What was unusual about Thoresby's attempt was the English companion that the bishop published alongside it. Written in verse by the monk John Gaytrick, this *Lay Folk's Catechism* was clearly aimed at a widespread readership, and this it certainly achieved. The catechism rehearses the Ten Commandments and fourteen articles of faith, as well as the several septimal fundamentals of Christian life: deadly sins and contrary virtues, sacraments, and works of corporal mercy. Very few bishops were as imaginative as Thoresby in their efforts to improve the standard and pastoral efficacy of their clergy but in general they acquitted themselves with similar care and industry during these post-plague years. To these men the epitaph inscribed on John Trillek's tomb might equally apply: each was 'gratus, prudens, pius'.[9]

It was in this spirit of pragmatism that one of the English church's longest-running disputes was brought to an end in 1353. The argument about which of the archiepiscopal sees of Canterbury and York had precedence in England had been going on since the first years of the Conquest. It would not be unreasonable to think that the renewed focus on the pastoral concerns of the church encouraged Simon Islip and the newly installed John Thoresby to come to a final settlement on the issue. For were there not now more important things to attend to than revisiting the squabbles of the past? There was one dispute, however, that the English church could not avoid, and that was between the king and the pope. It often fell to the metropolitans of England to defend the interests of the pope but, with Thoresby's election to York, Edward had ensured that both sees were occupied by men who owed their preferment entirely to him. This gave him the confidence to make another move against the papacy, whose interventions in favour of the French – and his clerical opponents at home – had increasingly irritated him.[x] Edward knew that he was not going to encounter any local opposition from the archbishop of Canterbury, whose ongoing spat with John Gynewell had resulted in that bishop appealing to the pope over his head; nor was Thoresby, only recently appointed, going to stick his neck out on account of the pope. So in 1353 the king introduced legislation – the so-called Statute of *Praemunire* – to restrict recourse to the papal courts. A hundred and eighty years later Henry VIII would cite *Praemunire* as a precedent in his first moves to break with Rome. This was not the intention at the time, however, and it should be seen for what it was – a device by which Edward could put pressure on an antipathetic Avignon pope to reverse his support for the king of France.

It was the success of the English fighting companies, rather than pressure on the papacy, that brought the French back to the negotiating table in 1354. John II agreed to a permanent (and, from the English point of view, very generous) settlement. Upon hearing the news, the Commons were asked for their approval, to which they replied 'Yes! Yes!', 'with one voice'.[10] Yet when the duke of Lancaster went to Avignon to seal the agreement, the French stood him up. So duke Henry had to return home, knowing that the news he bore left his liege with no choice but to resume the war, a decision confirmed by the great council at the end of March 1355. The campaign planned for that summer was cancelled, however, and when battle eventually came, it was not in France, but on the Scottish border, after a small Scots army – reinforced with gold and soldiers from France – marched into Northumberland in early October 1355 and, on 6th November, retook Berwick.

Edward headed north, wrested Berwick from the Scots, crossed the border and did the Lowlands much damage, but nothing was achieved

---

[x] Edward had been in dispute with John Grandison since 1349 over the crown's use of his parishes as sinecures for royal clerks.

there other than to refill the well of bitterness from which the Scots so eagerly drank. He was content to let Scotland go, however, for he was about to embark upon the largest campaign on the Continent that he had yet attempted. The Prince of Wales was already in Bordeaux, recapturing those possessions lost piecemeal to the French over the previous five years. In June 1356 a second army led by Lancaster marched hard towards the prince from the north-west: the king of France obligingly came between the two. The Prince of Wales met the French force in battle outside Poitiers, on 19th September 1356. This was a place of national sanctity for the French, for it was not far from here that Charles Martel had turned back the tide of conquering Islam in 732. On this occasion, however, it would be the French who were overcome. The Prince of Wales inflicted a terrible defeat on King John, who was captured alive at the battle's end. It was an audacious victory: much of the French warrior nobility was now in English hands – their ransoms alone, excluding that of the king, ensured that the campaign had more than paid for itself.

The prince and duke returned to England with King John II, who was received with due honour by ecstatic crowds in London. Edward now had in his possession both the king of Scotland and the greatest lord in Europe, the king of France, both of whom were imprisoned at Windsor. It was said that they rode out in the park with King Edward, these three sovereigns, and discussed how much better the castle would appear if it were to be extended onto higher ground. But this congress of kings was to be shortlived. With John in his custody, Edward could press the Scots for the ransom he demanded in return for their king. The Scots regent, Robert Stewart, and the great nobles of Scotland knew that their game was now up: they could no longer rely on the support of France in avoiding the demands of the English crown. So, on 26th September 1357, a council meeting in Edinburgh approved the payment to the English of a ransom of £66,666, to be made over in annual instalments spread over ten years. The sum was the equivalent of nearly two years' direct taxation from the whole of England: for the English this was an enormous prize; for the Scots it was a gargantuan penalty. It did, at least, allow the Scots to retrieve their king, unencumbered by the previous demands for fealty to the English crown that Edward had previously pressed. David crossed the border on 7th October 1357,

ten days before the eleventh anniversary of his capture at Neville's
Cross.

David's journey home cannot have been a happy one. The Lowlands
between the Tweed and the Forth still showed the scars of Edward's
spoliation a couple of years before, and the villages were still as empty
as they had been when David was last in Scotland, on parole, in 1352
– two years after the Great Death. From this ravaged land David had
to raise his ransom. Within a month of his release, a great council
was convened at Scone to discuss how this might be done. The crown
was to claim the profits of wool exports and customs were to be
increased. Royal lands given away in his absence were to be reclaimed.
A new tax assessment was to be undertaken, as the old one had been
rendered invalid by the mortality.

That these measures were successful was a tribute, in part, to the
assiduity of a clerk named Walter Biggar, whose achievement was
greater even that that of William Edington. For although both had to
deal with the dire effects of pestilence and war, the Scot had to contend
with the inheritance of an aimless regency (the accounts of some
sheriffs, for instance, had not been audited since before Neville's Cross)
and the long-lasting repercussions of brutal English raids on the most
productive parts of the country.

Credit must go to David as well, who had not idled away his days
in England: he had watched Edward and his treasurer at work, and
had made careful plans for his return. From the start he worked to
secure the support of the various constituencies that wielded power
in his realm. William Landel, the bishop of St Andrews and head of
the Scottish church, was brought within the inner circle of the king's
court. The men of the burghs, many of them freshly empowered as
had been the townsmen of England, were given enhanced representation in council and parliament, for which David gained the gratitude
and support of their chief representative, the substantial merchant
John Mercer. To the nobility he was careful not to challenge too many
of the grants of royal land made during Robert Stewart's regency,
against the wishes of the Scone parliament. Indeed, to the two
men in the country who posed the greatest potential threat, he
gave earldoms: the young William Douglas was made earl of Douglas
in recognition of his ascendancy in the western borders, and the
erstwhile regent was given the earldom of Strathearn, which had previ-

ously devolved to the crown. These were the actions of an astute politician, which did much to limit dissent during these years when the Scots paid heavily for the privilege of a present king.

The renewed vigour of the Scottish crown in this, David's third personal reign, was certainly impressive; yet what is more striking was the fact that Scotland was returned to its monarch in comparatively good order, despite the loss of the greater part of the Scottish baronage at Neville's Cross, despite the king's absence for eleven years, despite the ravages of the English, despite the deficiencies of the regent, and despite the calamity visited upon Scotland by the Great Death. This was all the more remarkable given that, unlike England, which had been united under one monarch for 400 years, the writ of the king of Scots had extended across mainland Scotland for less than a century.[xi] By the standards of English monarchs, the powers exercised by Scottish kings were still limited and weak. Nonetheless, the rulers of Scotland had, by the middle of the fourteenth century, developed many of the institutions (such as a Chancery, Exchequer and legal system) that were to be found south of the border. Faced with plague, this administration proved to be as resilient as the one in Westminster. In truth, the relative simplicity of the apparatus of Scottish government was a blessing, as there was – quite simply – far less that could go wrong when the bureaucracy temporarily shut down. There is a further reason for the persistence of the Scottish regency during the pestilence: in Scotland, as in England, there was considerable accumulated experience of governing in the king's absence. Ever since the premature death of Alexander III in 1286, the country had been plunged periodically into enforced regency, with senior nobles acting as 'guardians' of the realm in the monarch's name. Thus, by the time David left his realm for the second time, in 1346, there was a well-practised routine for governing in his absence, one that had already been tested in adversity, even in conflict; it was certainly a match for the pestilence. Indeed, one must wonder if in similar circumstances – the prolonged absence of the king, the interventions and disruptions by a foreign power, the natural fault lines between the different parts of the nation – the English polity would have fared so well.

On their own, these observations are not sufficient to explain how

---

[xi] Caithness was incorporated into the kingdom at the Treaty of Perth, 1266.

Scotland cohered during such testing times, especially given the structural deficiencies with which the Scottish realm was beset: there was a mixed nobility – native and immigrant; the country was divided into two languages; there was a messy admixture of customary and feudal law; and the powers of the king of the Scots were still restricted in large parts of his domain. Despite all this, Scottish society tended towards cohesion rather than fragmentation, a fact that undoubtedly ensured the survival of the nation through these years of war, regency and plague. The reason why this should be so must be found in the developing sense of national identity, the formation of which was greatly aided by the malicious omnipresence of the Sassenach, against whom it was not hard to define themselves. Indeed, the survival of the Scottish nation through these calamitous years was sure proof that the declaration made at Arbroath in 1320 was no groundless boast: 'for so long as a hundred men remain alive we will never in any way be bowed beneath the yoke of English domination; for it is not for glory, riches or honours we fight, but for freedom alone, that which no man of worth yields up but with life itself.' Pestilence had left rather more than this number in Scotland and done nothing to dampen the survivors' passion for independence. Edward III's acceptance that he had finally to jettison Balliol and adopt Bruce was a tacit recognition of the fact; it also exposed the gross hypocrisy of Edward's previous negotiating position with David, based as it was on an expectation that the Scots should assume exactly the same kind of vassal relationship with the English crown that Edward and his allies were fighting to adjure in France.

Unlike the Scots, the Welsh had long ago reconciled themselves to subjugation by the English. Centuries before Llywelyn ap Gruffudd's final stand, English lords had corralled the men and women of south Wales within their feudal manors – a good number on marginal land that had been difficult to farm and populate with tenants at the best of times. It was no surprise, therefore, that the pestilence had done considerable damage to English agriculture, industry, and townships in Wales – much of which had, in any event, been in decline for decades before the Great Death. The Prince of Wales's lead mines in Holywell in Flintshire, for instance, had suffered problems for decades, but by 1351 profits were diminished yet more because of the continued paucity of labourers. The English burgesses of Rhuddlan were granted a reduction of 25 per cent on the fees they paid the prince for the use of their mills, a rebate that was increased to a third in subsequent years 'until the said mills were of more value'. In simple, the fall in the population meant that far less milling was taking place. On his vast landed estate and in his towns, the prince was suffering so great a loss of tenants that his officials instituted a 'Great Roll of Debts' to record the arrears that had accumulated since the Great Death. Even where there were people able to take on new land, they were reluctant to do so, as there were now so many opportunities elsewhere, free of the harsh requirements of an English lord. Thus, in the lordship of Dyffryn Clwyd, held by Richard Fitzalan, it was found in 1356 that there were thirty vacant holdings where the heir was still alive, who had either not claimed the plot or had entered but had subsequently abandoned it. Much of this vacant land was simply let out to pasture. The population pressures of previous decades which made the colon-ization of marginal land in the March possible now no longer existed, so all over Wales land was returning to grass, to the state in which it had been before the Normans had come.

The result was an inevitable fall in the revenues that the English derived from their Welsh estates.[11] As was to be expected, the reflex reaction of most English magnates was to impose a solution on their despised Welsh subjects. One tactic was to extract out of tenants what could not be made in rents. Thus in 1352 the famously oppressive Humphrey de Bohun imposed an extraordinary fine on the men of his lordship of Brecon of £500, under the pretext that they had evaded seigniorial dues. This was at once a great revenue-raising exercise and a brutal reassertion of overlordship. The same year, the Prince of Wales, alarmed at the rapid transfer of so much land within Flintshire, ordered that all tenements purchased without his permission should be seized.

Yet, as in England, there was a limit to how far imposition could be used. The court roll of Clocaenog in Dyffryn Clwyd for 1359 shows how the officials of Richard Fitzalan (another well-known baronial tyrant) struggled to keep his tenants in order: four had to find friends or relatives who would pledge for them remaining in the lordship; warrants were sent out for the arrest of a further two who had already escaped; two more were fined for not doing the labour services they owed; others were ordered to explain why they did not hold bond land and do services. Fitzalan was clearly swimming against an overwhelming tide. Realizing this was futile, he accepted that leasing was inevitable, and by 1360 was taking £61 from the rent of vacant customary plots, ranging from single strips to whole tenements. Even the great Prince of Wales could not hold out against the wishes of his tenants. In 1359 he allowed the men around Holywell and Hopedale in Flintshire to buy and sell land without let, a privilege for which they paid £400. For Margam Abbey, long beset with financial woes, the pestilence forced the monks to break up their remaining granges into leasehold plots. Other lords found a different approach, allowing freemen to take on land that had previously been reserved for tied tenants, as at Chirkland, in north-east Wales – again in 1355. Similarly, the demesne attached to Beaumaris Castle was leased to the men of the town.

The most dramatic gesture the lord could make was to give freedom to his tenants held in bondage. For the Welsh, their freedom from English feudal lordship clearly had a double importance. Bondmen were winning their freedom on the estates of the bishop of St Asaph by 1355 – granted communal manumission either in return for higher rents or so that the bishop could let them the land that was lying untilled. This, of course, was a trend that predated the Great Death, but now the conversion of bond tenure to free tenure gathered pace. In the lordship of Bromfield and Yale, by Flintshire in north-east Wales, the lord in 1346 had been willing to grant land for life but only on his own terms, whereas after the Great Death he was forced to reduce rents by a third in order to retain tenants on the land. It was in the knowledge that some profit could be made from the grant of freedom that marcher lords were increasingly willing to loosen their grip on their tenants. Thus, when the men of Cydweli sought a charter of liberties from their lord, the duke of Lancaster, in 1356, he was willing to grant it so long as they paid a large fine.

The various responses of the English marcher barons did something to stem the losses in their lordships that followed the mortality.[12] However, the more significant outcome of so much leasing and manumission was the rapid change in the pattern of landholding across Wales. In the manor of Caldicot, whose lush shoreline pastures faced Thornbury across the Severn estuary, over 600 acres of customary and demesne land came on to the market between 1350 and 1362, a turnover that ensured that something like a third of new tenants had names which had hitherto not been recorded in the accounts of the lordship. In Neath, the lack of new English burghal tenants forced the town to concede the right of tenure to Welshmen, for the first time, in 1359. Whether it be in the towns or in the fields, the Welsh were definitely regaining something of their native land. It would be a mistake to over-state the fact, but it was surely the case that the appalling pestilence had done more to liberate the Welshman from English tyranny than had any of Llywelyn ap Gruffudd's heroic campaigns.

To the east of Offa's Dyke lay England's fields, which still gave visible evidence of the Great Death's impact. Much of the countryside was growing only weeds: from south to north land was lying uncultivated, for lack of tenants.[13] Untilled land becomes harder by the year to return to cultivation, so as time wore on it became more difficult to rent out those plots still left in the lords' hands. Nettle-strewn acres soon turned to thorny scrub and just as so many windmills stood motionless, the houses that went with unwanted tenements soon fell into disrepair. Villagers had long ago stripped empty buildings of their fittings; now the buildings themselves were seen as fair game. In Newnham in Worcestershire, villagers carried off whole timbers from empty houses and, despite the threats made by the lord's steward in the manor court, the villagers dismantled an entire cottage the following year. Lords too contributed to the changing landscape, in some cases substituting livestock for (now absent) humans. At Little Parndon in Essex two villein tenements, empty since the Great Death, were subsumed with the old customary meadow and pasture into a new park, where the lord grazed his livestock, while the deserted village of Tusmore in east Oxfordshire was entirely enclosed for sheep. By its repercussions, the pestilence could be read in the altered panorama of England.

The economic balance of the nation had also changed. For while England was still manifestly a feudal state, the fall in prices, rise in wages, monetary inflation, and collapse in rents and feudal dues had all combined to reduce manorial revenues and destroy landowners' capital. This had, in turn, already created subtle but perceptible shifts in social power: many peasants had been able to exercise a new-found economic strength, which threatened to thwart landowners' efforts to restore the profitability of their estates. The two impulses had collided in a rash of hasty accommodations and – on occasion – instances of feudal coercion, all of which continued through the 1350s. It was of course the case that peasants had been trying to free themselves of the dead hand of feudal constraint for decades, centuries even, before the Great Death – just as long as lords had sought to corral and control their tenants; but the mortality forced the pace of commutation and the leasing of land, thereby further fragmenting the structures of feudal ownership and control.

Landowners were exquisitely aware that all this was taking place; their instinctive reaction was to do all they could to make it cease. Their first recourse was to try to pretend that nothing had fundamentally changed. So, while the bishop of Winchester's officials permitted, even encouraged, his tenants to till and graze unlet tenements at a nominal price, simply in order to keep land in production and free of scrub, the licence was only given on a strictly temporary basis and the favour went unrecorded in the court rolls in case anyone should think that a precedent had been set: for the stewards and clerks were only waiting for the population to bounce back, at which point they would be able to commit the tenements to new villein tenants for customary works, just as they had done for hundreds of years previous to the Great Death.[xii] Likewise, they attempted to maintain the most obvious element of feudal landholding – the link between a family and a tenement – as best they could, going so far as to intervene in the peasant land market to ensure that villein tenements stayed intact.

Yet the reality was that land transfers had long ago begun to disrupt the pure land–family bond on which feudal tenure was based; the great ruptures inflicted on so many families by the Great Death only served to make the persistence of that bond all the more unlikely. Constantly frustrated, some lords continued to attempt to coerce their tenants to do their bidding – compelling villagers, for instance, to take on unlet land. This approach invariably caused more problems than it solved: when in 1357 the abbot of Ramsey ordered a villein to return

---

[xii] Not only did this preserve the purity of feudal tenure, but as customary services were legally attached to specific tenements, undivided holdings were easier to administer – in terms of manorial record keeping, the assignment of customary services and the calculation of tax obligations.

to his village and take up his holding once again, it had the effect of persuading other bondmen to flee the manor. Landowners soon learnt, therefore, that compulsion was almost always met with flight or resistance and consequently the instances of lords reimposing services or compelling entry into vacant landholdings were relatively rare.

Thus, even in the most oppressive of estates, lords were forced to trim their reactions to the effects of the mortality. In the palatinate of Durham, of all places – that famously severe estate – the bishop's officials were, by the middle of the decade, leasing demesnes to bondmen.[14] It was not a choice they made willingly: the villagers of Killerby were permitted to take on vacant land free of feudal obligations, so long as it was done 'in secret, because of the bad example it sets to the other villages'. Indeed, the need to make any accommodation with the bishop's tenants caused disagreements even within the management of the estate. When the arrangement with the men of Killerby was later put to the bishop's council, it was considered to be an unacceptable precedent and so in February 1356 the steward had to go back on his agreement with the villagers and insist that they pay rent and do services, 'as they were accustomed to do of old time'.[15] The matter did not finish there, for it appears that the increasingly frequent disputes in the palatinate boiled over in 1357 into some sort of revolt and the bishop was forced to appoint a special commission to hear the villagers' complaints against his officials – a clear indication that the seigniorial reaction was itself causing unrest.

The single greatest coercive tool available to landowners was, of course, the Statute of Labourers. The parliament of 1352 determined that the law should be vigorously enforced, and even before the session had ended the crown administration had despatched joint commissions for the keeping of the peace and for the enforcement of the Statute of Labourers throughout the country. The justices were drawn largely from the local landowning gentry and nobility and therefore had two interests in common with litigants – that labourers' wages should be kept down and that fines on miscreants, which went towards a reduction in local taxation, should be kept up.[xiii] Thus greatly encouraged, so many indictments were brought before the joint commissions that by the end of the year Westminster decided to send out dedicated

---

[xiii] The justices were promised bonuses for getting through a large volume of cases.

teams of justices to deal solely with offences against the Statute of Labourers. It was an enormous operation: between 1352 and 1359 over 250 commissions were issued to investigate and adjudicate on infractions of the statute, with more than 500 individuals sitting on these panels during that time.[16] In addition to the many thousands of cases brought before the justices of labourers, thousands more were presented to the two upper courts of the King's Bench and Common Pleas, while tens of thousands were settled in the local manor and hundred courts.

Every clause of the statute was enforced. In Rutland the justices heard in 1353 that all the labourers and servants of Greetham were refusing to answer charges of contravening the statute; during the same session the court set the maximum pay of a carter at 8s. per annum, enforcing obedience on pain of imprisonment. William Shipward, a ploughman of Byford in Herefordshire, left his employer before his contract had come to an end and in 1356 was fined 2s. 6d for this crime. The following year the justices in Warwickshire were presented with six smallholders who refused to work. Many of those arraigned before the justices had been indicted by their fellow villagers, like Roger Melbourne, a Derbyshire smith, who in 1358 was charged with refusing to work for his neighbours but giving his services to others instead at a higher rate. A village wrangle can be sensed in many of these indictments, just as the court records occasionally give a sense of the character of the individual labourers hauled before the bench. One can imagine, for instance, the collective elevation of eyebrows when it was explained that John Bishop, who was a digger, would not get out of bed for less than 5d. per day, with food – half as much again as a skilled labourer, such as a carpenter, might expect to earn – and even then Mr Bishop was unwilling to exert himself beyond digging up small trees.

The simple presence of the new law and its rigorous enforcement must have acted as a restraint on rates of pay; it was not possible that the considerable efforts of employers and constables, sheriffs and justices did not have some effect. However, the enormous number of cases brought under every clause of the statute is evidence enough that the labour legislation did not completely succeed in keeping wages down or enforcing terms of employment that were unfavourable to workers. Transgression of the statute was so widespread and habitual that it was a matter of note when no delinquents were to be found and all the villagers were compliant.[17] The records of the proceedings of the justices confirm the impression given by manorial accounts across the country: that everywhere workers were demanding and receiving wages greater than those allowed by law, and were working on short-term contracts, completely contrary to the statute. The average rise in wages paid on the estates of Westminster Abbey during this decade was 75 per cent; at Stallingborough in Lincolnshire workers making hay saw their wages increase by 100 per cent in the same period. The rate at which wages had risen was heavily influenced by local factors. On the Winchester estate, the average wage for building workers recorded in this decade was typically 20 and 50 per cent higher than it had been before the Great Death, although in some places, such as Wycombe and Esher – which were more affected by the competitive pull of London – wage rates had doubled. Here, as on the other side of London in Middlesex, those that gained most were the unskilled 'helpers' who accompanied carpenters, tilers and the like – precisely the kind of footloose young men who could easily make their way to the half-empty capital to find work and so had to be paid well to ensure that they stayed put.

This did not mean that labourers suddenly came into great riches. Although wages rose across the board, the cost of living had also gone up, so the amount of time that a labourer needed to work in order to pay for food and clothing was little different from how it had been in the years before the Great Death. In any case, although daily rates had risen, the seasonal nature of agricultural labour meant that there were few opportunities to increase the number of days spent labouring. It is telling that of 7,556 offenders fined in Essex in 1352, the average excess wage was only 22.9d. – no more than four to six days' legal labour. It was hardly a windfall.

More striking still is that far from fighting demands for higher wages, landowners willingly paid what they needed to keep labour on their estates. Many went to extraordinary lengths to hide their collusion, as lords too were liable to prosecution under the statute. The most common trick was to make additional payments in food or in kind. In some places the accounts themselves were fiddled. The ledgers relating to the bishop of Winchester's manor of Overton, in Hampshire, indicate no rise in wages between 1340 and 1359 – an improbability that more likely reflects fraud rather than the real payments made to local workers. Likewise, the wages quoted in the accounts of Ramsey Abbey after the Great Death show a new-found and deeply suspect uniformity, quite unlike the significant local variation in what labourers were paid on the abbey's estates before the pestilence. The great variation in enforcement within regions and counties suggests, moreover, that prosecutions were brought only where the landed interest demanded action, whereas in some parts of the country, where lords were prepared to pay high wages, the statute soon became a dead letter.[xiv]

The question remains, therefore, as to why the statute was so vigorously enforced if it largely failed to suppress wages and was manifestly broken by peasant and lord alike? Undoubtedly it helped employers enforce favourable contract terms, should they so wish, but this alone could not account for the remarkable industry with which labourers were prosecuted, especially in the first half of the 1350s. After all, the actions of so many delinquent labourers showed that there were many employers happy to accept the terms on which illegal labour was offered. The incentive came, therefore, not from a great reaction against excess labour, but from the offer of relief on taxation. For although each individual fine was small, the addition of so many produced a bounty for local taxpayers. The fines and excess wages in Essex alone came to £719 10s. in 1352, a figure which, after expenses, enabled £675 11s. to be paid towards the county's assessed contribution of £1,234 15s. 7¼d. In other words, in 1352, 55 per cent of the subsidy owed by Essex taxpayers was paid through the excess wages and fines of Essex labourers. This rebate was exceptional but the sums collected across the country were still impressive. During the period of the triennial grant of 1352–4, the penalties levied by justices of labourers came to around £10,000 which, net of costs, offset some £7,747 14s. 2d. (or 7 per cent) of the total assessed tax yield in those three years, which was close to £110,000.[18] This constituted a considerable and valuable reduction in

[xiv] In Essex, for instance, few cases were tried in the western half of the county, where the arable economy there depended on precisely the kind of seasonal labour that the statute forbade but which lords required; in the eastern part, however, the heaths and marshes supported a largely pastoral economy, whose labouring tasks were less seasonal, subject to annual contracts, and therefore less attractive to workers. Thus, in this eastern part, it suited lords to bring prosecutions, so that they might keep their labour force in place and their wages under control.

direct taxation. The crown made a paltry effort at redistribution, enough at least to head off calls for relief from certain towns and hundreds. Yet the local gentry were too involved in the distribution of the rebate to let money go out of their areas. As a consequence, most of the money collected was returned to those areas where the enforcement of the statute was most efficient and the receipt of fines was, therefore, greatest. The larger taxpayers in the counties, many of whom manned the commissions of labour justices and the panels that awarded relief, co-operated in the rigorous enforcement of the statute in these years, so that their payments of tax might be reduced. In short, the Statute of Labourers had become, by 1352, an *ad hoc* tax on rising incomes which was used by landowners to offset manorial incomes depressed through the effects of the Great Death. At its most fundamental, the rebate was no more than a mechanism by which lords might win back in a reduction of tax what they had lost in the increased cost of labour.

The diversion of the proceeds of labour prosecutions to local taxpayers served the crown well too. There had been many requests for tax relief due to the effects of the pestilence during the period of the triennial grant of 1352–4 but almost every one had been refused by the king's ministers, who fell back on the rebate as their excuse. When Hull pleaded impoverishment in 1353, for instance, even the king was moved to recognize that the town had suffered great 'waste and destruction' on account of storms and the plague, through which the survivors had been rendered 'so desolate and poverty-stricken in money'.[19] Yet Edward offered Hull no relief, other than an assurance that it would receive its share of the rebate. A rare show of leniency was made in the case of Northumberland, which in 1353 had very substantial difficulties in raising its tax: it was given a payment extension, yet still there was no reduction in the total amount owed. Only in extraordinary circumstances did the king's ministers relent. For the little extrusion of the Hampshire coast, Hayling Island, the assessment was reduced in 1352, although pestilence is cited as only one of four reasons given for the concession (the others including the attacks of the French and the damage done by the sea), and an ancillary one at that. It was only to the abbeys, who were persistent petitioners for relief, that Edward was generally sympathetic, if only out of a sense of obliged piety. Indeed, the crown granted the only known exemptions to the Statute of Labourers to two Carthusian monasteries.[xv]

With the end of the subsidy in 1354, however, the rebate lapsed and fines and excess wages reverted to the Treasury. Immediately there was a fall in the number of cases brought before the justices, as employers saw fines going straight to London rather than towards their tax bill. Responding to reduced demand, the king's ministers sent out fewer and fewer commissions and it was not long before the diminishing receipts of justice failed even to cover the expense of sending out dedicated commissions, so the commissions of labourers were re-merged in 1359 with the commissions of the peace in an effort to save on the duplication of clerks, justices and their expenses. The statute had become *de facto* another device of local justice, to be invoked at the direction of a litigant willing to bring a case to court.[xvi] For all the ingenuity of its conception, the Statue of Labourers had failed to counter the economic changes that the pestilence had wrought.

Neither peasant nor lord could change the weather, however, which was to have a significant influence on the fortunes of both through the course of the decade. A burning summer in 1351 produced an abysmal harvest and the drought the following year was remembered forty years later, when Henry Knighton recalled how 'cattle perished in their pastures for want of water, and marshes dried up so that they could be crossed where there never were paths before.'[20] Food prices shot up. Although the harvest of 1353 was good and prices fell back a little, the weather intervened again in 1356, pushing the cost of grains back to the highs of 1352. The extraordinarily low cereal prices of 1350 and 1351 were now a distant memory. Despite the fact that this significantly smaller population was fed by the same land mass, the prices of grains were now higher than they had been in the two

[xv] In 1354, Witham Priory in Somerset petitioned Edward to be allowed to pay wages above those set out in the statute and to be able to employ servants from wherever they might come. Charterhouses, exceptional in their austerity, were also entirely dependent on hired labour: they were also unwilling to break the law, even though it was more widely honoured in the breach than in the keeping. Doubtless mindful that Witham had been founded by Henry II in expiation for the death of Thomas Becket, Edward accepted its plea. A year later the Carthusian priory of Hinton, also in Somerset, received a similar dispensation.

[xvi] The crown only made two demands for direct taxation between 1355 and 1370 – a single tenth and fifteenth in 1357 and in 1360.

decades before the Great Death. Not everything was expensive: live-stock, of which there was still an abundance and whose pasture was now comparatively cheap, continued to be valued at less than it had been before the pestilence. This, however, was the exception, as most prices – even of fish – went up: the cost of herring was, by 1354, 50 per cent higher than it had been in the 1340s. Inflation continued to play its part, as Treasurer Edington's recoinage began, by the mid-1350s, to lift prices as he had intended. So, while a (relative) expansion in the money supply masked the fall in prices during the eighteen months that followed the plague, an (absolute) increase in coin exaggerated the rise in prices during the middle of the following decade.

Thus, peasant, lord and crown alike found themselves at the mercy of forces beyond their control in this aftermath of the Great Death. There could be no method in landowners' response to the consequences of the Great Death, therefore, just as there was nothing orchestrated or planned in the way that peasants chose to pursue their interests: both sides muddled along through these extraordinary years, grabbing opportunities when they saw them and rebuffing threats as best they could. For all that lords may have wished to maintain the full appa-ratus of feudal control, the need to retain paying tenants made compro-mise with peasant demands necessary; likewise, villeins may have been in a stronger position to negotiate, but they still had to deal with noble and ecclesiastical lords who owned the land and paid their wages. Everyone, meanwhile, had to live with exogenous influences on prices and the basic laws of supply and demand in the labour market, which the crown attempted – and largely failed – to command. Above all, plague had further confirmed that the case for feudalism – of tying bonded peasants to the land and extracting rent from them in kind through the products of their labour – was unequal to the manifest economic logic of commuting services for cash and hiring labour instead, selling the fruit of that labour in the market for a profit. It was a case that peasants were now able to make, in their many thousands of accommodations and acts of dissent, with unprecedented force.

The capture of John II could not bring so bitter and extended a conflict as the one that persisted between France and England to an end. Stunned by his defeat, the French king had agreed to everything that the English had demanded, yet nothing had been sealed, for the noble

Frenchmen who responded from across the Channel knew that all they could do was delay when their position was so weak. Besides, Paris soon erupted in uproar, bringing France closer to anarchy than at anytime save 1572 and 1789. So it was that proposals for peace continued back and forth, and John fretted the more in his gilded cell. After two years of prevarication, however, the French at last felt ready to resist their king's capitulation: when the Estates General received the details of the proposed peace on 19th May, they rejected it out of hand.

Edward's response was as expected. He left England with an army in September and made straight for Rheims, the place of coronation of the French kings. His purpose was clear: he had generously offered John a kingdom – if the French chose to refuse it, he would take the crown of France for himself. The king laid siege to the city, fully expecting the defenders to remember what he had done to Calais, thirteen years before. Behind their screens and palisades, the English could see little of the town except for its walls, and the towers of the great cathedral of Notre-Dame that stood within. These weeks presented Edward, long claimant to the French throne, with the denouement for which he had fought. But the king had begun to believe in his own myth. Winter was no time to keep a great army in the field – it had been a stretch in 1346 even when England was only twenty-one miles away over the Straits of Dover. Now he was isolated and his army was soon without food. Eleven days into the New Year the English were forced to lift the siege and go in search of pillage elsewhere. As the English host retreated from Rheims, Edward would have been forgiven a wistful glance over his shoulder. He had been within a couple of hundred metres of the French coronation throne, yet having come so close to the very thing for which he had fought so long, he had been thwarted. Edward had had the French crown within his grasp, yet his fingers had trembled, and then failed him, when the moment finally came. It was an achievement too far, even for him.

After the disappointment of Rheims, the resolution to this campaign could only be an anti-climax. The French successfully evaded the English forces for months and on Monday 13th April 1360 the exhausted invaders were scattered by a terrible storm, which caught them in the open plain that lay before Chartres Cathedral. Black Monday, as it became known, seemed to seal Edward's fate. He had embarked on this campaign under his own financial steam, thanks to the prodigious efforts of William Edington, who had been elevated to the chancellorship upon Archbishop Thoresby's resignation in 1356. But now even these resources were running low. Reports had come of attacks on the south coast and there were rumours that the French planned to send a force to England to spring their king from captivity. Black Monday had not only further demoralized his troops, it augured ill. So the English sat down and treated with the French, who had played a canny game and – given their poor hand – come out well. At Brétigny, on 3rd May 1360, Edward promised to give up his claim to the French throne in return for Gascony and further territories reaching north and east, deep inland, as well as Calais with its pale.[xvii] The ransom for John II was reduced to just over £500,000 and now included all additional prisoners that the English still held within their gaols. It was a permanent peace – at last – but nothing like the triumph conceded by John a year before, for it did no more than confirm the lands over which Edward already had control. On 24th October 1360, four years after his capture at Poitiers, John II found his freedom again, albeit in a much reduced realm; Edward returned home, his long sought-for settlement with France finally secured. His celebrations would be short-lived, however: for he was followed over the Channel by pestilence, which had returned.

[xvii] i.e. Guyenne, the Agenais, Armagnac, Saintonge, Poitou, Angoumois, Limousin, Périgord, Quercy and Rouergue.

14

Flowering amidst Failure

1361–1381

Our happy times of old have been rudely wiped out, for a bitter day afflicts the present.

John Gower, *Vox clamantis*[1]

The Second Pestilence had been working its way across central Europe since the middle of 1358, ravaging those villages that for some inexplicable reason had been spared during the pandemic a decade before. The pattern was not lost on contemporaries: Matteo Villani, brother of the Florentine merchant who had chronicled and then perished in the first plague,[2] heard from fellow travellers how 'it did not touch Flanders, where previously it had been very serious'.[3] It was not long before the epidemic had crossed westwards from the Low Countries into northern France, just as the English, French and Flemish warrior nobility were assembling in Calais for the formal return of the king-prisoner John to his subjects in France.

Before the disease arrived in London, however, Edward was able to present his treaty of Brétigny to parliament, which met in Westminster in January 1361. This should have been the moment of Edward's greatest triumph, the proof of the value of his exertions on the Continent over the previous quarter of a century. Yet the Commons had long tired of war with France, for which they had paid handsomely in their numerous grants of taxation, so the king's exultant declaration was met with restrained congratulation. Frankly, the county gentry represented in the Commons were more interested in gaining full powers over local justice, which they had enjoyed *de facto* since 1350. Confident in his realm and safe abroad, Edward acquiesced and it was

in this parliament that justices of the peace had their formal creation.[i]
With parliament done, Edward returned to Windsor, where in February
he married his fourth daughter to the duke of Brittany, an alliance
that gilded the treaty with France.

Within weeks, however, pestilence was once again in the capital,
having come over from Calais. Some attempt had been made to prevent
the epidemic taking hold: the king had commanded that all animal
slaughtering should be stopped at Smithfield and done only at Stratford
or Knightsbridge, for fear that the blood and entrails might pollute
the air and make the risk of infection worse. All precautions failed,
however, and by the end of Lent the pestilence had consumed London.
Edward himself heard news of one its early victims, for on 25th March
1361, Maundy Thursday, whilst riding in the park at Windsor, he received
a message that Henry Grosmont, the duke of Lancaster, had died two
days before. The duke had fallen ill with plague after parliament had
been dissolved; on 15th March he had made out his will. This strongest
of men held out as long as he could against his infection but finally,
on the morning of Tuesday, 23rd March, he succumbed.[ii]

Just as it had done twelve years before, the plague soon spread
out of London, forcing the king and queen to retreat to Beaulieu
Abbey, in the New Forest, where they spent the summer months.
Previously this semi-seclusion had afforded the royal family complete
sanctuary from the pestilence; perhaps the success of that experience had encouraged them to become lax in their precautions, as
infection eventually came: Mary, who had only just been married to
the duke of Brittany, died in the middle of September and her sister
Margaret, countess of Pembroke, was struck down shortly after.[iii]
Of the five daughters Philippa had given her king, one had died in

---

[i] The temporary derogation of minor judicial powers made to the county keepers
of the peace in 1350 was made formal, thereby confirming *de iure* their status as
justices of the peace, a role that the assorted gentry who made up the county benches
had for eleven years enjoyed *de facto*. Furthermore, the justices were given oversight
of weights and measures and, when their first commissions were announced on 20th
March 1361, over labourers too.

[ii] The duke's body was buried in his college of the Annunciation of St Mary in the
Newarke, Leicester. Among his executors were his sister, Lady Wake, who had seen
her husband fall victim to the pestilence in 1349, and John Gynewell, the dutiful
bishop of Lincoln, who had ministered to so many in that first mortality.

[iii] Both daughters were buried at Abingdon in Oxfordshire.

infancy, three had been lost to the plague, and now only one – Isabella
– survived.

By now the Midlands had been struck. As on the Continent the
plague was stripping out those places that had been left alone twelve
years before: the mortality among the priests in the hundred of
Barlichway in Warwickshire, for instance, was very severe, but had
been light in the Great Death twelve years earlier. By the middle of
October, York had been infected and it was not long before the whole
of the North was being ravaged by what Lancastrians came to call
'the forine dethe'; at the same time the epidemic was spreading through
the March and into Wales.[4] Eleven years before, Humphrey de Bohun,
the earl of Hereford, had successfully sought refuge from infection
by shutting himself away in his castle at Brecon. In 1361 he died.
Whether this feudal tyrant had on this occasion failed to evade the
plague is not clear, although his tenants can have cared little how this
feudal tyrant perished.

By Christmas 1361 the Second Pestilence was leaving England and
entering neighbouring nations. In Ireland it killed one of the native
kings, while in Scotland, according to John Fordun, 'the form of the
disease and the number of deaths were just the same as in the first
outbreak in the jubilee year'.[5] The instinct, for those that were able,
was to flee – a tactic that had been shown to be effective last time
round. Walter Bower, writing eighty years later, recalled how David
II 'accompanied by many of the more wealthy and more noble men
of the kingdom, withdrew to the northern parts of the same kingdom,
partly because of the horrible sights and sounds of the multitude of
ill and dead, partly because of fear and alarm at that pestilence which
was then spreading in the southern parts of that kingdom, and
which he planned to escape in good health'.[6] Yet eventually the disease
made its way through the Highlands of Scotland, just as it went up
into the Cambrian Mountains and across the bogs of Ireland, coming
to its conclusion – as it had done twelve years before – in the most
remote extremes of the British Isles.

The harrowing of the British Isles was not quite over, however. For
as the light drew in on Saturday, 15th January 1362, St Maurus' Day, a
wind started to blow from the south-west. Within a few hours the
gusting had turned into a gale, which howled so hard that trees, even
though they had no leaves, were ripped from the ground. Everywhere

there was destruction: windmills were 'thrown down', tiles stripped from roofs, fences flattened and hedges demolished.[7] The cathedral tower in Norwich toppled over and in Dublin, nearly 400 miles away, the steeple of St Saviour's Dominican priory was torn away. This 'fearsome wind',[8] following hard on the heels of the second epidemic of plague, still inspired awe several decades later: William Langland's 'Reason' saw no accident that the two catastrophes were visited on England together:

> . . . this pestelences was for puyre synne
> And the south-weste wynde on a Saturday at euene
> Was pertliche for pruyde and for no poynt elles.
> Pere-trees and plum-trees were poffed to þe erthe
> In ensaunple, segges, þat we sholde do þe bettere.
> Beches and brode okes were blowe to þe grounde
> And turned vpward here tayl in tokenynge of drede
> That dedly synne ar domesday shal fordon hem alle.[iv]

At Ashwell, in Hertfordshire, an inscribed record was made of the storm in the soft clunch of the church tower, possibly by one of the masons brought in to strengthen the structure after the storm. Just beneath an earlier scrawl, which plainly states that 'the first plague was in June 1349', the Gothic graffito described what had taken place. It is a less literate account than Langland's, yet none the less striking in its author's lament:

> A pitiable plague departed in 1350, leaving a wretched people to witness another plague, and in the end a mighty wind, Maurus, thunders throughout the world in [1362].[9]

Pitiable indeed: the villagers of Ashwell, and those across the British Isles, must have wondered when their extraordinary afflictions would come to an end.

★   ★   ★

[iv] . . . this pestilence was for pure sin / And the south-west wind on a Saturday evening / Clearly had no cause other than pride. / Pear trees and plum trees were puffed to the earth / As a warning to men that they should do better. / Beeches and broad oaks were blown to the ground / And their roots turned upward as a dreadful sign / That deadly sin shall destroy them all on Doomsday. (Langland, *Piers Plowman* (ed. Pearsall), Passus V, ll.115–22, p. 103; my translation.)

William Hutton the Younger,[v] the head mason of York Minster, spent a good part of the pestilential year of 1361 kneeling in a room above the vestibule that linked the church with the canons' chapter house. The floor had been specially skimmed with plaster, so that Hutton could set out in ruled and compassed charcoal the final details of the new choir. Eleven years earlier, Thomas Sampson had bequeathed £20 to this project in expectation that building would begin within the year; but the plague that took his life also delayed the completion of the nave roof, which had to be finished before the new east end was begun. By 1360, however, the final weatherproofing had at last been done, thereby completing a project that had been started in 1291. Hutton gave the word that he was ready to start with the choir. So the cathedral clergy came together, processing under the mason's tracing room to their chapter house, and gave the order to proceed: Archbishop Thoresby laid the foundation stone on Friday, 30th July 1361. It was only a month and a half since he had ordered prayers and processions as a precaution against the plague; the dean and chapter, it seems, would not allow pestilence to postpone their plans this time round.

As the walls rose from the ground, it was clear that the new choir conformed to the plans that had been laid out by Hutton's predecessors long before the pestilence of 1349 intervened; all, that is, apart from the tracery that filled the aisle windows, the design and execution of which was left until last. These were the subjects of Hutton's sketchings – neat but unadventurous renditions of the rectilinear style that was becoming popular in the South. Not that the older, curvilinear, 'Decorated' forms were already dead: they were here, at York, carved in the stones raised around Hutton's windows, just as they were to be seen in recent additions to England's most southerly cathedral – Exeter – and northernmost, in Carlisle. However, if by the 1360s the influence of William Ramsey and his work at St Paul's Cathedral and Gloucester Abbey was yet to be felt in Carlisle, in the South his 'Perpendicular' patterns could be found in almost every new building that was being put up. The continuation of so many building projects already in progress before the Great Death was critical to this

---

[v] Commonly given as William de Hoton the Younger. Hutton's father had briefly (1349–51) been master mason at the minster after the death of Thomas Pacenham, for which see Ch. 10, p. 226.

diffusion of this new style. Indeed, the delay at York was a rare hiatus: in most instances, carpenters, masons, tilers, plasterers and glaziers all got back to work almost as soon as the first pestilence had ceased: the rebuilding of the nave vault at Tewkesbury Abbey, started in the 1340s, continued through the 1350s, whilst further north construction of the new roof of Lichfield Cathedral, briefly halted by plague, had resumed by 1352. This practical continuity had stylistic implications, for although the champion of the Perpendicular, William Ramsey, had died, the continuation of projects for which he had formerly been responsible, like Lichfield and Gloucester, helped to maintain the momentum of the emerging style. Thus, far from retarding the progression of the Perpendicular, the Great Death pushed new men forward who built – in every sense – on what Ramsey had begun.

No better example of this exists than the convent of Bonshommes, founded by William Edington in his home village of Edington in Wiltshire, and the first major church to be started after the Great Death. Begun within a few years of the plague and substantially complete by 1361, this extraordinary building was more like a nobleman's house than a college for priests, being all plain walls topped by merlons, a squat tower, corner turrets, and windows that resembled arrow loops.[10] The anonymous mason who built this showed considerable imagination, yet it is clear that the buildings that informed his thinking had Ramsey's mark upon them – the chapter house at St Paul's, the south transept at Gloucester and, most striking of all, Sir John Pulteney's palace at Penshurst Place, all of which predated the Great Death. Thus, through the completion of his work and the survival of his pupils, the great mason's style outlived the plague and quickly progressed beyond what even he had achieved.

Despite the early adoption of the Perpendicular throughout the South of England, the Decorated and Perpendicular forms of English Gothic continued to rub shoulders for decades after the Great Death, just as they had coexisted for some years before the epidemic. Some masons were able to work in both idioms, building in whatever form that they felt to be appropriate. The pre-eminent master mason of the late fourteenth century, Henry Yeveley, followed a consciously old-fashioned form in his nave at Westminster Abbey, begun in 1376, whilst two years later embarking upon a new nave at Canterbury Cathedral, which today stands as the single greatest achievement of early Perpendicular Gothic. In York, Richard Patrington adopted a rectilinear approach for the upper parts of the choir begun by William Hutton, his predecessor, yet it was deployed with a flamboyance that more closely accorded with earlier, Decorated, phases of work at the minster than with the restrained Perpendicular that was by then predominant in the South.

It is difficult to assess, therefore, whether the Great Death made any material difference to the widespread diffusion of Perpendicular Gothic or the corresponding decline of the Decorated style. Certainly, these related trends had their origin in the years before the Great Death and would most probably have played themselves out even had plague not intervened. Yet the crisis in manorial revenues and the sharp drop in the population altered the priorities of those who were building churches. Now economies were more desirable, extensions and enlargements less necessary. The refurbishment of existing structures suddenly seemed more attractive, something for which the Perpendicular, born of the challenges posed by giving a Gothic skin to the Romanesque Norman bones of Gloucester Abbey, was especially suited. For the chief quality of the Perpendicular form was the flexibility it afforded the mason. Not only did this make a caprice like the church at Edington possible but it also made easier the refurbishment of old buildings, as at Edington's cathedral at Winchester, where work remodelling the giant Norman nave was restarted in the 1360s and completed by Edington's successor, William Wykeham, thirty years later.[11] Moreover, Perpendicular was emphatically English – an advantage in the times when England was at war with France, which had hitherto been the fount of architectural taste for English patrons and English masons. So while the pestilence did nothing to create one style or suppress another, it helped to accelerate the adoption of Perpendicular Gothic, an emergent style that – by pure chance – responded to the changed demands of these dramatically changed times.

Whilst there was a demonstrable evolution of a new architectural style through the central decades of the fourteenth century, other building trades showed a surprising degree of continuity, something the pestilence did little to change. Certainly it did nothing to diminish the quality of what the finest English craftsmen and artists could achieve, as the extraordinary painting schemes of St Stephen's and Windsor – executed respectively in the 1350s and 1360s – made clear; for here were some of the earliest examples of large-scale perspective in England. On the other hand, there had been a decline in the output and fineness of London brasses some years before the Great Death and the mortality does seem to have encouraged brassmakers from Tournai to enter what was a promising market. The competition clearly had a beneficial effect, for within fifteen years two new workshops were turning out excellent products, even if they were not yet of the standard produced half a century before.

Brassmaking was just one of the artisanal trades that had benefited from the increasingly diverse means by which the wealthy sought to preserve their memory after death; if not a brass, then it might be a commemorative window or – for the most wealthy – an effigy. Yet the complete absence of a boom in these memorials after the Great Death probably indicates that the supply of these products was seriously constricted by the deaths of so many skilled craftsmen. There are, however, outstanding examples of each of these disciplines still surviving from the three decades that followed the first pestilence, which demonstrate that even if a large number of practitioners had died, sufficient artisans survived to pass on their skills to a new generation. The tombs of Edward III and his son Edward, the Prince of Wales, were among the finest ever created for the English crown while William Edington's likeness in his alabaster effigy captures, despite its subsequent mutilation, the bishop's features and purposeful gaze as well as any good portrait should. To be sure, these were commissions from a very narrow elite, who could procure the services of a correspondingly small pool of the finest sculptors – some of them foreign. Glassmaking, on the other hand, depended on a greater number of craftsmen, not only because the scale of each window was large but because the market for coloured glass included virtually every parish church in the land. Although glassmakers had to make do with a more limited palate, the result not of the mortality but of the embargo on trade with France which restricted the supply of suitable colour, what was generally true of other crafts was also true of glassmaking: for large commissions, quality could still be bought. The great east window at Gloucester Abbey, which commemorates the English fallen of Crécy, was installed by the early 1360s and at the time was the largest coloured window in England.

The vandals of the Reformation removed almost every trace of the windows – the 'poor man's Bible' – that filtered coloured light on to those painted walls that have since been scraped, scoured and lime-washed away from every medieval church in England. The distinction of that glass, and that painting, was not in its artistic merit, which was variable, but in its meaning and the ease with which it could be understood. The little fragment at Hurstbourne Tarrant in Hampshire, painted around the time of the Great Death, was part of a far larger scheme that the villagers of Faccombe Netherton, from nearby, will have known well. It is of simple ambition, yet in its simplicity and in its message it is still a thing of great beauty. The subject was the popular legend of the 'Three Living and the Three Dead', which had emerged out of the French court in the late thirteenth century. Three young men – a prince and his two noble friends – encounter three terrible cadavers. When challenged by the haughty youths, the first Death pronounces: 'What you are, we were, and what we are, you will be.' The second goes on to remind the young men that mortality treats rich and poor alike, while the third warns that no one escapes the clutches of death. Through the early fourteenth century the story became a popular subject for wall painting, and it is not hard to see why: not only did it playfully expound three profound truths of mortality, the painted setting for the legend provided good decoration for a church wall. Thus, whether the example at Hurstbourne Tarrant was executed before or after the Great Death is of little significance, as there were depictions of this legend that predated the plague. There is some fractional evidence, however, that very few of the better examples of English parish art were produced in the decades after the Great Death. This should be no surprise, as the halving of the population meant that, for a while at least, few churches were rebuilt and extended; there was less need for new wall paintings, therefore, and new windows. Those new paintings and windows that were produced continued to use subjects that had been popularized long before the Great Death – such as the Passion, the Last Judgement, and the Three Living and the Three Dead.

Even so, it cannot be doubted that these visual portrayals of death and the dead, both in their rubric and in their visual meaning, held an additional significance for a population hugely sensitized to the mortality of man. For even if the Great Death caused no substantive change in the depiction of the mortal and the morbid in parish art, we can be sure that these paintings carried a fresh, immediate and frightening significance. This, at least, was something shared by prince and pauper alike, so it was fitting that Edward, Prince of Wales, chose an aphorism for his epitaph that repeated the captions painted on so many humble church walls: 'As thou art, so once was I; as I am, so shalt thou be.'

Building work was going on at Westminster Abbey almost as soon as the plague had left, with a new cloister surrounding the grave where so many of the abbey's brothers lay. Within a few years, the new abbot – Simon Langham – began the wholesale redevelopment of the abbey's Westminster estate, beginning with the almonry, a building beside the open ground that lay before the west front, which for centuries had been the place where the local poor received food doles – normally a hunk of bread and splash of ale. (Edward I had endowed an annual distribution of alms in memory of his queen, Eleanor of Castile, which on one occasion attracted as many as 36,000 people – the equivalent of a third of the population of London.) The development was completed by the mid-1360s and consisted in part of a range of shops on the south side of the almonry's open square. It was a shrewd speculative move: by investing when property prices were low, the abbey benefited when rents rose again, as they did in the 1360s. However, there was another part to Langham's plan: fences and gates were erected on the other sides of the almonry square, thereby restricting access to the almonry itself. This did not mean that the almonry ceased to function: quite the reverse – it spent proportionately as much on its charitable operation as it had done before the Great Death. The only difference was that now the monks could control whom they let in to receive doles and alms, and whom they chose to turn away.

The enclosure of the Westminster Abbey almonry reflected a growing tendency to differentiate between the deserving and the undeserving poor. This was somewhat at odds with the liberal and indiscriminate charity of earlier decades (of which Edward I's bequest to the abbey almonry was a classic case). True or not, there was now a common perception that as wages had risen and labour was scarce, there was no excuse for the able-bodied to beg. It was a sentiment enshrined in the labour legislation of 1349 and every one of its reiterations. By the 1370s, William Langland was writing that the sturdy beggar should receive no more than dog biscuits until he had taken up work; only then would he deserve a tasty meal. Yet Langland was not unfeeling, nor was he cruel: the false beggar, he claimed, 'defrauds the needy', because they take alms from those that truly need them and make donors suspicious of giving anything at all.[12] This was a sophisticated argument but one that was nonetheless widespread. For instance, at much the same time as Langland was composing his poem, a painter was working to cover the west wall of Trotton church in Sussex with a tableau that included a large exposition of the Seven Acts of Corporal Mercy. This was a simple depiction of charitable acts, the performance of which eased the path to Heaven: clothing the naked, feeding the hungry, giving drink to the thirsty, tending the sick, giving hospitality to the stranger, visiting the prisoner, and burying the dead. The tight definition of these works of charity was entirely deliberate: the acts were good precisely because the recipient was in need. There was nothing new in this teaching, of course, but the proliferation of paintings such as this one at Trotton, in huge technicolour on the wall of an unremarkable parish church, demonstrates that the instruction received by the illiterate peasantry on the nature of charity accorded precisely with the rationale of Langham's almonry project and the logic of Langland's verse.

Criticism of the unworthy pauper was the corollary of growing unease at the tastes of the ill-deserving newly enriched. Within two years of the Great Death, the aldermen of London were legislating against the showy wealth of the city's prostitutes, who had presumably done well out of the immigration of so many young men and the many husbands who had lost their wives. According to the city fathers, these women had latterly 'assumed the fashion of being clad and attired in the manner and dress of good and noble dames and damsels of the realm', and so should cease wearing expensive furs but dress only in simple clothes.[13] Clearly this ordinance had no effect, as in 1355 it was repeated, this time ordering the women to wear red or striped hoods, and clothes turned inside out, so that people might better recognize their profession.

These ladies were not the only ones to have prospered after the mortality. In the countryside as well as in the towns, there were a good number who had benefited from the openings created by so many deaths. As sure as night followed day, the new prosperity of these *arrivistes* aroused the resentment of those who had already arrived. The provincial knights of the Commons were especially alarmed by this perceived distortion of society, not just because they objected to the accumulation of competing wealth but because their new-found riches allowed these *nouveaux riches* to ignore the will of their lords. Many found the taste of the moneyed peasantry particularly objectionable: it was galling enough to be challenged by an upstart peasant, even more so when his wife had been poured into a crass travesty of noble dress. For lately a few prosperous countrymen had been walking about in tightly worn gowns, pointed shoes, hose and vulgar belts, not in the loose-fitting smocks and simple caps that they had worn before. The fresh flush of wealth shown off in the wake of the second pestilence seems to have been the final straw for many and in 1363 parliament persuaded the king to pass a statute against 'the outrageous and excessive apparel of many people, contrary to their estate and degree'. For peasants, the law regulated not only clothing but the amount of fish and meat that they could eat, and forbade their use of gold and silver vessels. The legislation was not aimed solely at labourers and tenants, as it divided the landed interest into several parts and graded the clothing they should wear appropriately. So the wives of gentlemen beneath the rank of knight whose property was worth less than £100 a year were not permitted to wear garments with turned-back facings or fur linings, whereas the children of a knight worth more than £133 per annum could wear miniver, but not ermine. There was a predictable prejudice against urban wealth: a merchant had to be worth at least £1,000 in order to be able to dress like a country gentleman with an income of only £200. Inevitably, this ludicrous statute was found to be completely unworkable, not least because it hit the burgeoning trade of so many mercers and tailors in the towns, so eighteen months later the legislation was repealed. From now on, the king said, 'all people shall be as free as they were before.'[14]

According to more-censorious observers, men and women were already indulging in licence of a different kind. For the first time in several hundred years the fashion was for women to wear their hair up but uncovered, exposing the flesh of their neck for men to see. Inevitably, the monk-chroniclers were horrified by such revealing dress and disapproved of the fashion for men to wear short jackets and close-fitting hose, which left little undefined; 'the Lord's vengeance will follow,' intoned the monk of Malmesbury.[15] John of Reading pointed out that tight clothes made it difficult to kneel in prayer; it was, he posited, yet another sign of the degeneration of society, where men 'considered to deflower virgins and violate the chastity of wives and widows was doing them a favour, not an injury. Men did not have coitus with their wives, or married women with their husbands, but preferred to beget bastards with strangers.'[16] While the outrage of these frustrated monks was exaggerated, their claims that there had been a slackening in social morals and inhibitions does suggest a hangover from the well-chronicled sexual abandon of those who lived through the Great Death. The fear and chaos of the epidemic had made libertines out of the most strait-laced: the philtre they had tasted then was hard to put aside once normality returned.

The mortality made more profound alterations to the structure of society than these conspicuous, but ephemeral, issues of fashion and sex. The effect of early promotion of so many young men, by inheritance and through the advancement of the church, surely changed perceptions of youth. The young were certainly more mobile, as the dislocation of families and the changes in landholding patterns encouraged young women and men to move from failing manors to flourishing villages, and from the countryside to successful towns.[vi] It was for this reason that the vast majority of abandoned villages lost their last inhabitants not during the plague but in the decades and centuries that followed: for these sad settlements it was a slow death where gradually the young, mobile and fertile moved away, leaving only a few established villein tenants, together with the elderly, the exceptionally poor, and the infirm, all of whom had little option but to stay put. Thus, when lords so often cited the 'poverty' of the village in explaining why rent receipts were so diminished, it was not because the place had suddenly become impoverished but because only the poor were now left.

The aged struggled all the more to cultivate their land and live. It was one of the beneficial features of a tight land market, as had existed before the Great Death, that the elderly and widowed could pass on

[vi] Differential migration helps to explain why complaints of flight by lords seemed more acute in some areas than in others, even between manors within the same estate.

their lands when they could no longer till them, receiving a place to live and a retirement income from the beneficiary in return. In places this practice continued after the Great Death, as in Wooton Underwood in Buckinghamshire, where a widow was in 1358 given the use of the bed chamber beside the door to the hall in a house, in return for which her host took on the tenement she was no longer able to farm herself. However, with so much empty land and so many plots going cheap, it must have been hard for old people to make such agreements. On the bishop of Durham's estate, where there was a tradition of managing retirement agreements through the manor court, land owned by frail old people had increasingly to be forced onto more-able people in the village. So at Warden Law, just east of Houghton-le-Spring in Durham, all but twelve acres of land was taken from Agnes Holbeswick, because she was judged to be incapable of managing it, and forced onto another villager, William Morton. That the villagers themselves could not come to a voluntary arrangement suggests that no one wanted Agnes's land; it must be hoped that she was looked after by her fellows, nonetheless. However, to have land at all was still an advantage, as for those landless peasants with nothing to hand over old age was an especially terrifying prospect, all the more so if they no longer had family to care for them. The loss of so many children in the plagues took away this insurance from many poor parents, although the fact that there was no perceptible increase in the destitution of the elderly after the pestilence suggests that, in most instances, the existing communal arrangements for the welfare of the decrepit continued to suffice.

It is an inadequacy of medieval history that the lives and prospects of women are not better chronicled or understood. Yet it is undeniable that the Great Death and subsequent plagues had a significant, if subtle, effect on the status and fortunes of women. As women seldom held land solely in their own name, it is rare to have a consistent record of a woman in a manor account, except for those instances where she married or was caught fornicating outside marriage. However, the lack of good and consistent information should not be taken as *prima facie* evidence that women possessed no rights at all and were, as a group, oppressed. Many women made money out of those chores – spinning, weaving, cooking and brewing – which they were already doing for their families in the home. This was no guarantee of independence but the money brought in was a valued contribution to family income. Moreover, although men answered for their wives and daughters in court, women were afforded considerable protection under the law and enjoyed property rights that, whilst not equal to those of men, permitted them to hold land of their own. Yet it cannot be denied that women, especially poor women and single mothers, might suffer considerable hardship, especially when available labour exceeded demand, as it had done in many places before the Great Death. Those who had no family, or whose family had no money, were often forced to become itinerant workers; at worst, some girls were pushed into vagrancy, which led all too easily to prostitution.

In women's employment prospects at least, the pestilence made a beneficial change. Women benefited from the disproportionate increase in the wages gained by the unskilled: it had always, where possible, been acceptable to substitute the (cheaper) labour of women for that of men, but with manorial incomes under pressure the temptation to do so was that much greater. As the Malmesbury monk reported, the shortage of male servants meant that 'women and children had to be used to drive ploughs and carts, which was unheard of'.[17] More young girls were sent into the service of wealthier peasants – those villagers who retained one or possibly two live-in labourers to help in the household. Perhaps 10 per cent of adults were servants of some kind or other, mostly to other peasants, and there was probably a proportional increase in the number of women taking on this role in the aftermath of the Great Death. Service was right at the bottom of the scale of jobs, yet women were also taking control of land as well, either in their own right – as spinsters or widows – or in joint tenure with their husbands. The deaths of so many male offspring forced parents to pass land to daughters, which led in turn to a *de facto* improvement in female inheritance rights. Very occasionally, a woman used an inheritance to create a more considerable landholding, like the lady villein of Winterbourne Earls, a few miles north of Salisbury in Wiltshire, who by 1363 had doubled her initial fifteen acres through the addition of a number of small parcels of land. The increased incidence in female landholding did not simply represent a nominal improvement in status: it allowed women to dispose of their land and their assets as they wished. Alice Inkpen, a married woman of Adderbury in Oxfordshire, made a number of grants of land to female kinswomen

in 1361, perhaps in an effort to support them in recent widowhood.
Some older and financially independent women used their savings to
pay their own marriage-fines, sometimes with no specific husband
intended but merely so that they could enjoy the right to marry whom
they desired, when they so wished. Further evidence of an improvement in the status of women can be found in the presence of women
in many of the small rural parish guilds and religious fraternities that
grew up at the end of the century. It would be a mistake to overstate
this change, not least because it is doubtful that it persisted in the long
term; in the aftermath of the Great Death, however, it is clear that
the mortality had precipitated a limited improvement in the wealth
and status of many women.

Although some women did well in the countryside, a far larger
number moved to the towns – so many in fact that by the late 1370s
women made up over half the population of some cities (52.5 per cent
in York, 54 per cent in Carlisle), a ratio that had moved in women's
favour since the Great Death, before when male labour had been more
plentiful. Girls, some as young as twelve, would be packed off to work
as a live-in servant for a craftsman or shopkeeper, often one known
to the girl's family through kin or trade connections. Most of these
female servants worked in selling and victualling, and in clothmaking,
leatherwork and the like; indeed there were a very few, although more
than before, in heavier work, like metal smithing. Typically, female
servants would work in these places well into their twenties or even
later.[18] Those who made enough money (and did not get married)
might set up on their own, moving to one of the poorer suburbs of
their adopted town and taking on piecework or casual service, such
as the two 'spinsters' living and working in Beverley in 1367. This was
very much in a pattern of employment that had developed before the
Great Death, but it is clear that the labour shortage accentuated the
feminization of urban service, which accounted for perhaps a third
of all jobs in the towns; in addition, a significant number played a
more important role in business and trade than before. Those that
married often continued to work, commonly as alewives in taverns
and inns – a traditional position for a woman that the pestilence did
little to change. There was a growing number, however, who worked
with their husbands in other trades, a good few of whom carried on
their husbands' businesses in widowhood, even enjoying their

husbands' civic privileges. It was a sure measure of this change that some poll tax assessments from the late 1370s differentiated between those women who were dependent on their family or master and those who had gained their financial independence – a telling distinction that would have been unlikely had the assessment been made a hundred years earlier.

Yet if this were a 'golden age' for medieval women, it is only with the benefit of hindsight that it can be identified as such. In most instances women could still not set up on their own in trade and were still excluded from most of the urban guilds that controlled business in the towns. By and large, women still occupied the least well paid and most poorly skilled jobs in the economy, and their legal identities were still framed by their relationship to a man – whether he be their father, master, or husband. And while the pestilence may have increased the incidence of early widowhood, the medieval romantic notion of the proud widow (partly drawn from the idea of regained chastity) was just that: in reality the frequency of remarriage shows that the lot of the widow was not necessarily a happy one. Other than to cite marginal improvements in prosperity and independence here and there, the primary and over-riding role of women remained the begetting and bearing of children. If some enjoyed greater freedom and a few saw an improvement in their wealth, it did nothing to change this fundamental fact. Yet even in childbirth, subtle changes to the lives of women would have a wider impact on English society.

Medieval marriage was an informal affair. The only sacrament not made by the church, a couple were espoused in the house of the bride's father or legal guardian, often after union had been consummated; consecration by the church took place at some point later. This is as it happened to Katherine, a serving-girl in York, when she married John Dene in the house of her master, who provided a crate of wine for the celebrations. Indeed, there is little that is unfamiliar in medieval marriage: one man declared to his bride that, before meeting her, he had never found anyone whom he was able to love, while the bride of John Astlott of Hull was worried that her father would disapprove, whereupon John assured her that he would take the old man a goose and convince him over dinner. Just as we might expect today, couples – especially in the towns – brought their own savings and incomes into the marriage, women retaining the rights to their previous property if their husband should die.

The age at which people married and in what numbers, were both critical determinants of the fertility of the medieval English population, as the bearing of children outside wedlock – although not uncommon – was by no means the norm. Any change to the pattern of marriage, even if it was very subtle, had implications for the size and increase of the population as a whole. There is good reason to think that the Great Death, by making specific and local changes to the status and economic independence of some groups of women, had just such an effect. The impact was most visible in the towns, which were unable to sustain their populations without immigration – a situation only accentuated by the socio-structural changes brought about by the Great Death. The employment of more women in early life as servants delayed the time at which they married, and the increase in the proportion of female-to-male town dwellers reduced the chance that a woman would get married at all. By the end of the 1370s, for instance, no more than 55 per cent of the adult female population in Hull was married, and marriage was taking place slightly later than it had done in the past: women were normally betrothed in their mid- to late twenties, to men of roughly the same age. Even if this were a change, over the average, of only a year or two, it had profound implications for the fertility of urban populations, which was already low. As a result, while successful towns grew, they did so less by their own internal resources and more by sucking migrants in from the countryside around. Conversely, those towns where there were few opportunities soon saw their numbers fall, as they attracted few immigrants to make up for the insufficient growth they generated internally.

Although towns only constituted about 10 per cent of the English population, this drawing in of country folk, especially the young, meant that they had a disproportionate influence on the population as a whole through the resulting negative effect on rural fertility. Even for those who stayed – who were still the vast, vast majority – the pestilence altered patterns of marriage. The marginal increase in female service in families delayed marriage, just as it did in the towns. Moreover, as labourers tended to get married later than smallholders (smallholders settling earlier and having greater use for children than did wage-labourers), the relative increase in the labouring population acted to delay marriage too – a trend only confirmed as labourers' wages steadily went up and many of the meanest smallholdings were subsumed into larger plots. So although marriage and fertility remained far higher in rural populations than in the towns, both were reduced through the effects of mass mortality.

Everything else being equal, these slight changes to the pattern of marriage and child-bearing would have changed the rate of population growth by small degrees; but everything else was not equal, for the Great Death inaugurated a period of recurrent plague that lasted well into the seventeenth century. In the first instance, the population was reduced by half; in the second, any infinitesimal recovery achieved in the 1350s was reversed, and the population may well have fallen by a further 10–20 per cent. Later plagues were successively less deadly, but they were increasingly concentrated in the towns, and were more frequent, making the replenishment of urban populations through immigration all the more necessary and urgent, thereby attracting more and more young, fertile people from the countryside to places which were more at risk from future infection. All the while family after family was dismembered by plague, further disrupting marriages and the bearing of children.[19]

Although the succeeding bouts of pestilence were less lethal, they were particularly dangerous to children, most probably because infants had none of the select immunity that their parents and elder relatives possessed. 'At first it killed infants in huge numbers,' said the chronicler of Grey Friars in Lynn, 'from which circumstance it is commonly called "the boys' pestilence",' wrote a monk of Louth Abbey.[20] The effect of this was to retard the recovery of the population still further, for while the birth rate might increase in the years immediately after a plague as couples bore children to make up for those that were lost, pestilence soon returned, causing a disproportionately high mortality among this vulnerable group, well before they had reached a fertile age.[21] So although overall mortality fell in each repeated round of pestilence, its effects were felt most by that cohort of the population that would provide future population recovery and growth.

Everything conspired, therefore, for the pestilence to have a particularly pernicious effect on the ability of the population to recover.

Coupled with subtle alterations to nuptuality and fertility, recurrent plague was enough to prevent a recovery in the population during the century after the Great Death. Indeed, the population of England (and, we must assume, Ireland, Scotland and Wales) continued to fall through the later decades of the fourteenth century and only began to grow again towards the end of the fifteenth century. In some places, like much of East Anglia, rural populations did not recover their pre-plague numbers until the nineteenth century.

There remains a conundrum, therefore: why did the rural population not repeat the extraordinary increase that it had shown during the twelfth and thirteenth centuries? Clearly something more significant than the marginal age of marriage, or occasional spikes in plague-induced mortality, or indeed small differences in the climate, had changed. The answer, perhaps, can be found in the century before the Great Death, when population growth first slowed and then stagnated. That it did so was not primarily the result of famine, or anything to do with disease, but because of economic restraints on fertility. Although the population had halved, these factors persisted and intensified after the Great Death.

Feudal agriculture promoted fertility: it benefited lords (more tenants, more revenue) and their tenants (labour services were less burdensome if families were large). However, the resulting increase in the population inevitably defeated the limited financial advantages of customary labour, as hired workers were more efficient and, as they became more abundant, cost-effective. Thus, population growth helped undermine the feudal structures that had helped to cause it, which in turn produced a 'feedback' effect on population growth; for labourers and peasant farmers had less incentive to have very large families than did bondmen who fed and housed themselves through their family's combined labour. The newly enlarged population discouraged fertility in other ways too: as land got more scarce and partible inheritance left many with ever more tiny tenements, the number of poor smallholders – those landowners least able to support children – increased. The chances of marriage for landless men were even worse: these most extreme poor, who certainly did not vanish with the pestilence, had few children, as much by force of circumstance as by choice.

These economic and social trends were well entrenched by the time of the Great Death. Although the reduction in population and consequent freeing up of land removed a key constraint to fertility, the ongoing disintegration of feudal agriculture should be afforded some responsibility for the failure of the rural population to recover and increase after the Great Death, for the same forces that had slowed and then flattened the growth of the population before the first pestilence continued to act on the families that survived this and subsequent plagues. It is arguable, therefore, that even if the effects of recurrent pestilence and changed marriage patterns were to be omitted, for pre-existing reasons the population would not have bounced back. At the outside there would have been a very gradual recovery, but certainly not at the remarkable rate of population growth England experienced two centuries before. Indeed, this is precisely what happened in later centuries, when plague only had a negligible impact on overall mortality.

In his dying weeks, the duke of Lancaster had been attended by his own doctor, Richard of Ireland, and two Italian physicians, Richard Gouche of Florence and Pascal of Bologna. It is not unlikely that the efforts of these men prolonged Henry's life beyond the usual three or four days from the first appearance of symptoms to death. Later in the year the abbot of St Alban's, Thomas de la Mare, contracted the plague but, miraculously, survived. Like Lancaster, the abbot had access to the very best medical advice. De la Mare was one of the ecclesiastics who had travelled to Avignon in the previous pestilence and while there he doubtless met Guy de Chauliac, the great surgeon. Of the Great Death de Chauliac commented: 'for previous plagues there were remedies; for this one, nothing.' De Chauliac was to change his mind, however, for he too was infected in the second epidemic and, through self-medication, he survived. In his seminal work, *The Great Surgery*, of 1363, he not only made detailed observations about the epidemiology of the pestilence (including the susceptibility of children to the second epidemic) but went on to describe the many remedies that he had used, applying poultices to his buboes and inflicting several courses of blood-letting upon his ailing body. He had, thereby, 'evaded God's judgement', even though his fellows had concluded that he was 'about to die'.[22]

Two years after de Chauliac penned his treatise, John of Burgundy, a doctor from Liège, circulated a plague tract that soon spawned copies all over Europe. Burgundy relied on a classical explanation of plague, involving the same deified Galenic system that had informed the first responses to the Great Death. Yet his tract also offers sensible advice ('above all, sexual intercourse should be avoided') which, if followed, may have reduced the risk of infection.[23] Writing at the same time, Jean Jacmé, a physician of Montpellier, advised his readers that company should at all costs be avoided, 'lest some man be infected by infectious breath' and, when isolation was impossible, that a sponge soaked in vinegar be held before the mouth and nose, 'because all sour things stop the way of humours and suffer no venomous things to enter into a man's body' – precisely the technique Jacmé himself had used when visiting patients during the epidemic and by which he believed he had 'escaped the pestilence'.[24] It was in the same spirit of practical medicine that medical treatises proliferated during these decades and made their way into English hands, so that by the end of the fourteenth century plague tracts had acquired a wide lay audience among the literate classes.

Much of the advice given by physicians was already commonplace, in particular the (correct) observation that bad smells and disease were somehow linked. It was no surprise, therefore, that civic authorities all over England made moves to improve the hygiene of their cities, fearing that the disgusting state of the butcheries, the foul riversides and open sewers, might increase the risk of future infection. Immediately after the pestilence had left Bristol the aldermen sent out an ordinance requiring people to remove their night-soil and rubbish from the street within three days; a few years later they banned citizens from throwing urine and foul water into the thoroughfares, householders being made responsible for that portion of street in front of their property. In 1351 the university of Cambridge petitioned the king to do something to ensure 'that the townsmen should be compelled to clean the streets, then very noxious to all persons passing, as well as the inhabitants'. In 1367 there were orders to clear the river banks of the Yare in Norwich, and in 1371 the same was commanded for the Ouse in York, the butchers of the city being prohibited from throwing offal into the river, except downstream from where water was drawn for brewing and baking. Remarkable foresight was shown by the councillors of Hereford who, realizing the danger arising from strangers coming into the city carrying disease, moved the market place a mile outside the western wall, so that traders and merchants from other towns did not come within the walls on market day.

It was in London that the most concerted efforts were made to improve public sanitation and hygiene. Even while the first epidemic was at its height, Edward III himself had ordered that 'human faeces and other filth' should be cleared from London's streets and lanes, as it was causing the air to be 'infected' and 'poisoned to the danger of men passing, especially in the mortality by the contagious sickness which arises daily'.[vii] In 1357 the king wrote again to the mayor, recalling the city's once famed cleanliness and explaining how he had been 'passing along the water of the Thames' and had noticed the 'dung, and laystalls, and other filth . . . upon the bank of the river'.[25] This, he pointed out, caused 'fumes and other abominable stenches' to rise up, so that 'great peril will, it is feared, ensue, to the persons dwelling within the said city and to the nobles and others passing along the said river, unless some fitting remedy be speedily provided for the same.'[26] The king deigned to offer some suggestions: to clean the place up forthwith, and to impose penalties on those who fouled the streets and river again. The mayor and community certainly made an effort to clean up the city in the decades that followed: the disposal of dung and ordure in the river was tightly controlled, poultries and butcheries inside the city were moved outside the walls, and the city's small ditches and streams were thoroughly dredged. It was not simply out of a sense of decency that all this was done but a sincere belief that the risk of disease – of all kinds – was heightened by the smell that emanated from the muck left around. There was surely a commercial incentive too: just down the road in Westminster, the only properties that the almoner was finding it hard to rent out in his redeveloped site were those by the open sewer, 'on account of the stench of the public latrine'.[27] A thorough clean-out ensured that the shops were soon let.

Thus, within a few years of the recurrence of plague, physicians were making concerted efforts to identify the means by which pestilence spread and the methods by which infection might be prevented, and were researching and testing cures for the disease – theories and ideas that were then distributed widely. At the same time, urban author-

vii On 8th April 1349. *Calendar of the Close Rolls*, Edward III, Vol. IX: 1349–54, pp. 65–6. See p. 110 above.

ities were acting to keep their towns free from infection. Although much of this had little effect on the transmission of pestilence, the associated improvements in hygiene, however slight, must have saved many lives. And when plague did come, there was a growing body of knowledge and experience about how best to prevent infection and the spread of the epidemic. These efforts were not only impressive in themselves; they were in part responsible for the diminishing virulence with which plague attacked, slowly but surely, with every successive epidemic.

The Second Pestilence laid waste the decade of fitful recovery that had followed the Great Death. A return to profitability even before this second epidemic had been very patchy indeed. The estate of the Durham Priory provides an excellent example, for some of the priory's manors had recovered and even exceeded their pre-plague output, whereas others – especially the smaller settlements – had seen very serious decline. Now, villages already halved in size had to contend once again with the desolation left by epidemic disease – the mass graves, the forlorn survivors, the misshapen families and the land left to grow weeds – and as if that had not been enough, villagers across the South of England then had to deal with the fallen trees and wrecked windmills left by the St Maurus' Day storm.

Landowners did not wait for the pestilence to take hold before they acted to head off the problems they now knew the epidemic would soon send their way and the parliament of 1361 hastily updated the provisions of the Statute of Labourers. The maximum legal rate that a master carpenter could charge was increased by a third – from 3d. to 4d. per day – with a corresponding rise for 'others'. However, these rates were already being exceeded on many manors, even on those of the chancellor, William Edington. As had become clear, the purpose of the legal pay scale was not to try to control wages *en masse*, which had failed from the start – not least because most employers were complicit in the widespread defiance of the law; rather, it was a legal mechanism by which landowners could prosecute wilful labourers, should they so wish, and to retain labour, which was now even more scarce. It was largely this last over-riding concern that troubled the parliament of 1361 most, as was clear from the new clause they added to the statute, which provided for the branding of the letter 'F', for 'falsity', on the forehead of any man who left their lord's service without permission.

As parliament correctly anticipated, prices and wages soared once pestilence spread. At the end of October, Edward instructed the mayor of London to regulate the price and sale of bread within the city. The expectation that the crown would intervene to control markets was now so entrenched that, when unscrupulous roofers sought to turn a quick shilling out of the ruination left by the St Maurus' Day storm the following year, the king ordered tile manufacturers not to charge more than they had done at Christmas, and tilers not to levy wages higher than they had done before the storm.[viii] Yet neither these micro-restrictions nor the more general clauses in the amended Statute of Labourers had any consistent impact as prices, and wages continued to increase. As in the early 1350s, rates were driven not solely by the mortality but by an unhappy concomitance of appalling weather. A dismal harvest in 1363 pushed prices up so much that by mid-1364 they were higher than they had been at any time since the Great Famine. The harvest of 1364 was exceptional, however, and the following two years were also good. Yet prices did not fall, as inflation continued unabated – the result of the further reduction in the population, repeated re-coining, and the inflow of money in ransom payments and export sales. Inflation further increased the price of livestock, which was rising for the first time since the Great Death, when the glut of heriots had forced prices for sheep, pigs and cattle to rock-bottom. Now they were on their way up again, a result of the sheep murrain that was widespread through the 1360s, and the more meaty diets of those peasants who had done well out of the mortality and had more cash to spend on meat.

Increased prices and good harvests ensured that manorial revenues once again showed tentative signs of recovery, and wages remained high, untroubled by the Statute of Labourers, which landowners had little incentive to use when manor incomes improved. This brief period of recovery did little, however, to stop the transformation of feudal manors: commutation continued apace and leasing was more and more widespread. Indeed, the market forces that had for so long been slowly undermining the apparatus of the manor for centuries were essentially unchanged; they had merely been stimulated and concentrated by the transforming effect of the mortality. Thus, changes that might otherwise have happened gradually, over decades and generations, were now compressed into single seasons.

This is a picture painted with broad brushes, however: each lord, each peasant, each manor responded to the challenges and opportunities of these years in different ways. For all the instances of success, there was also continued decay, which itself could act as a spur to a change in landholding, as at Wharram Percy in Yorkshire, owned by the insane Eustachia Percy until her death in 1365 and then by her son, Walter, until his death without heir in 1367. The tiny manor was then subsumed within the great Percy estate. It is doubtful whether the baron, Henry Percy, ever took an interest in little Wharram and who could blame him: the population had shrunk considerably as a result of the plagues and the management of the estate had hardly been assiduous as it had long been in the hands of uninterested trustees. The manor house was falling into dereliction and the church, extended early in the century, was already in disrepair.[28] It is probable that Henry Percy's official turned what was left of the demesne over to pasture and leased agriculture, and thus reduced the village to a mere rump, comprising perhaps only thirty households in all – a number of labourers and a few tenants, farming the land they had inherited from their villein forefathers but now holding it on simple leases.

It need not have been like this. The monks of Glastonbury, for instance, worked hard to maintain the profitability of their manors of Longbridge Deverill and Monkton Deverill. It had not been easy, however, for while Longbridge produced an income not that different from the pre-plague years, revenues from Monkton Deverill, with its poorer land, had declined considerably. Clearly people were moving out of Monkton, like John Maggestone, and were making their way to larger villages elsewhere, leaving a few remaining tenants behind and many more sheep. Nonetheless, the abbey's careful management of these two manors, helped by the high prices of the late 1360s, ensured that the two combined were still returning a considerable income, with the healthy return from Longbridge offsetting the substantial fall in income from Monkton.

High prices and good harvests in the mid-1360s may have permitted some landowners to put off more commutation and leasing, but this

Indian summer would represent only a brief respite, for the weather once again intervened. First, there was a widespread sheep murrain, which in turn had caused the price of wool and cloth to soar. Then the harvests of 1368 and 1369 were utterly ruined, by incessant rain in one year and terrible drought the next. Prices shot up, past even where they had reached five years before, and – in 1370 – even exceeding the previous peak achieved during the Great Famine; any advantage that landowners might have was offset not only by a corresponding increase in wages but by chronically low yields. So, unlike during the Great Famine, the shortage was felt not by the peasantry, whose poorest members still managed to get by, but by landowners, whose finances showed the effects of the squeeze. Predictably, the Commons started banging the legislation drum all over again and – after much petitioning – finally persuaded the king's ministers to turn full and perpetual legal responsibility for the enforcement of the Statute of Labourers over to the justices of the peace, whose ranks were filled almost entirely by the same country gentry making the complaint.

The effects of the appalling weather were compounded by a third bout of plague. The epidemic must have started, once again, in the South – most probably by Christmas 1368. It was in the North by the summer of 1369 and still present in the East Riding of Yorkshire in October. It was, a Northern chronicler noted, 'great beyond measure, lasted a long time and was particularly fatal to children'.[29] Indeed, while less than a sixth of the clergy in the diocese of York died, it may well have been the case that across the North as a whole a greater proportion of the population perished, greater even than during the epidemic of 1361.[30] By now, plague was becoming an awful fact of life, so less was recorded than had been in the first and second pestilences. It is clear, however, that the disease again reached across the breadth of the British Isles.

The passage of the Third Pestilence coincided with the death of Philippa of Hainault, who in the middle of August 1369 gave up her last breath. Edward had lost his most loyal companion, a remarkable consort whose record was one entirely of praise – a rarity in England, where foreign queens were more often the subject of envy and scorn. This remarkable woman had bade him farewell before each of his foreign campaigns, accompanied his Scottish prisoners to London in 1346, watched his near defeat from atop a cliff by Winchelsea in 1350, and had borne him twelve children, of whom only five survived her. Two of Philippa's sons – Prince Lionel and John of Gaunt – were forefathers of those Lancastrian, Yorkist and Tudor dynasties that were to dominate English politics through the following 230 years. Edward, heavy with his loss, waited until the plague had passed before commencing her funeral. Over the course of a number of cold January days the queen's body was moved solemnly by road from Windsor, via Kingston, St Mary Overy in Southwark and St Paul's, to Westminster Abbey, where she was buried, near the shrine of St Edward the Confessor.

The plague levelled all men, for the king shared in a grief repeated in homes all over the British Isles. It was probably late in this Third Pestilence that the Welsh poet Llywelyn Fychan lost four of his 'gentle darlings', to add to the one he had lost in the epidemic nine years before. 'Our lives are never free of grief', Fychan lamented, when 'a pestilence of terrible ferocity has come into our midst like a great rage' – 'an eradicating phantom infamous for its greed'. Then, in a remarkable passage, the bard describes the course of the disease in his sons, in closer detail than anyone had so far achieved:

> It would be hard to find, despicable little thing, a more pitiless tumour.
> Woe is me, stuff of evil treachery, from the shilling under the armpit.
> It is a most evil vein of inflammation where it strikes, a bead which causes loud lamentation; accompaniment of agony, it would provoke an outcry, a lad with whom there's no use pleading; a swelling under the armpit, grievous sore lump, white knob, poisonous misfortune, pommel of a sword of swift strife, punishment for an evil burden of sins.
> It caused grief and fury everywhere, shape of an apple full of pain, bitter head of an odious onion, a little boil which spares no one.
> Smouldering like a hot coal, a tiny thing which brings about man's end.
> Misery of the world, ashen-grey colour, it becomes inflamed, it's incessant.
> Evil provision of grief quite openly, a reaping of black pangs, ugly pox, dreadful in its haste, is it not similar to seeds of black peas?
> Inflamed burning of brittle coal fragments, tempestuous host like studs; crowds from the brink of death, a heavy sickness produces them, horrible to us.

A shower of peas giving rise to affliction, messenger of swift black
   death; parings from the petals of the corn-poppy, murderous
   rabble, evil omen; black plague, they don't come with any good
   intent, halfpennies, seaweed scales, a grim throng, humble
   speech, berries, it is painful that they should be on fair skin.
A sad business for all, by Christ and my faith, the sight of them was
   grief to me.

Llywelyn Fychan ends only with a quiet request: 'give me here God my
Father, gracious sense, recompense of hope, my payment for my family.'[31]
For the third time in two decades, survivors across Wales, Scotland,
Ireland and England were whispering a similar, desperate, refrain.

Yet one more calamity was to befall the benighted people of
England, to add to the manifold misfortunes they suffered in this
terrible year of animal disease, record prices, drought and plague. For
all through the spring of 1369 great bonfires burned an awful warning
on the cliff tops of the south coast. The French were patrolling the
Channel – in advance, it was feared, of an attack. The ninth anniversary of the treaty of Brétigny had not yet been reached but the peace
inaugurated in 1360 was now all but dead.

The king of France formally repudiated the peace in May 1369; Edward
III, in response, resurrected his claim to the crown of France. Yet while
the French had every intention of ending the peace, Edward had few
means of defending his claim. The halcyon years of the 1360s had been
entirely wasted: the French and Scottish ransoms had been frittered
away on show-castles but not on defence; the king's administration, so
finely honed by William Edington, had since been in the hands of less
able men; and the government of the new English dominions in France,
which had been entrusted to the Prince of Wales, had achieved little
other than to incite resentment amongst Edward's Continental subjects.

The concern of Edward's subjects came to a head in the parliament
of spring 1371, where Edward endured the most difficult assembly
he had experienced since the near rebellion of 1341. The Commons'
anger was the product of the wasted peace. They were particularly
incensed by the king's administration, which they believed to be incom-
petent and corrupt. As the bureaucracy was almost entirely staffed by
priests, the Commons' invective broadened into a more general attack
on the church; some, indeed, advocated a wholesale disendowment

of the English church. The Commons demanded that the chancellor, William Wykeham, and the treasurer be removed. Despite his affection for the unctuous bishop of Winchester, Edward's priority now was for cash, so he was forced to comply. Yet when the king asked for a subsidy to fund the war, the Commons did not immediately assent, even though no direct taxation had been asked of them since 1357.[ix] They complained that the old 1334 assessments were now completely unusable, as the country had been so greatly changed by three rounds of plague. Moreover, they wanted to reprise the idea of the rebate, last used in 1354, which was meant to ensure that the more wealthy parts of the country paid more than did those that were suffering. The Commons' solution was a parish tax, to be levied on every parish in the land, according to its ability to pay. The clergy would contribute half, the laity the other part. Happy to have any kind of grant at all, the king did not object and adopted the Commons' proposals as his own. Thus, for the first time in over a decade, tax collectors were sent out to every corner of England, charged with finding the money to keep Edward's enfeebled armies in the field.

Even with weapons and soldiers, it was an army that lacked generals. Edward, Prince of Wales, was incapacitated by illness, the king himself was old, and almost all his warrior companions – Lancaster, Mortimer, Northampton, Suffolk, Beauchamp – were now dead, struck down either by old age or by plague. The one remaining captain of the former French wars, Sir Walter Manny, was well past his fighting days; besides, he was now involved with less temporal affairs. On Friday, 28th March, the day before the testy parliament of 1371 was prorogued, Manny set his seal upon the foundation writ for a new charterhouse at West Smithfield, by the cemetery he had established there at the height of the Great Death, twenty-two years before. The grizzled old war dog had had to do battle with the full bureaucratic might of the church to see his plan through but now, finally, he had secured the site for his priory. Here the brothers of St Bruno would pray in solitude for the souls of the founders and the more than 50,000 plague victims buried on the other side of their priory church.

★   ★   ★

[ix] Excluding the special local subsidy of 1360, raised for self-defence, which was largely repaid to taxpayers when, in the end, it was not required.

The charterhouse in Smithfield was an incongruity. This was the meat market of London, beyond whose shambles were the stews of Cock Lane: here the Carthusian brothers, those most ascetic of monks, were supposed to lead their life of silent contemplation, just yards from the butchers and traders, beggars and whores who filled this bustling corner of the city. Yet it was, in a sense, entirely appropriate, for Manny's charterhouse took its place in Smithfield just as the pestilence had occupied a place in the public mind: for whilst life in Smithfield had in time returned to all it had been – noise, grit, misery and pleasure – there now was added the unvanishing memory of the Great Death, and a trepid resignation to future plagues – a silent ever-present pestilential death amidst the unchanged vitality of medieval life.

William Langland must have spent many hours in the streets and side-alleys of Smithfield, watching carefully as the world and his wife went by. Here was the material for his tavern of the Seven Sins, with Gluttony – having drunk himself into a stupor in the company of loose women and a rabble of ne'er-do-wells – pissing two quarts and loudly farting before vomiting as he swayed towards the tavern door. This was the rude world of Langland's *The Vision of Piers the Plowman*. In rich, alliterative English, Langland presents his audience with a panorama of society – the famous 'fair field full of folk'.[32] It is into this Gomorrah that he thrusts his protagonist, Will, and hero, Piers, a simple and taciturn ploughman who shows, by example, how all should live: he is safe in his social estate, hard-working and devout. Taking his cue from Piers, the poet encounters personifications of the various virtues and vices, and thereby discovers the means by which the true Christian life might be achieved.

Pestilence plays its role in Langland's dreams, but as with Manny's charterhouse at Smithfield, it stands on the periphery of an ongoing human drama. The plague had had its effects: Langland claims that since the pestilence many a marriage had descended into 'foul words', rancour and blows, that the disease had encouraged priests to abandon their churches, and given the friars licence to indulge in irrelevant debate.[33] Yet these were just incidents; the substance of Langland's polemic is concerned with the more general degradation of society. Properly ordered, each estate should do as God has assigned: the king should rule in justice, the nobility protect the realm, the church show the way to salvation, and the common people work to provide food and shelter for all. Now, however, all was corrupted: venality infected the court and parliament was a sham; the king and nobility had perverted justice; the common people were divided between malingerers and those 'on the make', who fought against feudal authority and were ambitious beyond their station; worst of all were Langland's fellow churchmen, especially the friars, who undermined conscience and disrupted the work of worthy parish priests. Yet the poet did not claim that any of this was the work of pestilence; rather, it was the other way round:

> Resoun reuerentliche tofore al þe reume prechede,
> And preuede þat this pestelences was for puyre synne.[x]

Langland assures us that it had not always been thus: the church, for instance, had once shared its patrimony with the poor. He offers no analysis of how this degeneration progressed, however: it was of no consequence, as an explanation did nothing to advance his narrative message, which was the search for the good Christian life and how it might be pursued.

Langland's despair at the state of society echoed the voices of those around him: preachers deplored the collapse in morals and laymen bemoaned the misfortunes of the realm, among them Langland's famous contemporary, John Gower – a lawyer, perhaps, and certainly a minor landowner. Gower's first work – the massive *Mirour de l'omme* – was written in courtly Anglo-Norman French and begun just as Langland completed the first recension of his *Vision*.[xi] Gower, like Langland, saw sin as the cause of this corruption, and sin was the fault of Man. Disturbances in the world (and therefore, by implication, plague) resulted from the disruption to nature that was the consequence of human sin. Man, therefore, was solely responsible for the miseries of the world. Nonetheless, the pestilence for Gower was still a defining moment in the degeneration of society. Although he was too young to remember life before pestilence came, he willingly believed what

---

[x] Reason reverently preached before all the realm, / And showed that this pestilence was for pure sin. (Langland, *Piers Plowman* (ed. Pearsall), Passus V, ll.114–15, p. 103; my translation.)
[xi] The so-called 'B' text.

others told him: that things were far better before the Great Death, when each of the orders – king, knights, priests and commons – had respected their place and obligations to others; now, however, every part of society had resiled from their God-given responsibilities, especially the peasant classes, which were corrupted by sloth and greed. Gower would return again and again to this imagined, former, happy time. In his final large-scale work, the giant English poem *Confessio Amantis*, completed in the 1390s, he wrote:[34]

> What shal befalle hierafterward
> Got wot, for now upon this tyde
> Men se the world on every syde
> In sondry wyse so diversed,
> That it welnyh stant al reversed,
> As forto speke of tyme ago.[xii]

The contemporary renown of Langland and Gower attested to a gradual increase in lay literacy, advanced by a proliferation of popular books, both spiritual and secular, which reflected the interests of a predominantly noble audience. Thus, Chaucer's *Book of the Duchess*, written – like the 'B' revision of Langland's *Vision* and Gower's *Mirour* – in the 1370s, was most probably a commemoration of Blanche of Lancaster, daughter of Henry Grosmont and John of Gaunt's wife. Yet for all its aristocratic provenance, *The Book of the Duchess* expounds a universal theme – of loss, and grief: for it is an elegy, in which a Black Knight mourns for his dead lady 'White'.[35]

> 'I have of sorwe so great won
> That joye gete I never non,
> Now that I see my lady bryght,
> Which I have loved with al my myght,
> Is fro me ded and ys agoon.' [xiii]

[xii] What shall happen in the future / God only knows, for at present / Men see the world on every side / In many ways so different, / That it stands amost all reversed, / As from times past.

[xiii] 'So great is my sorrow / That I will never again experience joy, / Now that I see my lady bright, / Which I have loved with all my might / Is dead and from me gone.'

Chaucer's was just one of a number of late fourteenth-century works of 'consolation'; another was *Pearl*, a profoundly moving allegory by an anonymous poet, stricken with a 'desolating sorrow' for the loss of his daughter, the 'pearl without blemish'.[xiv] It is easy to see how these works met with a receptive market and indeed played upon contemporary anxieties, for everyone – no matter who they were – had suffered repeated and heavy bereavement at the hands of the plague. But the antecedents of works of 'consolation' lay long before the Great Death, and the popularity of this literary form ran parallel with the growth in personal devotional texts, from the works of Richard Rolle before the Great Death to those of Julian of Norwich, Walter Hilton, John Thwing of Bridlington and the anonymous author of the *Cloud of Unknowing* in the decades that followed.

The king among these first princes of English verse was Geoffrey Chaucer – sometime soldier, customs official, ambassador and prolific court poet. During the 1370s Chaucer lived in rooms above Aldgate, which gave him a good view of the great concourse of London, barging, weaving and shuffling in and out of the capital all day. As with Langland, it was in observations of London folk that Chaucer assembled his material, which would be used twenty years later to famous effect in his own great satire on society, *The Canterbury Tales*. Chaucer's concept is unique, but it has elements in common with the work of Langland and Gower. On the one hand, the *Tales* present a number of ideals, in the irreproachable Knight, poor and devout Parson, and the hard-working Plowman; the other pilgrims, however, are caricatures of a different kind – a corpulent monk, dishonest friar, corrupt pardoner, and fraudulent doctor. This is Langland's 'fair field full of folk' in pointillist detail, with characters – like the Host (Harry Bailey) and Cook (Roger of Ware) – who were quite possibly real people. (Indeed, the depiction of the Man of Law might well have been a chummy dig at Chaucer's friend John Gower.) Even the action had a factual basis, for the famous pilgrimage to Canterbury was at this time more popular than ever before.[36]

It is all the more striking, therefore, that pestilence plays so small a part in the *Tales*, meriting no greater mention, in the main,

---

[xiv] Written, most probably, by the anonymous poet of *Sir Gawain and the Green Knight*.

than as a casual curse. Plague's sole cameo comes in the Pardoner's Tale:[37]

> Ther cam a privee theef men clepeth Deeth,
> That in this contree al the peple sleeth,
> And with his spere he smoot his herte atwo,
> And wente his wey withouten wordes mo.
> He hath a thousand slayn this pestilence.[xv]

Yet even here plague plays little role – it is more a backdrop to the narrative: pestilence claims none of the protagonists, whose deaths were instead brought about through their own greed. Thus, far from providing the premise for the whole drama, as it did in Boccaccio's *Decameron* (from which Chaucer drew inspiration), pestilence had become, in the world of the *Tales*, part of the general scenery of life. Plague was almost a commonplace, familiar to Chaucer's characters just as it was to his public. So the tavern-keeper in the 'Pardoner's Tale' warns his drinkers to be careful where they go, just as many must have done in reality when the epidemic was about:[38]

> for [pestilence] hath slayn this year,
> Henne over a mile, withinne a greet village,
> Bothe men and womman, child, and [labourer], and page;
> I trowe his habitacioun be there.[xvi]

Like those listening to the tavern-keeper's words of warning, Chaucer and his audience were clearly habituated to plague and how it should be avoided. The extraordinary coincidence of these men – Langland, Gower, Chaucer – is proof enough that the pestilence had done nothing to diminish the quality of English literature. For this golden age of English writing was the first full flowering of a language that had been in evolution long before the Conqueror came. Evidence for this

---

[xv] There came an unseen thief called Death, / That slayed all the people thereabouts, / And with his spear he smote their hearts in two, / And went his way without another word. / He had killed a thousand during this pestilence.
[xvi] for this year pestilence has killed, / Over a mile hence, within a large village, / Both men and women, children, labourers, and pages; / I am sure he has his habitation there.

could be found beyond the realms of great writing: a petition put before parliament in 1362 asked that all cases in the king's courts be tried in English, as French was not now known well enough, while the parliaments of 1362, 1363 and 1364 were all opened with speeches in English. It was not long before the vernacular started to creep into official use: the first legal instrument written in English was issued in 1376, parliament was petitioned in English in 1386 and the earliest English wills to be found in London's Court of husting appear the following year.

It is true that the increasing adoption of this rapidly maturing language was ascribed, by some, to the influence of the mortality. John Trevisa, writing in the 1380s, commented that after the first pestilence it was increasingly common for grammar school masters to teach their charges to translate Latin into English, rather than French. Trevisa saw the advantage in this – that children learnt grammar far more quickly – but also the disadvantage – that 'they conneþ na more Frensch þan can here lift heele.'[39] There may indeed have been some problems in grammar education. In York, for instance, the chancellor of the minster found it impossible to find a suitable master for the cathedral school and so had to appoint a spare cleric in 1368 on a short-term contract, merely as a stopgap.

There were other reasons, however, for the decline of French and emergence of English in these years. Spoken French had become increasingly unfashionable among the educated classes as the war with France drew on. In any case, the French spoken in England was a distant (and rather less sophisticated) cousin of the Continental language: for centuries Anglo-Norman French had been the butt of joking French sophisticates. Yet since the end of the thirteenth century, enough of the crucial military and courtly French vocabulary had been integrated into Old English to make the resulting amalgam useful and acceptable to English nobles and knights. Now that these men were fighting for England in foreign France, it seemed all the more appropriate that they should cultivate the English language. Gone were the family ties that had once bonded the Anglo-Norman nobility to their French cousins, and gone were the estates in Normandy that their great-great-grandparents remembered so well. It was no surprise, therefore, that there was a growing insistence on the use of English in parliament, and a deliberate propagation of the native tongue in the English court. It was a court that now spoke English fluently, which it had not done fifty years earlier. Edward III, it was said, could only swear in English; for his grandson Richard, English was his mother tongue. It was in this transition that English emerged in the last quarter of the fourteenth century as the common language of the English people, for reasons quite unconnected to the pestilence with which it coincided.

In their desire to decry the ills of the world, both Langland and Gower ignored what Chaucer saw in his Knight's Yeoman – the peasant made good through simple hard work. John Smith, of Brightwell Baldwin in Oxfordshire, was one such. Smith first appeared in the village records in the mid-1350s: he was a typical smallholder, with a few acres and a share in a house. He was clearly respected (serving on a jury) and ambitious (taking on a flock of sheep). Within fifteen years, John had put together a small portfolio of properties and land, including a cottage and three separate tenements which had most likely been vacated through death. There were very many men like John across England – lucky survivors from successive plagues, who turned their wit and their energy towards making best use of these grief-laden times. John Maggestone, the labourer and sometime brewer from Monkton Deverill, was another. After the Great Death John had moved to Longbridge Deverill, where opportunities were better. He carried on brewing and working but it was only in 1369 that he got the break for which he had been waiting and saving for many years. Perhaps through a lucky inheritance, he felt able at last to invest his savings in land of his own, paying 106s. 8d.[xvii] – a substantial sum for a man like John – to enter 23⅓ acres at Crockerton, a village a little further down the Wylye valley from Longbridge, towards Warminster.

For most landowners, however, this was a time of tribulation. The crisis of the late 1360s was a prelude to plummeting profits in the early 1370s. High prices were counteracted by astonishingly low yields, falling rates and receipts of rents made worse by ever-rising wage costs. Tellingly, the variation in the rent rates was narrowing, a reflection of the decreasing importance of the quality of land, now that it was

[xvii] Approximately £5.33.

available in such quantities and that labour inputs were more of a consideration than yields. In some places the damage done by the Great Death had still to be repaired, as at Tutbury in Staffordshire, where seven shops had stood empty since 'the first pestilence'; but everywhere, however, manor accounts told of how more recent vicissitudes had made things so much worse.[40]

With revenues from rents depressed by the mortality and profits eroded by rising wage-bills and low yields, lords had to resort, once again, to coercion in order to shore up their margins. The obvious first response was to bring prosecutions under the Statute of Labourers (which had lain almost in abeyance since the settled years of the mid-1360s), and commissions were sent out throughout England during the early 1370s to enforce the statute with renewed ferocity.[xviii] Yet, just as in the 1350s, labour legislation was found to be of only very limited utility, so lords concentrated on raising revenue instead. As most were not in a position to raise rents, they resorted to milking the dues of feudal tenure. Even though ever-increasing numbers of peasants rented their land and hired out their labour for cash, very few had been formally freed from feudal obligations. They were still liable, therefore, to those feudal exactions – such as chevage (paid by villeins on leaving their manor), merchet (on marriage), and heriot (on death) – which attached to their holdings and to their status as bonded tenants. It was these trappings of feudal control that lords now sought to exploit, in the absence of anything else they could do to sustain their revenues at former levels.[41]

Unsurprisingly, tenants reacted with a new determination to resist landowners' feudal will, bringing to an end a decade of comparative peace. The efforts of the justices in the early 1370s to enforce the Statute of Labourers were met with brazen recalcitrance, while the once sporadic instances of outright disobedience became increasingly common. Robert Hagham of Willingham, by Stow in Lincolnshire, had already been arraigned before the justices; when they came for his wife, Joanna, in 1373, he 'totally hindered the constables of this

---

[xviii] It was a mark of how serious landowners considered the situation that even the bishop of Durham, who already ran one of the more controlled feudal regimes in England, despatched a commission in 1372 specifically to enquire into excess wages – presumably because Bishop Hatfield felt that the control of wages was now beyond even his local control.

[area] in performing their duty'. Similarly, villagers strove to avoid the strictures of the manorial court. Take Robert Grys of Tibberton, a village a few miles outside Worcester: Robert was one of the many tenants of the bishop of Worcester who had accumulated holdings left vacant by plague, each one replete with a house and outbuildings which were unlikely ever to be filled again. The population of Tibberton, as in most villages, was now far smaller – perhaps half the size – than it had been when every dwelling was needed. Yet the bishop's steward insisted that the buildings, which were still the bishop's property, be maintained and the feudal dues that were still attached to the house be paid, even though they had long been empty. So, in 1370 Robert Grys took a torch to one of his unused houses in the village, hoping no doubt that it would be thought to be an accident and he would be relieved of the burden. Robert was not a particularly competent arsonist, however, and only half the house burned down. The evidence was there of the fire so Robert was ordered to rebuild the lord's property, which will have cost him dear: to rebuild a house cost between £2 and £4, equivalent to the annual income of a fairly well-to-do peasant.[xix] Robert's attempt to defy his lord was not isolated, for there was something of a movement gathering pace in 1370 across the bishop of Worcester's estates, as the tenants decided *en masse* to withdraw their remaining labour services from their lord.

The work of the justices of the peace and the increased impositions of landowners were all the more resented for the fact that tax collectors, mercifully absent since 1357, had reappeared in 1371. The burden of this tax was uncommonly large, not least because there had been a massive over-estimation of the number of villages in England – the result, in small part, of the abandonment of settlements that had taken place after the plagues. So parliament reverted to the old assessment of the tenth and fifteenth in 1372, and also in 1373 and 1374. Taken together, these subsidies represented an intensity of taxation that had not been experienced by the English since the 1340s. The demands of the crown might have been forgiven, had the war been going well, but the opposite was the case. By the end of 1374, the English had lost almost every acre of land won during Edward's reign,

[xix] It is remarkable that the cost of the actual construction of a house in 1370 as a proportion of annual family earnings is not so far off what it is today.

and the most-southern parts of England itself were under increasing attack. For so long fortune had looked kindly on this flawed but brilliant king; now she laughed at his wrinkled face. To heap misery on his humiliation, plague arrived, once again, on the south coast in late 1374; within a few months it had taken hold of the capital. One chronicler claimed, now almost by rote, that the epidemic killed 'a large number of Londoners', including a good number in royal administration, which will have done nothing to aid Edward's increasingly sclerotic organization.[42] Crushed abroad and afflicted at home, the country had been brought to its knees. The king was forced to sue for a truce with France, and on 27th June 1375, at Bruges, the French agreed to keep the peace for a year. The only consolation for the English – and it was a small one – was that the pope was prepared to grant a plenary indulgence for every person in England who died during the current, fourth, pestilence – the same indulgence that Clement VI had refused in 1349.[xx]

It is quite possible that John Smith, the smallholder-made-good of Brightwell Baldwin, died in the epidemic of 1375. He was probably quite old already and expected his end to come fairly soon: he had commissioned a brass to preserve his memory in the parish church of the village where he had spent his life. This was a luxury which very few peasant-farmers could afford, for this small plate of metal cost as much as twenty-five times the annual rent on one of the tenements he had acquired of late. Yet the epitaph inscribed thereon makes plain how little John thought of his new-found wealth:

> Man come and see how all the dead shall be.
> When you are called and carried away we take nothing when we
>   away fare.
> All that we care for is then other men's.
> Except for that which we do for God's love we have nothing there.
> Under this grave lies John the Smith: God give his soul heaven's
>   greeting.[43]

It was the prime failing of Langland and Gower that, for all their excoriation of peasant society, they could not see how the ambitious

---

[xx]The benefit of the indulgence lasted for six months – an interesting stipulation, for it showed that it was now commonly understood how long the epidemic would last.

and self-advancing villager might be just as capable of the humility and piety possessed by the self-denying paragons they imagined should fill the ranks of the labouring class.

After a sudden illness, David II of Scotland died on 22nd February 1371. The hapless king was only forty-six, but despite two marriages and a third engagement, he had produced no heir to whom he could pass on the Bruce line. With David's last sigh the dynasty begun by David's father, Robert – saviour of the Scottish nation and its greatest king – came to an end.

David had proved himself a far more competent ruler in peace than he had been a leader in war. Despite the heavy imposition of ransom payments (which David skilfully avoided paying between 1360 and 1365), a near rebellion in 1363 and several recurrences of epidemic plague, David passed on the Scottish crown to his heir – his nephew Robert Stewart – in a better state than he had received it upon his return from English captivity in 1357. Crown revenues in 1371 were four times the income of the Scottish crown fifty years before,[44] an extraordinary achievement and one for which David's chamberlain – Walter Biggar – should take much credit. Between them, king and chamberlain reformed the management of royal finances and the collection of customs and subsidies, centralized the bureaucracy of the crown at Edinburgh, and forced the Scots parliament into the habit of making regular grants of direct taxation. In return, parliament was called more often, given an audit function over the Exchequer, and was granted additional judicial powers. David showed similar tact in his treatment of the mercantile community, whom he described in 1364 as 'our beloved Scottish burgesses', handing them a monopoly as wholesalers to the clergy and laity of Scotland, as well as to all foreign merchants.

By these measures, David II and Walter Biggar considerably improved the state of the crown finances. However, the accounts of the Treasury gave an inaccurate picture of the health of the Scottish economy as a whole, which was far from strong. Inflation was rampant, even more so than in England. Forced to hand over a large portion of Scotland's national product to the English during the period of the ransom – a sum not even remotely compensated for by the country's export trade – Biggar had to devalue the coinage. On the basis of face-value alone, the Scottish pound fell by 35 per cent in value during the latter part of David II's reign, although the real fall was probably far greater. Taken together with impressive receipts from the wool and hide custom (the result of strong Continental demand), chronic inflation flattered the crown finances – and by extension the performance of the national economy. In reality, however, income from agriculture, which was by far the largest component of the economy, was severely depressed. The royal estate, for instance, returned only a quarter of the income it had provided fifty years before,[45] and a tenth of the amount generated in the previous century. It is true that the king's patrimony had been eroded through alienation but a good part of this decline could be put down to the agricultural depression. Thus, when the kingdom was reassessed for taxation in 1366, it was found that the properties of the church, which had in aggregate been worth over £15,000 in the thirteenth century, were now valued at £9,396 – a fall in value of 37 per cent. This was the truest reflection of the depression that beset Scotland in these years.

Just as it had done south of the border, the decline in agricultural incomes accelerated the erosion of the feudal economy: James Douglas of Dalkeith, for instance, had by 1376 leased his lands at Kilbucho in the borders and Aberdour in Fife, while the estate managers of the earl of Strathearn and of Cupar Angus Abbey were increasingly renting out their demesne. Also, as in England, some more adventurous peasants were making use of cheap land. On the Douglas estate the larger tenants now typically rented around fifty acres, which was two times what they might have farmed a hundred years before. This figure is by no means accidental, for with half the population now gone, the amount of land available for cultivation had, in effect, doubled.

The problems in the rural economy were reflected in the state of the burghs. As Scottish towns were essentially mercantile, most burghs suffered from the contraction of their markets. So although Edinburgh and Dundee did well while wool exports remained strong, most burghs experienced stagnation or decline. Continuing rivalries between towns, such as the mid-Angus towns of Brechin, Forfar and Montrose, pointed to competition for dwindling business. Auchterhouse was crushed by neighbouring Dundee, while Scrabster, on the extreme north of Caithness, failed entirely when its already small hinterland was so drastically reduced. Despite the considerable advantages conferred by burghal status, fully twenty towns failed to develop into anything in the decades following the Great Death, despite being designated as burghs.

The impression of stability given by strong royal finances was, therefore, far from real. So, although a half-century later Walter Bower would write that these years 'were made prosperous by way of great abundance of provisions, fruits and animals, and especially the tranquility of peace', the pestilence had in fact done structural damage to the Scottish economy, damage that was hidden, for the time being at least, by good government and a strong export trade.[46] The illusion was maintained for a while under the new regime of Robert II. Walter Biggar remained in post until his death, sometime in 1376 or 1377, and so in 1374 the crown produced a healthy surplus of 13 per cent.[47] However, once Biggar was gone Robert was shown to be as feeble a king as he had been regent: the administration was allowed to slide and direct taxation was foregone. Beyond his control was the collapse in customs revenues, which followed the decline of the Continental wool trade and a number of local sheep murrains. By the mid-1380s, the export of unprocessed wool stood at less than half what it had been a decade before, while during the 1380s the number of hides shipped had slipped by 15 per cent.[48] The impact on royal revenue was immediate and damaging: from now on the Exchequer regularly recorded a deficit. It was a trend that would continue well into the fifteenth century, incapacitating an already ineffectual Scottish crown – a decline in which pestilence had undoubtedly played a part.

In halving the Scottish population and substantially reducing the home market, the pestilence had one further consequence, whose effects would be felt for hundreds of years to come. The kingdom of Scotland had always been an amalgam of Highland and Lowland – each with differing customs, farming methods and languages. However, in the century before the Great Death, Lowland farms edged into the foothills of the Highlands and the trade in wool and hides depended, in part, on Highland pasture. Slowly but surely, commerce was blurring the line between the two communities. Yet with the retreat of Lowland agriculture after the Great Death and the turning over of Lowland arable to pasture, the gradual integration of the two economies ceased and went into reverse. There was less and less reason for the Highlander and Lowlander to speak, or to involve themselves with each other. All of this fed a growing sense of cultural difference, of antipathy even, to the point where John Fordun felt able to describe the Highlanders as 'a savage and untamed race, rude and independent, given to rapine . . . and exceedingly cruel'.[49] This prejudice soon seeped into Scottish government: the first surviving reference to the difficulty of governing the Highlands dates from 1369 and from that date the claim would come to be repeated more and more often. While there were other factors at work (not least the resumption of border warfare and the consequent reorientation of Edinburgh to England), by reducing the opportunities by which the Highlanders might be able to participate in the Lowland commercial economy, pestilence played a role in pushing these two parts of the Scots nation away from each other. It is from this point, therefore, that tension between the crown and Highland society increased and a growing lack of sympathy between Lowland and Highland Scots can be traced.

As in England and the borders of Scotland, depopulation and the vagaries of cereal and labour costs did much to precipitate the disintegration of the feudal manors of the southern plains of Wales, a decline felt worst of all by the once great Cistercian houses that dominated the lands further west. Here the plagues had made a previously challenging situation hopeless. By 1380 both Neath Abbey and Margam Abbey were in arrears on the payment of their clerical tenth, the result of the continuing demands of taxation, decimated revenues, and the inundation of their coastal lands which was the inevitable outcome of a failure of maintenance on the sea wall because labour was short. Those remnants of the Cistercian granges which had not already been leased were now farmed out. Few houses recovered from this position of slow decline and it is little surprise that as soon as a papal ban on appropriations came to an end in 1376, abbots reached once again for this favourite device of shoring up monastic income. By reducing the number and salaries of vicars in appropriated parishes and foregoing maintenance work on the fabric of the church, vicarage and tithe barns, the abbeys were able to cut costs and take more of the income themselves, doing further damage to pastoral care and causing much resentment at the behaviour of the

monks. Most scandalously, some priories farmed out their parishes to
third parties, thereby abdicating all their powers over the cure of souls.
There was, of course, a precedent for this before the Great Death,
but the struggle to maintain incomes in these remote monasteries
after the pestilence encouraged the more widespread abuse of their
clerical privileges.

Such despair was not the universal experience of Welsh landowners.
The fortunes of the manors near the English border had been helped,
to a limited extent, by the several large towns nearby in which they
could market their goods,[50] whilst for those farming sheep high wool
prices ensured, as in Scotland, some good profits. Thus, in contrast
to the straitened Cistercian houses of Glamorgan, the remote abbey
of Strata Florida, nestled at the feet of the Cambrian Mountains, still
had in 1379 an active demesne on which grazed some 1,327 sheep and
428 cattle. It was because of sheep that most marcher lords had been
able to continue to extract income from their Welsh lands, despite the
death of so many of their tenants. The de Bohun estates were in one
sense a model, for not only did the earl's officials ruthlessly impose
feudal dues on those tenants that remained but they also diversified
into farming sheep, which allowed them to generate an income from
land not only vacated by dead tenants but also on high ground that
would otherwise be unproductive waste, like the Epynt Mountains in
Brecon, where the earl had three thousand sheep. While wool prices
remained high and livestock was cheap, this was a highly successful
strategy – so much so that the earl's officials started renting land from
the impoverished Cistercian monks of Dore in order to extend the
lord's pasture. This concerted shift to pastoral sheep farming meant
that by 1373 the Bohun flocks produced 18,500 fleeces, returning an
increase in income some 40 per cent over what had been achieved in
the mixed farms operated prior to the Great Death. Although this was
the most impressive of sheep-farming enterprises in the March, the
earl's flock was just one of the many that now populated the hills up
and down the March.

As in Scotland, an economy sustained by a high price of wool was
particularly vulnerable when, from the mid-1370s, that price collapsed.
Between 1372 and 1375, the de Bohun estate saw its value decline by
almost a quarter – just in the space of three years. This was no
temporary anomaly: the fall in revenues was mirrored in most marcher

lordships and continued towards the end of the century and into the next. The contraction in sheep farming that followed left large tracts of upland uncultivated and ungrazed. Many of the bond tenants who had survived the plagues had either fled or purchased their own freedom: the number of serfs in one community in Dyffryn Clwyd, for instance, had by 1381 fallen from 212 to 47. This depopulation of the Welsh March and abandonment of so much land encouraged the mountain Welsh to nudge back down from their highland fastnesses, where they had been contained for so many decades. A similar process was underway in south Wales, where the Welsh were moving back down the valleys towards the Glamorgan plain, and at the other end of the principality, in Denbigh, Welshmen were nibbling at the edges of failed English manors, reclaiming gradually what they had not owned for several hundred years.

In truth, the abandonment of land in the March had been taking place before the Great Death and the widespread but temporary expansion of sheep-farming in the aftermath of the plague had only served to stay that process. It was a similar situation in the English colonial towns that encircled Wales, where Welshmen had been trying – successfully – to gain a foothold before the pestilence came. The emptying of so many burgage tenements undoubtedly opened the door to the Welsh, and the remaining Englishmen could not afford to be so picky about whom they let in. So Welshmen were now establishing themselves in Oswestry, Monmouth and Ruthin, through marriage or the illicit purchase of land. Indeed, while wool sales were strong those towns connected with the trade enjoyed a brief florescence – places like Denbigh, Wrexham and Brecon, along the March; Rhayader – the only new town to be established in Wales in these years – owed its success to its position on the droving pass between the Radnor forest and the Cambrian Mountains. These, however, were the towns able to attract enterprising incomers; there were many small towns in Wales which, with shrinking markets, offered few prospects. Several English towns, like Harlech and Criccieth, some of them still less than a century young, were in trouble, while others, like Bere in Merioneth and Cefnllys in Maelienydd, had disappeared altogether, as what remained of their populations gave up and sought a fresh start elsewhere. At least nine boroughs were deserted in the 150 years after the Great Death and even significant places like Caerphilly,

Cardiff and Tenby went into decline as their southern lowland markets dwindled.

The infiltration of Welshmen into the upper reaches of the March and the burgage tenements of English colonial towns accelerated the process by which the Welsh adopted English legal practice, such as primogeniture and written judgements, in defiance of Edward I's original settlement that obliged both communities to keep to their own legal customs. Some English settlers started using the Welsh mortgage, which proved particularly useful when there were restrictions on the sale or alienation of land, yet by and large the process of acculturation went almost entirely one way, with the Welsh taking on the habits and practices of their English occupying neighbours. The fact was not missed by contemporaries. Ranulf Higden remarked that the Welsh were beginning to till not only the fields but their gardens too; they were increasingly living in towns; some wore stockings and shoes, unlike their ancestors who were proud of their bare legs; some of them were even sleeping under sheets:

> So they semeth now in mynde
> More Englische men than Walsche kind.

There was some predictable concern among the minority English that their much-reduced communities were somehow threatened. Back in 1366 the burghers of Beaumaris asked that their charter, first granted by Edward I, be confirmed, especially those clauses that excluded Welshmen from the privileges of the town. The disquiet was felt most keenly by English churchmen, who saw themselves as a bulwark against Welsh barbarism and moral degeneracy. The poverty of the Welsh church had been greatly exacerbated by the pestilence, which made the recruitment of English clergy and religious into the church in Wales all the more difficult. In an effort to do something about it, the bishop of Bangor, Thomas Ringstead, bequeathed money to support five poor scholars from the diocese to study at Oxford and Cambridge. The donation came with one condition, however: the beneficiaries had to be English. It was in the same vein that Ringstead attached a rider to his generous gift of £100 to Bangor Cathedral – that no Welshman should be appointed his successor.

The actions of reactionary Englishmen fanned the embers of Welsh resistance, which had never been fully extinguished, even after a century of unchallenged English rule. Complaints rarely rose above petty resentments – like the protests of the Welshmen of north-east Wales who, during the 1370s, grumbled repeatedly about the privileges accorded the English burghers of Rhuddlan and Flint. Yet the English had fought the Welsh for several hundred years: they knew well that a Welshman's grievance was rarely forgotten and grudges allowed to compound might erupt into a violent response. With the return of war with France, English nervousness increased. The royal castles of Wales, many crumbling through years of neglect, were garrisoned again in 1370, 1372 and 1377, while English burgesses of the north Wales settler towns were ordered to 'to keep their town at their own peril'.[51] The fear was not without foundation. For although there were many large Welsh landowners who co-operated in the English rule (one of them – Sir Rhys ap Gruffudd – had fought as a captain to the English on the Scottish border and in France), the suspicion remained that the descendants of the Welsh princes might one day try to exploit English weakness and seek to regain what had once been theirs. In 1372 that fear was realized, when Owain ap Thomas ap Rhodri, or Owain Lawgoch, great-nephew of Llywelyn ap Gruffudd, made an attempt to emulate his ancestor and wrest Wales from English control. Supported by Charles V of France, Lawgoch made a half-hearted attempt to sail on Wales but was repulsed; before he could try again, an assassination was arranged.[xxi] His was a warning that the proud spirit of the Welsh nobility might yet pose a threat to the English domination of Wales. A note written in one late fourteenth-century translation of Geoffrey of Monmouth's *History* laments that the Welsh 'to this day suffer pain and deprivation and exile in their own land'.[52] It was that humiliation that propelled one Welshman to lead a rising as the fourteenth century drew to a close. Yet this was no mountain rebel but an anglicized great lord, who owned lands from Cardigan Bay to the Shropshire hills and whose grandmother was a Le Strange: Owain Glyn Dŵr. By loosening the grip of English lords and burghers over Welsh land, pestilence had, by subtle degrees, helped to create the circumstances by which a Welshman might make one final, heroic, bid to release his countrymen from the heavy weight of English chains.

*   *   *

[xxi] In the town of Montagne sur Mer in Poitou in July 1378.

The English had never shackled the Irish as they had the Welsh. The indifference of successive English monarchs, not least Edward III, meant that by the time plague came to the island in 1348, the colony was already in grave distress. The near collapse of colonial government after the death of Sir Thomas Rokeby in 1357 was exacerbated by the first return of pestilence in 1361, which left the colony – already disabled by the absence of so many of its great lords – further denuded and all the more open to attack. That second, pestilential, year, had marked the nadir of the colony's fortunes: the empty royal Treasury and Exchequer had to be moved from Dublin to Carlow because the shrivelled eastern English exclave was now completely cut off from the largest part of the dismembered colony, which lay along the south coast. Crown tenants in Dublin soon followed and in 1362 vacant lands had to be leased out to whoever would take them on. No better evidence could be produced to show the degree to which the Anglo-Irish colonial enterprise had become unstuck.

No longer distracted in France, Edward had belatedly recognized that he had to intervene. In his own words, the colony was 'now subject to such devastation and destruction . . . that it will soon be plunged into total ruin'. Answering the colonists' call that he send them 'a good well-endowed leader, well stocked and fortified with men and treasure', Edward had appointed his son, Prince Lionel, as his satrap across the Irish Sea.[53] The young prince arrived in September 1361 with a larger force than the island had witnessed for several decades. Although the capture of Art Mac Murrough, king of Leinster, in 1361 and his subsequent death removed one of the finest antagonists of the Anglo-Irish, Lionel achieved little by his efforts or the large sums that he spent.[54] The lack of progress and the continued reluctance of absent lords to contribute to the protection of their lands, either in person or in treasure, forced Edward to decree in 1365 that a year's worth of revenues from their possessions should be seized in order to pay for the colony's defence. Yet Lionel was persuaded that there were more fundamental reasons for the failure of the colony: that many of those who were supposed to defend the March and the English way of life had instead gone native, behaving like petty kings in their own lordships and obeying the English administration only when it suited, as a consequence of which all of Lionel's attempts to co-ordinate a response to native Irish attacks had been frustrated.

The prince's answer was to legislate for success. In 1366 he called a great council of the principal Anglo-Irish lords and their English administrators, whose product – the Statute of Kilkenny – would become an infamous symbol of English oppression in Ireland. The statute incorporated the bulk of Rokeby's ordinances of 1351, seasoned now with a good dollop of English prejudice. The document ascribed all the problems of Ireland to the degeneracy of the settlers who, 'forsaking the English language, dress, style of riding, laws, and usages, live and govern themselves according to the manners, dress, and language of the Irish enemies and also had contracted marriages and alliances with them whereby the land and the liege people thereof, the English language, the allegiance due to our lord king, and English laws are put in subjection and decayed . . .' The result was that the Anglo-Irish colony was 'decayed and the Irish enemies exalted and raised up'.[55] The cause being diagnosed, the cure was simple to prescribe. As in earlier ordinances the Anglo-Irish council reserved to itself the right to declare war and treat for peace, while the primacy of common law was restated. All exogamous marriages were once again banned and the fostering of children across community lines was prohibited. While these clauses comprehended the legal and familial separation of the two nations, the statute also aspired to enforce the complete cultural division of Gaelic and Anglo-Ireland: the Anglo-Irish were only to speak English, name themselves by English names, and ride in the English manner; Irish musicians and games were banned; even insulting an Anglo-Irishman by claiming that he was 'an Irish dog' was no longer permitted. Most shockingly, priests 'of the nation of the Irish' were no longer allowed to minister to the colonists, nor to enter their religious houses. In promulgating this hierarchy of priests, the colonists implied that the native Irishman was somehow incapable and inferior in the bestowal of the sacraments to people of English stock.

For all its appalling language, the Statute of Kilkenny made plain the inadequacy of the Anglo-Irish position. The origins of this slowly unfolding calamity lay, of course, long before the coming of plague, but it is certainly true that pestilence helped to reinforce the supremacy of the native Irish over the floundering English. For the colonists, each successive plague made life that much more unbearable, further reducing the numbers of people who were able to fight and fund the protection

of the colony against Gaelic Irish guerrilla attacks, which only intensified as the colonial ability to resist became depleted. Limerick was
burnt by the O'Brien[xxii] and the Macnamara in 1369, while a few years
later Kilmaclenine, a tiny borough north of the River Blackwater in
county Cork, was completely overrun. In 1375 the once-proud port of
Waterford was plundered: the mayor, bailiff and coroner of the city
were killed, as were twenty-six of the leading men of Waterford and
eighty merchants from outside, including traders from Coventry and
Bristol. The raiders returned six weeks later and killed a further
twenty-four of the city's leading citizens. No wonder that by the end
of the century a French visitor, Jean Creton, would comment that
Waterford was inhabited by 'wretched and filthy people, some in rags,
others girt with a rope – had the one a hole, the other a hut for their
dwelling'. With the countryside between the towns emptied by plague
and plundered from raiding, the few remaining colonial settlements
were reduced to disconnected merchant patriciates, the pathetic
remnant of a once considerable colony. Of Dublin, Creton said: 'I
should have been heartily glad to have been penniless in Poitiers or
Paris, because here there was no amusement or mirth, only trouble,
toil and danger.'[56]

Prince Lionel was gone before 1366 was out: the March soon
dissolved into disorder and the native Irish threatened the interior of
the colony once again. Cultural separation was shown immediately
to be a failure and it was now more clear than ever that without a
radical change in royal policy, the best that could be hoped for was
that the inevitable destruction of Anglo-Ireland could be delayed.
Edward sent William Windsor, a former lieutenant of Lionel in Ireland
and close friend of the king's mistress, Alice Perrers, to attempt this
near-impossible task; the unfortunate man arrived just months before
Ireland was engulfed in its third round of epidemic plague, 'of which
many nobles and citizens and especially young people and children
died'. It was an ominous start to a turbulent posting. For it was not
long before the new justiciar had antagonized the colonists who, while
recognizing that strong leadership was needed, disliked following
commands – which Windsor was not reluctant to dispense. Their
disputes set a dangerous precedent, for the crown was increasingly

---

[xxii] Anglicized from Ó Briain – prominent family clan of Thomond.

doing battle not with the native Irish but with the colonial settlers, who came together into something approaching a party. Their petition of 1376 said as much: the protest of the Anglo-Irish, they claimed, was against the justiciar's attacks on the 'liberties, privileges, rights, laws, and customs of the land of Ireland'.[57] It was the final damnation of Edward's disastrous policies in Ireland, for the English crown now had not only the resurgent Gaelic Irish with which to contend but also a renegade rump of a bankrupted colonial estate.

The arrival of the fourth pestilence in 1375 elicited an almost elegiac response from the current archbishop of Canterbury, Simon Sudbury:

> we are assailed by plagues or epidemics, by the horrors of war, the unhealthiness of the air, the scarcity of crops and the diminishing of livestock, all of which leaves us more than usually bewildered and depressed. We cannot even take pleasure in our independence, for foreigners find ingenious excuses to plunder our possessions and make frequent attacks on our men, and other troubles increase daily – as it is perfectly obvious to informed observers.[58]

Such were the fruits of Edward's reign. Yet he was hardly able to perceive them: the king now viewed the world through a rheumy eye, and his ears heard little other than the sweet nothings whispered there by the siren who attended his geriatric concupiscence.

Trouble piled upon trouble. The 'Good' parliament of 1376 impeached Alice Perrers and others in what they called the 'covyn' that was controlling the king; the Commons' attempted seizure of the crown administration was only narrowly averted. Then, on 8th June 1376 – Trinity Sunday – the Prince of Wales died at Westminster Palace. England was now left with a senile king, a nine-year-old heir, Richard of Bordeaux, and a deeply unpopular regent, John of Gaunt. Only Edward's reputation now kept him immune from direct attack, while the faction and failure that gripped his government allowed restiveness to grow in his realm.

It was a measure of the depth of England's travails that two extra-ordinary harvests, in 1375 and 1376, did not ameliorate the rising sense of unease. For the first time in living memory, the direction of prices and wages diverged. Grain prices, built up over the two decades after the Great Death, began to unwind as the abundant harvests had their effect, but the cost of labour – which since the Great Death (and before) had run a roughly parallel course with prices – held firm and, in some areas, continued to increase. So whilst labourers, once again, benefited, their lords – especially the smaller landowners who lacked the clout of the great barons – saw their profits further diminished.

A profound sense of grievance thus filled the Westminster air when parliament assembled in spring 1377, summoned to discuss the crown's demand for a subsidy in order that it could respond to the threatened French invasion. For almost every member of parliament was paying his labourers more than ever before, and their tenants were doing well out of good harvests and historically low rents. Indeed, the process of commutation had allowed many peasants to escape paying tax altogether, as on many estates the share of the tenth and fifteenth was related to the services owed by tenants. So, the members asked, why should these newly enriched peasants not contribute to the defence of the realm as they once had done? Their solution, once the session was underway, was a flat tax of a groat – 4d. – on every man and woman over the age of fourteen. Not only was this affordable for anyone who was not a genuine pauper (who were in any case exempt) but the tax was simple to assess and easy to collect. More important for many was the symbolic virtue of the new tax: like Langland and Gower, these men had seen what had happened in the two decades since the Great Death, and their diagnosis of England's problems was much the same. By creaming off some of the new wealth of the peasantry, they might do something to restore the dignity of the land-owning estate. The concept was voted through on 19th February 1377, and the assessment of every adult in England for this new 'poll tax' duly began.

The same day that the Commons were voting on the poll tax, there was a near riot at St Paul's. John Wyclif, until recently an obscure Oxford academic, had been preaching – at John of Gaunt's behest – public sermons in the capital attacking the authority of the pope and the endowment of the church. Summoned to appear before Simon Sudbury, the archbishop of Canterbury, and William Courtenay, the bishop of London, in the Lady Chapel at St Paul's Cathedral, Wyclif had appeared with his patron in support. First they had to run the gauntlet of an angry crowd, which had gathered after news had circulated that some of Gaunt's allies in parliament had proposed the abolition of London's privileges, including the mayoralty, only that morning. Matters only got worse once proceedings finally got under way. As the bishops put their questions to Wyclif, Gaunt lost his temper and threatened to drag Courtenay out of the cathedral by his hair. The crowd erupted in fury and Gaunt fled the tumult, from which Wyclif had to be saved by his accusers. The night-time curfew did little to cool the crowd's anger and the following day the duke was forced to leave his supper on the table when the mob surrounded his palace of the Savoy; only Courtenay's intervention stopped them burning the place down. London had not seen a disturbance like this since the days of Edward II: it did not bode well.

Wyclif may have been only a minor entry in Oxford's annals had it not been for his deposition as master of Simon Islip's new foundation of Canterbury College by Simon Langham, Islip's successor, in favour of a Benedictine monk. Despite Wyclif's appeal to Avignon, Langham's decision was upheld by the pope. The whole affair greatly embittered the man who – for all his brilliance – was possessed of an angry person- ality. His disappointment drove him to launch increasingly strident attacks on the papacy and on the religious. Nevertheless, he was toler- ated by the Oxford authorities: academics were given considerable licence to engage in theological dispute – even when it was potentially heretical – but only within the closed intellectual compound of the university. Before the public, churchmen were expected to abide by what was orthodox. By setting out his views in public, Wyclif had most definitely crossed that line. In May 1377, three months after his appearance at St Paul's, Wyclif was formally censured by the pope. The case against him was written by Adam Easton, who was working in the curia at Avignon, and it was Easton's friend, Thomas Brinton, now bishop of Rochester, who informed the errant cleric of the pope's decision. So the lives of these three Oxford contemporaries, who had gone up to Oxford in the years immediately after the Great Death, now came together again – this time in rancorous dispute.

Wyclif's opponents were as conscious of the need for reform as was the irascible Oxford don. William Courtenay was a vocal critic of 'chop- churches', while a year after Wyclif's censure Sudbury sent out a stiffly worded ordinance attacking 'greedy and pleasure-seeking' priests that hired themselves out for excessive rates, who 'vomit out the enormous salaries with which they are stuffed'.[xxiii] These sybaritic clerics, Sudbury claimed, worked themselves into a 'lather of lechery over various fleshy delights' and were, therefore, 'a detestable scandal to the clergy and the worst possible example to the laity'.[59] This was a lashing of which Wyclif's keenest firebrands would have been proud, yet it came in this instance from the head of the church in England.

The bishops knew very well that words alone would not suffice. The challenges posed by mass mortality persisted, although by their strenuous efforts much progress had already been achieved in rebuilding the pastoral mechanisms of the church. Where congregations had collapsed, parishes had been united, as in Cambridge, where the churches of All Saints and St Giles were brought together in 1365. Simon Langham, who was then bishop of Ely, gave his reasons plainly: the parishioners of All Saints were for the most part dead because of the pestilence and those that survived had gone to other parishes. The nave was falling down and the bones in the graveyard were exposed to gnawing dogs and pecking ravens. As St Giles had lost parishioners as well, it made sense to bring the two congregations together. It was, however, not all like this. In the Hereford diocese, for instance, ordinations were increasing, albeit only slightly, after the protracted fall that had started within a few years of the Great Death. Indeed, in some places the situation was markedly better even than it had been before the Great Death: in the diocese of Lincoln, some rectories that had, before the pestilence, been put in the charge of a cleric in minor orders now enjoyed the service of a fully fledged priest. Moreover, efforts continued to improve clerical education, as was so clearly shown by Wykeham's new foundations in Winchester and Oxford, which were explicitly charged with correcting the lack of educated priests that was one result of the mortality. While the universities only dealt with a tiny minority, their patronage must have reflected a wider, less documented, concentration on clerical education, for there is little evidence to corroborate the view of some contemporaries that standards overall had slipped. Finally, the English church had responded

---

[xxiii] Both must have noted the hypocrisy of Wyclif's position, for he was every inch an absentee rector, having exchanged Ludgershall in Buckinghamshire for the far richer living of Lutterworth in Leicestershire in 1374.

with some enthusiasm to the papal demands, enshrined in the 1366 bull *Consueta*, which controlled pluralism, and his other initiatives of that year to put a break on the appropriation of parishes by monasteries.

Thus, for all the faults identified by Langland, Wyclif, Sudbury and others, the church was certainly not utterly corrupted; had it been, then it could hardly have inspired the kind of devotion and piety that the laity demonstrated in these years. Chantries were still being founded, albeit at a more modest rate, which was unsurprising given the smaller population. Pilgrims, on the other hand, were flocking in greater numbers than ever before to the holy places of England, at least if the evidence of the cathedral shrines is representative. Westminster Abbey, for example, took £103 at the shrine of St Edward the Confessor in 1372–3, six times the income generated in 1346–7. This absolute increase in pilgrim numbers was all the more remarkable for the reduction in the population from which they were drawn. The pilgrimage was an ancient form of personal spiritual exercise; new forms of devotion also demonstrated the vitality of Christian life in England. Parish fraternities – rare in the 1350s – were, by the 1370s, increasingly common. In Essex, for instance, at least six village fraternities were founded between 1363 and 1379,[60] a trend that would continue well into the next century, to the point where almost every village would have a fraternity of some sort or other. Not only was this a reflection of the increased prosperity and ambition of the rural peasantry but it was an endorsement too of the hierarchy's efforts to maintain the integrity of parochial life.

This, then, was the true picture of the church three decades after the Great Death: untidy but vital, blessed with more virtuous leadership than it was beset with corpulent abuse, and responsive to the needs of the faithful, for whom it provided succour. Indeed, it was from the pulpits that the first early warnings of social ferment were to be heard, and not from Wyclif's vituperative tongue, but from a bishop – Thomas Brinton, the new bishop of Rochester, who started preaching in London when his Oxford contemporary first took to the stump.

Many of Brinton's targets were familiar: false merchants, extravagant clothing, the lack of devotion in the people. However, the prelate was also prepared to fire political broadsides, the power of which were all the more surprising given his rank. As early as 1375, only two years after his election to the Rochester see, Brinton was lamenting the state of the nation:

> Let us look at what is happening now. We are not strong or fortunate in war. We are not stable in faith. We are not honourable in the eyes of the world – on the contrary, we are of all men the falsest, and in consequence not loved by God. It is undoubtedly for that reason that there exists in the kingdom of England so marked a diminution of fruitfulness, so cruel a pestilence, so much injustice, so many illegitimate children . . .[61]

As the months wore on and the situation at home and abroad deteriorated, the bishop only became more outspoken: 'our modern rulers – those overthrowers of truth and justice – wishing to raise their lords to the altars, as they know how, have proclaimed the coward a hero, the weak man strong, the fool a wise man, the adulterer and the pursuer of luxury a man chaste and holy' – all observations that could, with very little imagination, be applied both to members of the royal family and to a number of their supporters. His assault on Alice Perrers was hardly covert: the 'keys of the kingdom . . . hang at the girdle of a woman'. He did not reserve his opprobrium for the court and royal administration, however: the bishops had failed to stand up for justice and too many of their clergy were 'unfit and unworthy'. The greatest fault, however, lay with the lords, who live, 'for the most part, upon the goods of other people', whilst they 'hardly pay their servants their proper and appointed wages'. Even the heathen princes of India treated the poor with greater respect. The rich would do well to remember that 'in death all, both rich and poor, find the like end; as hired actors on a stage when their parts in the play are over, all return to the position from which they had been raised.' It was, in short, 'the rich people and the nobility who are the main cause of our afflictions'. He urged action, lest some calamity befall the kingdom: 'let us be not merely talkers, but doers.'[62]

'The truth shall make you free' was the motto of this magnificent prelate, but the rich did not wish to hear it.[63] It was Brinton, the orthodox radical – not Wyclif, the refractory heretic – who was the true prophet of the age.

★   ★   ★

On 21st June 1377, after many months of false warnings, king Edward III died in his palace of Sheen. Alice Perrers, who tended him until his last breath, then yanked the rings from the dead man's fingers and fled.

The new king, Richard II, was only ten years old. Three days after his grandfather's death, the French launched their most devastating raids on the south coast since the Conquest, in which they were met in a remarkable defence by the abbot of Battle. Despite his monks' best efforts, Rottingdean and Lewes were taken, Portsmouth, Dartmouth and Plymouth were sacked, Hastings and Rye were plundered, and then, for much of August, the Isle of Wight was occupied. Towns burned from Southampton to Gravesend.

Any attempts to renew the peace were frustrated by the instability of the papacy. On 17th January 1377, Pope Gregory XI, nephew of Clement VI, had entered Rome, bringing the 'Babylonian Captivity' of the church in Avignon, which had lasted since 1309, to an end. The election the following year of an Italian pope, Urban VI, should have initiated a realignment of papal sympathies in England's favour – a rare crumb of comfort for the stricken English. Yet by the end of August 1378 word reached England that the French cardinals had already fallen out with Urban and on 20th September they elected a rival pope, Clement VII, who immediately re-established a papal court in Avignon. The schism of the Western church would, in time, have more profound consequences for the English church than the plague ever did; for the moment, it made the chances of reconciliation between France and England all the more remote.

Catastrophe was soon compounded by calamity: in 1378 pestilence attacked once again, the fifth time it had come. On this occasion it seems to have bypassed the south of England, entering in at York directly from the Continent and – in the words of Thomas Walsingham – 'almost the entire whole region was rapidly stripped of its best men.' It was an opportunity the Scots felt they could not miss. Enriched by the receipts of wool (they had stopped paying the ransom as soon as they had heard of Edward's death) and emboldened by the crisis in England, they launched massive raids over the border. No doubt the accounts of the Scots' brutality were enhanced by repeated telling, as the tales made their way south: by the time they got to St Albans, Walsingham – always in the market for a good story – was able to relate how the raiders 'beheaded many people and then – carried away by their savage nature – were not ashamed to kick the heads backwards and forwards as though playing football with them'.[64] A petition was sent from Lancaster to the king, asking that he 'consider this very great hurt and damage which they have suffered, and are still suffering, both by pestilence and by the continual devastations of the Scots enemy'.[65] Not that the presence of plague deterred the invaders, who religiously crossed themselves before they waded the border stream, in so doing invoking the protection of their patron saints:

Gode and Seynt Mungo, Seynt Romayne and Seynt Andreu, scheld us this day fro Goddis grace, and the foule deth that Yngleesh men dyene upon.[66]

It had now been so long since the Scots had attempted such an invasion that they had forgotten what had happened the last time they sought to capitalize on the presence of plague. The raiders took the disease back over the border with them and, as a result, pestilence had gone through Scotland by the close of 1380. A later chronicler remembered it as a powerful epidemic, killing a third of the people there.[67] Not that the Scots' infection was much comfort to the English: assailed from both south and north and beset by pestilence, the people of England surveyed a pitiful scene. To think that just ten years before, the English king ruled half of France; now he was forced to defend the frontiers of his own realm. There was an even greater threat, however, within.

During the harvest of 1377, a 'great rumour' whipped round the villages of Berkshire and Hampshire. Apparently, it was said, Domesday Book showed that the villeins hold their land not of their lords but direct from the king. If so, this would accord them all the ancient privileges of living on the king's land, as well as a chance of manumission, just as he had granted his bondmen at Windsor in 1369. Some villages had already collected enough money to apply to Chancery for copies of their entry in the Domesday Book. Hopes were running high: some were so confident of a validation of their claim that they refused to render services and court dues to their current lords. The tenants of the abbot of Chertsey had even risen in revolt. Yet the rumour turned out to be precisely that, and very few of the villein tenants found the satisfaction they sought. However, the speed with which this 'great rumour' spread, the excitement it caused, and the investment that villein tenants were willing to make in order to discover its truth, were testament to the considerable pressures that were building up within so many manors.

The problem was one of fundamental economics. Prices had in no way recovered since the bountiful harvest of 1375 but wages continued to go up, reflecting sustained pressures on the labour market as a result of recurrent plague. Although some of the largest and best-run estates had suffered a decline in income of as little as 10 per cent in the thirty years since the Great Death, their margins had been considerably eroded by rampant inflation; most small manors, which did not have the power to corral tenants or reap the rewards of large economies of scale, fared far worse. To those lords who had completely manumitted their tenants and rented out their lands on a straight lease, there was almost nothing to do but sit and wait for the market to turn; for those who had retained some vestigial feudal control, however, there was still the option of tightening the screws on their tenants. So the Statute of Labourers was enforced with ever-increasing determination and vigour and more and more old feudal dues were resurrected, while old by-laws of the manor court, which in some cases had become a dead letter, were suddenly invoked anew as if the decades had simply not passed. For a generation that had seen such extraordinary change, within the space of a lifetime, since the Great Death of 1348–9, this was a sharp reminder indeed that most peasants still lived in a state of servitude, even despite the advances that some had made in their income and status during the intervening years. Indeed, it was a measure of landowners' desperation to keep the old feudal distinctions intact that the Commons attempted, in 1379, to resurrect the failed sumptuary legislation of 1363, the better to *show* the prescribed division of the social order upon which the lords' claims were founded and built. Most sensibly, Richard's ministers kicked the idea into the long grass.

The nervous assertiveness of landowners was unsurprisingly met with increasing peasant resistance. In some places it was the justices who bore the brunt of peasant disobedience: by 1378, for instance, it was apparent that a large part of Essex was resisting the enforcement of the statute, although the problem was clearly not isolated to Essex, as the same year parliament asked the new king to reaffirm the statute, a request that he granted. Yet it was in the manor courts and in the villages that the lords found their will most sorely tested. In Blackmore, south-west of Chelmsford in Essex, the tenants 'utterly refused' to elect a rent collector from among their number in 1375, for which they were fined. This was not only a ruse to avoid paying what was due, but a test by which the tenants probed how far they could assert their demands. The court held on 11th November 1377 at Harmondsworth in Middlesex was a picture of disobedience: Robert Baker shouted at the jury in front of everyone, telling them they had handed down a false verdict, while Walter Brewer followed with a tirade of abuse all of his own, and would not be silenced despite the calls of the lord's seneschal. The tenants of the bishop of Worcester went one step further, rising in 1378 in something approaching a rebellion. Their complaint was the level of labour services that the estate still levied, and the tenants' reaction brought a favourable response, as the officials commuted *opera* permanently into money rent. Countless incidents like these encouraged peasant hopes that they might be able to throw off the exactions imposed on them by their lords.

Whole tracts of the English countryside had been set on edge by unanswered grievances and frustrated ambitions; in many towns also, the atmosphere was becoming increasingly uneasy. Although the circumstances differed from place to place, in almost all the often testy relationship between striving newcomers and the established civic elite was the cause of dissent. In Norwich there was a successful attempt by the more powerful burgesses to consolidate their control over the city, turning the city into what was, in effect, a medieval civic corporation.[xxiv] While this was an astute move on the councillors'

[xxiv] In 1378 the burgesses obtained from King Richard a new charter which gave the merchant oligarchy similar powers in justice and the creation of by-laws as enjoyed by the aldermen of London. Emboldened by this, and by the Statute of Gloucester which reinforced the rights of urban leaders across the country, the twenty-four councillors raised a local tax from Norwich citizens and used the proceeds to buy up all the plots in the market square and the landing stage by the river, thereby municipalizing the trading assets of the city and turning the regular deficit of the council into a profit.

part, it was also deeply unpopular among minor merchants and traders, who resented the stranglehold on trade, legislation and justice that the great merchants of Norwich now possessed. It was a similar situation in York, where by the 1370s the wealthy merchants who organized the city's international trade, especially in cloth, had come to dominate the government of the city, much to the exclusion of the small traders, craftsmen and property-owners who had wielded more power in the past. On Monday, 26th November 1380, a claque of the men of York – mostly representing the lower orders of the commercial community – came out against the mayor, John Gisburne, stormed the guildhall and ran the merchant out of the city. In his place they installed Simon Quixley, allegedly against both his own will and that of the leading men of York. News of this 'horrible thing' was passed quickly to the parliament then meeting, with the king, at Northampton.[68] The king's ministers pursued a gentle approach to the situation: the rioters were dealt with leniently, investigations were announced, and Quixley was installed by normal election in February 1381. That, they must have hoped, would be the end of the fractious atmosphere in the capital of the North.

The main business of the Northampton parliament was to consider the crown's desperate pleas for money, as the beleaguered English armies on the Continent were unable to move for lack of funds. The Commons offered another poll tax, but this time the rate was set at a shilling per person – three times the rate imposed in 1377 – although collectors were given some freedom to levy the tax according to the ability to pay. When the receipts started to arrive back at the Exchequer in April 1381, it was apparent that nothing like the amount expected was being paid. The collectors were under no illusion as to why this might be: hardened by an exceptionally cold winter and resentful of this onerous tax, people across England were simply refusing to hand over the money. John Waleys of Sparham in Norfolk even threatened to decapitate the village tax collector. Desperate for cash, the crown officials sent out commissions to collect what was due. It would be the efficient spark that lit the pyre of bitterness and complaint, pre-fuelled by feudal imposition, labour legislation and oppressive taxation over recent years, thereby starting one of the greatest conflagrations of civil disobedience ever to have been seen in the British Isles.

The moment came on Thursday, 30th May 1381, when John Bampton, one of the commissioners charged with the investigation of non-payment, arrived at Fobbing, between Basildon and the mudbanks of the Thames, where he planned to root out those who had refused to pay. He was soon chased off by the villagers, who threatened to lynch him if he did not go. A royal justice, Robert Bealknap, was quickly despatched to deal with this flagrant affront to the authority of the crown, but the Fobbing men intercepted the judge at Brentwood and accosted him. Meanwhile, on the other side of the Thames estuary, a group from the village at Erith attacked their overlord, the abbot and monks of Lesnes. It may well be that the men of Erith had heard via the ferry of what had happened at Fobbing; perhaps it was pure coincidence – another of the local peasant revolts that had become increasingly common in recent years. Yet what is certain is that when news reached Kent of the disturbances in Essex, the rioters took heart. They roamed from Dartford to Rochester, taking on angry men at every turn, until they came to Maidstone. There they chose a local brigand, Wat Tyler, as their leader and under his orders sprung the prisoners from the archbishop's gaol. Among the absconders was John Ball, a wild priest, who for twenty years or more had caused irritation to the church authorities in Kent. While one group headed off to Canterbury, where they did great damage to the abbey and the archbishop's quarters, the main bulk of the *turba* made for London. By Wednesday, 12th June 1381, they had set up camp on Blackheath, overlooking the Thames.

In Essex, meanwhile, the rebels were going from village to village, breaking into manor houses and burning the court rolls, believing that if they destroyed the evidence of their servitude, they would be freed of the fines with which they had been increasingly oppressed. But it was not only the villeins who joined in this protest: there were freemen too – angry at the rents they were charged and the restrictions placed on the labour they could hire; there were even some minor gentlemen farmers among the crowds, who doubtless saw it as safer to join in the revolt than try to resist it themselves. Like a bushfire the rebellion whipped through Essex; soon it had crossed the Stour into Suffolk and gone westwards into Hertfordshire and Cambridgeshire. Once they had ransacked the manor house, there was very little left that each of these small bands of rebellious villagers could achieve, other than to do as others were and make for London, where they could impress their demands on the king. So by the same Wednesday that the Kentish men were congregating at Blackheath, a whole multitude of Essex men had assembled at Mile End, on the main road from the county into the capital.

The following day, Thursday, 13th June, the rabble entered London – the Kentish men over London Bridge and the Essex men through Aldgate, under the room that Chaucer rented. Some headed for the Temple, where they knew the lawyers to be – those who, by clever argument and suasion, had rebuffed the poor peasants' many appeals for freedom and feudal restraint. Others looked for the treasurer, Sir Robert Hales, whom they held responsible for the poll tax. The Kentish men, many of whom were free tenants, sought out Simon Sudbury – their liege lord on his estates in Kent. The chaos gave Londoners the opportunity to settle some of their own disputes. A number of them set on and murdered Flemishmen, whom they had long blamed for taking their trade; others, not forgetting Gaunt's slight, stormed the Savoy at last, and threw the riches of the duke – who was treating with the Scots on the border – down from the windows into the street.

Before any more damage could be done, young Richard (who, it should be remembered, was still only fourteen years old) decided to act. The next day, Friday, 14th June, he rode to Mile End to meet the Essex rebels – who were probably the larger contingent of insurgents but had so far been the more restrained. Their demands were fourfold: that villeinage be abolished; that a man's labour be his own, unfettered by law; that land be rented out at no more than 4d. per acre; and that the oppressive servants of the crown be arrested and tried. In his desperation to ensure the dispersal of the crowds, the king granted all of these demands and ordered clerks to set up tables, there and then, so that charters of manumission could be produced.

With the king's party out of the capital at Mile End, however, the Kentish men realized that they had London to themselves. The Londoners having let them in, they stormed the Tower, where they found both Hales and Sudbury together with William Appleton, a physician who was known to be a close councillor of the young king. All three were taken out onto Tower Hill and, before Tyler and Ball, were beheaded. Like a common criminal, the archbishop of Canterbury's head was placed on a stake over the gate to London Bridge.

The Kentish rebels drank to their success through the night, bringing anarchy to the capital: smoke plumes rose from burning buildings, and terrified Londoners hid from the rampaging mob. The unexpected success of the insurgents was a problem for both parties: the king and his advisers were at a loss as to how to stop the revolt, whilst Tyler and Ball – with London at their mercy and the head of Sudbury on a stick – had no greater target left than the crown itself, an objective too far even for this lunatic pair. The instruments of government, however, were fair game. So, early on the Saturday, Tyler and Ball led the Kentish men to Westminster; however, on their arrival, their intoxicated followers were distracted by reports that the hated governor of the Marshalsea prison was hiding in the abbey. Breaking into the sanctuary, they found the poor man clinging to a pillar by St Edward's shrine and, after wrenching him clear, dragged him outside – in full view of the king – and thence to Cheapside, where he was beheaded in front of a jeering crowd.

Now was Richard's chance. He summoned the rebel leaders to Smithfield, not far from Cheapside but outside the city walls, where he promised them a conference. With Tyler at their head, the rebels arrayed themselves on the west side of Smithfield. The king and his entourage rode between them and St Bartholomew's gate. The gables of Manny's charterhouse provided the backdrop to the north; no doubt the monks – coaxed out of seclusion by this great event – had come out to watch. Wat Tyler repeated the demands made the previous day by Essex rebels at Mile End, adding – at John Ball's behest – that the church should be stripped of its property. For some time Richard and Tyler talked together, the king calmly ignoring the brigand's surly replies. But Tyler was drunk, and after a while he called for some more ale, which prompted a hot-headed valet on the king's side to shout at him derisory abuse. Insults flew between the two men, at which the mayor of London, William Walworth, who was standing by, finally lost his temper, and ordered Tyler to show the king's presence more respect. The rebel leader shot back an obstinate response, so Walworth attempted to arrest him; Tyler drew his dagger, but Walworth got to him first, and ran him through.

As Tyler lay dying on the ground, his followers shifted and shuffled on their feet, their makeshift weapons held more tightly in their gripped palms. Sensing the moment, the young king – with extraordinary bravery – rode forward, and addressed the rebels himself: 'Be still – I am your king, your leader and your chief, and those of you who are loyal to me should go immediately into the field.'[69] With the king's life in their hands, the Kentish men followed him from Smithfield northwards, past Manny's charterhouse, over the mass grave of those Londoners struck down in the Great Death and towards the fields of Clerkenwell. A force soon came from London to rescue the king, who had distracted the remaining rebel leaders in conversation. Yet, although he was now in a position to do so, Richard refrained from a massacre, and allowed the aggrieved labourers and peasants to make their way peacefully home. So the crowd broke up and the rebels went back to the villages and fields they had sought to seize for themselves. In that attempt the rebels had failed, but their lords had been given a sharp lesson in the fragility of their power, and they did not dare levy the poll tax again.

Epilogue

The Great Rebellion, or Peasants' Revolt as it would later be known, did not end with the dispersal of the crowds from Smithfield: the men of Norfolk converged on Norwich which, fraught with the tensions built up over previous decades, exploded into violence, while the northern towns were once again thrown into upheaval. It did not take long, however, for each of these revolts to be suppressed and despite the continuing rumbling of protest, the authorities – both by force and by tact – prevented a repetition of those extraordinary events.

The Peasants' Revolt was not some final and dramatic result of that now distant catastrophe the Black Death. For the uprising was as much the result of immediate difficulties – a deeply unpopular and regressive tax, political crisis, foreign failure, the cumulative effect of a series of remarkably variable harvests and the economic volatility that followed – as it was the consequence of that first, unprecedented, mortality. Indeed, as time wore on, the unambiguous influence of plague is increasingly difficult to discern. By the 1390s there were very few left who could remember the first pestilence. Plague had become endemic, a feared but nonetheless accepted part of life.

Yet the Great Death had had a dramatic impact, if only because of its terrible suddenness and unparalleled extent. It is a natural affliction of historians to link specific momentous events with social change, if only because the alternative – to deny the wider importance of the great moments of history – seems so unsatisfactory, even incredible. The connection need not exist, however, even if it comforts the historian to think that it does. The study of the Black Death has been distorted perhaps more than that of any other great calamity from this conceit. It is important therefore, to ask first what might have changed had the Great Death *not* taken place.

Some effects are undeniable: for instance, the temporary but substantial change in the status and fortunes of some women would not otherwise have occurred. Similarly, it is possible that the tentative strengthening of the relationship between Highland and Lowland Scotland would have continued, had not massive depopulation reduced so significantly exchange between the two. Indeed, Scotland as a whole would surely have enjoyed greater prosperity had it not been dealt so great a blow by plague. More speculative must be the assertion that the Welsh insurrection of the late 1390s would not have occurred had not the English colonial project been so damaged, both in the towns and in the March, by the plague; it is, nonetheless, a perfectly reasonable speculation to make. More certain is the effect the disease had on medical study and the actions of city councils to control public hygiene. Indeed, it is not outlandish to argue that the mechanisms by which plague was eventually defeated – isolation and quarantine – had their beginnings in the first panicked responses of those terrified men and women of the middle of the fourteenth century.

Conversely, there is much that would not have changed, plague or no plague. It is difficult to find evidence, for instance, to support the old argument that the course of architectural history would have been significantly different had there been no pestilence, or that the flowering of English literature at the end of the fourteenth century would have been delayed. Perhaps there would have been more numerous, and more exceptional, examples of English art – whether in glass, wall painting, or brass – but the difference can only have been marginal, especially given the incomparable quality of what was produced during the fifteenth century. Similarly, it is hard to see how the pestilence did much to alter the intellectual isolation of England in the late fourteenth century, which had already set in by the time the first plague came. Nor would it have altered the outcomes of Edward III's disastrous engagement with France. In all these instances, pestilence had negligible long-term effects.

For the greater part, however, the Great Death confirmed, accelerated, and accentuated those changes and trends that had other origins elsewhere. The ruination of the Anglo-Irish colony, for instance, would without the plague have continued, albeit at a less precipitous rate. Medieval government would surely have taken on greater competencies and become more complex, if over a longer period of time. Late fourteenth-century concern at clerical abuse may have been given piquancy by the effects of the mortality, but it would no doubt have existed nonetheless. Indeed, it is arguable that the Schism of 1378 had a far greater effect on the English church than did the Great Death. The idea that somehow there was a causative connection between plague and the Reformation is, therefore, absurd; Wyclif and his phenomenon were *suigeneris*. Most importantly, we can discount conclusively that traditional argument that the feudal economy was undone by the Black Death. For it is certain that the disintegration of the feudal economy was well underway before the first pestilence. The basic economic flaws in the feudal model guaranteed that its dissolution would continue, whether the Great Death had happened or not. However, it is indisputable that the precipitate rebalancing of the rural economy altered the pace of the reordering of feudal landholding, even if a hastening of commutation and leasing was often offset by a hardening in the reaction of landowners. Certainly, the mere compression of so much change into so few generations had social repurcussions, if only because men and women saw privileges won earlier in their lifetimes later withdrawn.

So while the Black Death affected the pace of change in many aspects of medieval life and forced into a tight compass the inevitable decay of feudalism, it was not the spring of action. It is an unsurprising conclusion. For disease and death create nothing, except grief. The greatest power of pestilence and mass mortality is not their own, but the reaction they provoke in the hearts of those who remain behind – the will to survive, the instinct for increase, and – for many – the desire to seek something better. A true account of this time is, therefore, not just one of disaster but also of triumph, for the final conclusion must be that even this greatest of all pandemics, this most calamitous of crises, this Great Death, did not alter in any fundamental way the manner in which people lived their lives, nor crush the spirit of those who survived.

*   *   *

Take Notice:
O lamentable Death, thou dost plunge multitudes into the lowest pit!
Now these, now those, now everywhere thou ravagest, O Death!
Death withers children and to wretched old men it brings an end.
Neither those who wear horns nor those who wear veils are saved by their lot.

Therefore:
Harden thyself to the world and seek pardon with a pure mind
Pray, reflect, for death makes no delay, and worship!

From a fifteenth-century wall painting in Acle Church, Norfolk.[1]

Appendix 1

The Epidemiology of the Black Death: An Overview

In their separate discoveries of the plague bacillus in 1894, Shibasaburo Kitasako and Alexandre Yersin claimed to have identified the agent that had caused the great plague pandemics of history, whose nature still remained unknown. The symptoms of bubonic plague – fever followed by the appearance of black buboes in the groin, armpits and neck – were all too similar to the oft-reported symptoms of the ancient plague, which had scoured Europe in Justinian's time, again during the mid-fourteenth-century, and then periodically until it vanished in the early eighteenth century. Four years after Kitasako and Yersin's discovery, Paul-Louis Simond identified the extraordinary route by which the plague bacillus entered the human bloodstream in the predominant form of the disease – bubonic plague. He observed that while the rat population provided the reservoir for the disease, something that had been known for centuries across southern and eastern Asia, it was the rat-borne flea that actually transmitted the bacillus to human beings.

These were sensational discoveries and it is no wonder that European historians quickly believed the first assertions of scientists that they had discovered the plague of centuries past to be definitive. By the time Cardinal Gasquet published the second edition of his classic popular history of the Black Death, in 1908, he too was able to suggest the link between bubonic plague – which was by this time causing horrific mortality in India – and the fourteenth-century pandemic. Since then Gasquet's suggestion has become the hard fact of most Black Death histories. For a century schoolchildren have learnt that men and women in the middle ages were killed by the terrible combination of the plague bacillus (Yersinia pestis), the black rat (*Rattus rattus*) and the rodent flea (*Xenopsylla cheopis*), or by associated infections – pneumonic and septicaemic plague. However, the last two decades of the twentieth century have seen this dogma challenged.

Ironically, it was a promoter of the rat-flex nexus that first made plain how spurious was the notion that the Great Death was bubonic plague. For in his enormous history of the epidemic in the British Isles, published in 1970, J. W. D Shrewsbury claimed – rightly – that the mortality must have been far lower than the medieval chroniclers had claimed, had the infection been bubonic plague, perhaps as little as 10–15 per cent of the population. Yet none of the evidence supports this conclusion, so the reverse must have been true: that the mortality was somewhere between 30–50 per cent but could not have been caused by bubonic plague. The first positive blow against the rat-flea dogma was made in 1984 by the zoologist Graham Twigg, who made the crucial observation that the black rat was hardly established in the British Isles in the mid-fourteenth century, a point confirmed by Gunnar Karlsson in 1996 when he demonstrated that the rat was entirely absent from Iceland, which nonetheless suffered from the Great Death.

The zoologists would only lay the foundations for a far wider attack on the rat-flea dogma. In 2001, Susan Scott and Christopher Duncan exposed the manifest inconsistency between the epidemiology and biology of bubonic plague and what we know of the fourteenth-century epidemic, whilst two years later James Wood, Rebecca Ferrel, and Sharon DeWitte-Aviña demonstrated, using ecclesiastical records, the speed with which the Great Death moved. By now it was clear that by its pattern of spread alone the Black Death could not have been the bubonic plague discovered at the end of the nineteenth century. The extraordinary work of George Christakos et al. (2005 and subsequently) in modelling both epidemics shows beyond doubt that the two could not possibly be the same. Meanwhile, Samuel Cohn has, by careful textual analysis, demolished the casual and inaccurate association made by historians and scientists alike of the symptoms of modern plague and those symptoms described by medieval chroniclers; moreover, Cohn has credited contemporaries with rather more insight than more prejudiced commentators have yet been given to allow.

None of this is to say that the controversy is now settled. Michel Drancourt has used samples of bodies retrieved from plague pits in Montpellier (2004 and subsequently) to suggest that DNA discovered in victims' teeth is that of bubonic plague. His analysis, however, is fraught with technical difficulties and has since been challenged; moreover, it is impossible to prove that the bodies from this singular example were not from much later, seventeenth-century, plagues, which may well have been caused by *Yersinia pestis*. In truth, there has not been a convincing rebuttal to the central arguments made by Twigg, Christakos, Scott, Cohn and others. Rats were neither present in sufficient quantities, nor capable of covering such remarkable distances, to have been vectors for the disease; nor was there any plague of rats reported at the time – which is all the more telling considering how observant of natural phenomena medieval people were. Besides, temperatures were too cold for plague to prosper in northern Europe: the slowing of the epidemic during the winter is attributable not to the disease itself (whatever it was) but to the hibernation of medieval markets and slackened pace of village life. In the spring and summer, when the Great Death was at its most virulent, it was covering up to five kilometres per day, while bubonic plague in India could travel as slowly as fifteen metres per week – and that with all the railways and trade which India enjoyed. Finally, bubonic plague has never achieved a mortality rate comparable to the Black Death, even though it was present among communities in Victorian India whose poverty and living conditions were at least as bad, if not worse, as those endured by town-dwellers in fourteenth-century England. In short, rats could not have been the carrier of the disease, the plague bacillus – in all its forms – could not have prospered in the temperate north and was never sufficiently virulent to have caused so rapid and terrible a mortality.

The demolition of the case for bubonic plague re-opens the question of what pathogen carried the Black Death. It is important that speculative diagnoses are made with extreme care and with strong caveats attached, for if one thing is certain in all of this, it is that historians are often poor interpreters of science and scientists indelicate handlers of historical records. Some have suggested a form of anthrax, others a haemorrhagic fever: all of these explanations have their difficulties, however. What is clear is that this disease had an incubation period of about a month, showed its symptoms for only two to four days, and almost in every instance resulted in death. Contemporaries thought it infectious and contagious (which bubonic plague is not) recommended avoiding diseased people and, if possible, flight.

It may well be that their understanding was very much better than our own, because at some point in the centuries that followed, medieval plague eventually became extinct. Whether this was the result of cumulative immunity, community action, or both, it is impossible to tell; what is also uncertain is whether such a disease might reappear, and whether in that case we would all be as helpless as those who faced that previously unknown pandemic, which came upon them with only a few days' notice and was gone within a matter of months. A little more humility in the face of that threat might serve us well.

Appendix 2

The Spread of the Black Death in the British Isles: Mapping the Epidemic

It was Elisabeth Carpentier who made the first serious attempt to map the spread of the Black Death, with the map included in her seminal article 'Autour de la peste noire', of 1962.[1] This showed the progression of the pandemic across the Near East, the Maghreb and Europe, as it advanced year by year, with a line indicating the extent of the pandemic at the close of each of the years when the Black Death was present. Ole Benedictow gives a refined version of this map in his book *The Black Death 1346–1353*, published in 2004.

The considerable gaps in recorded information concerning the spread of the disease through much of Europe, and the concentration of data in very specific places, have meant that these attempts to map the progress of the epidemic have had to be made with broad brushes. However, the advent of powerful computer mapping software has given epidemiologists a new tool, one realized to brilliant effect by George Christakos and his colleagues. Using stochastic prediction methods, where the complex calculation of numerous probabilities allows unrelated and irregular data to be given form, Christakos has been able to build a comprehensive map of the spread of the Black Death through continental Europe and the British Isles. The maps presented overleaf are based on Prof. Christakos's work, after some refinements made in conjunction with this author. Furthermore, the maps relating to the British Isles show the major roads and waterways used in the mid-fourteenth century in the British Isles, based in part on the evidence of the Gough Map of *c.*1360. It should be stressed that these maps are based on models and, as such, are not definitive or certain. However, they are without doubt the most accurate representation of the spread of the epidemic made to date.

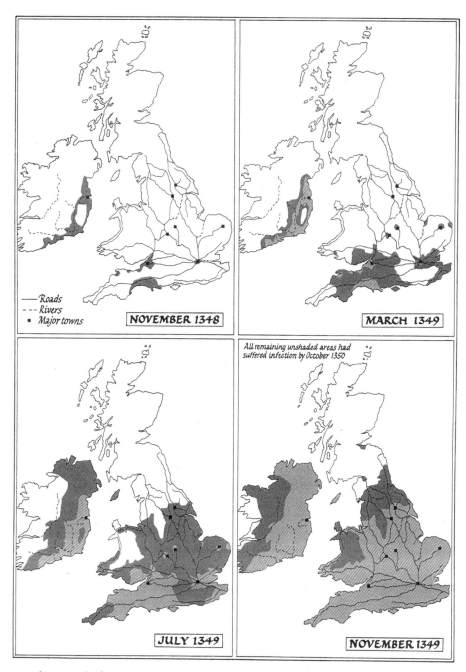

The spread of the Black Death through the British Isles, shown in four month intervals. Heavily shaded areas indicate where infection was present; lightly shaded areas show those regions where the epidemic has passed; unshaded areas had yet to be infected. By October 1350 the disease had penetrated every corner of the British Isles.

Notes

I have relied upon a simple rule in annotating this book. A note is provided when additional detail is of tangential interest; an assertion is made that requires justification; a direct quotation is made, in which instance a full reference is given; and a measurement requires a metric conversion (which is necessarily approximate). All the authorities that have directly informed the text are listed in the Select Bibliography on p. 463. Except where stated otherwise, all biblical references are from the 1611 Authorized Version.

1. *Missale ad usum insignis et præclaræ ecclesiæ Sarum* (ed. F. Dickinson), col. 886*; my translation.

1. Galling the Gleaned Land

1. 'Sir Gawain and the Green Knight', in *The Poems of the Pearl Manuscript* (eds. Andrew and Waldron), Fit II, l. 504, p. 226; my translation.
2. Langland, *Piers Plowman*, Passus VIII, ll. 116–17, p. 151; my translation.
3. Bartsocas, 'Two fourteenth-century Greek descriptions', pp. 395–6.
4. Ex. 7:8–13:16; Ex. 8:1; 1 Sam. 5:1–6:1.
5. 2 Sam. 24:15–19; see also 1 Chron. 21:14–19.
6. Rev. 15–16.
7. Rev. 6:8.

2. The Fruits of Peace

1. Thomas Hardy, 'The Convergence of the Twain', vs. V–VII.
2. *Poems of Laurence Minot* (eds. James and Simons), Poem IX, ll. 8–10.
3. Jean Froissart fancifully states that the Queen went with the English to

the battlefield. Most historians have rejected this, but given the chronicler's proximity to the Queen, it is likely that this is simply an exaggeration of what actually did happen. The Queen was probably in York,
overseeing the repair of the walls – a detail from Froissart that suggests
a good source-line. No doubt she also sent messages of support to
Zouche and the other English leaders, which Froissart later embellished
into a great pre-battle speech. It would have been entirely appropriate
for the Queen to accompany the Scottish king south to London.

4. He arrived sometime in January 1347.

5. *Chron. Johannis de Reading* (ed. Tait), p. 89. Trans. Horrox, *Black Death*.
    p. 131.

6. *Knighton's Chronicle* (trans. and ed. Martin), pp. 92–4.

7. *Chron. Johannis de Reading* (ed. Tait), p. 89. Trans. Horrox, *Black Death*,
    p. 131.

8. Fra Michele da Piazza, *Cronaca*; trans. Horrox, *Black Death*, p. 36.

9. I have chosen to take Louis Heyligen's (see below) reference to storms
    as the explanation for the delay in the Genoese galleys being expelled
    from Messina in October and arriving in Genoa in December.

10. Heyligen states that the infected boats arrived on 31st December. I have
    employed a loose antedating of some of the dates stated by the chron-
    iclers, to take account of an incubation period of which they were not
    aware. See Appendix 1.

11. Gabriele de' Mussi, *Historia de Morbo*; trans. Horrox, *The Black Death*,
    p. 19.

12. Schevill, *History of Florence*, pp. 239–40.

13. de' Mussi, *Historia de Morbo*; trans. Horrox, *The Black Death*, pp. 24–5.

14. Boccaccio, *Decameron*, pp. 11–12.

15. Petrarch, *Canzoniere*, 'Morte à spento quel sol ch'abagliar suolmi' (no.
    363), p. 303.

16. Louis Heyligen of Beeringen; trans. Horrox, *Black Death*, p. 45.

17. 'Regiment de Preservacio' (trans. Duran-Reynolds and Winslow), p. 65.

18. By the early fourteenth century feudal services were being commuted
    all over the country: at Rockbourne in Hampshire twenty-three out of
    forty-eight villeins had had all their labour services commuted to a cash
    rent by 1300; at Teddington in Middlesex *opera* were first sold in 1313;
    and in Porlock in Somerset free and commuted rents increased by nearly
    70 per cent between 1319 and 1345, while the corresponding value of
    services still claimed from villein tenants fell from 60s. 6d. to 10s. in the
    same period.

19. In Porlock the area of demesne land fell from 287 acres in 1319 to 146
    acres in 1345, while in Shropshire, where grain prices were particularly
    low owing to the distance to major markets, demesnes on the estates

of the earl of Arundel and of Wenlock Priory were all leased out by the early 1300s. In Corsham, in Wiltshire, the entire demesne had been let to the villein tenants as early as the mid-thirteenth century.

20. At Redgrave, a couple of miles east of Hinderclay, there were normally about 65 transfers of land a year between living tenants. In 1316 this almost tripled to 188; in 1317 it was more than double the average at 135.

21. In the manor of Harthill, on the edge of the Peak District in Derbyshire, the lack of any significant markets saw villeins abandon the more marginal land, so that by 1337 only two thirds of the manor was being tilled, the rest lying 'uncultivated for lack of tenants'. The problems experienced by the Augustinian abbey of Lilleshall in Shropshire were attributed directly to cattle disease, which forced the area of demesne to be reduced for lack of oxen to pull ploughs. These very specific problems should not be allowed to overshadow the success of most manors, which returned healthy profits throughout these years. For instance, the many pleas of poverty in the inquisitions on the levying of the ninth should be put against the increase in income from rents that was also evident in many parts of the country.

22. Such as in Langenhoe at Essex.

23. Thompson, 'Registers of John Gynewell', p. 309.

3. Pestilence Arrives

1. Langland, *Piers Plowman*, Passus XXII, l. 100, p. 366.

2. Chaucer, *The Canterbury Tales*, 'General Prologue', l. 400, in *Riverside Chaucer* (ed. Benson), p. 30.

3. ibid., l. 389, p. 29.

4. *Historical Papers and Letters* (ed. Raine), p. 396. Trans. Horrox, *Black Death*, p. 111.

5. The *Anonimalle Chronicle* claims the pestilence arrived at Bristol around 1st August 1348; the chronicler – who was probably writing in the north of England – does not mention Melcombe Regis. Ralph Higden, in his *Polychronicon*, claims that the pestilence arrived in the Bristol area on 24th June 1348; Higden was writing in Chester and, again, this seems to be a generalization of events. The chronicler of the *Eulogium* was far nearer, however, as he was writing in Malmesbury Abbey, just over twenty miles to the east of Bristol. This anonymous monk was very clear that the disease arrived at Melcombe, that it did so around 7th July 1348, and then came to Bristol. Robert of Avesbury, who like these other chroniclers was a contemporary, records that the pestilence first

broke out in Dorset around 1st August. Geoffrey le Baker, writing in mid-Oxfordshire around the time of the pestilence, states with certainty that the disease began in Bristol on 15th August 1348.

6. *Register of Ralph of Shrewsbury* (ed. Holmes), p. 555. Trans. Horrox, *Black Death*, p. 112–13.

7. I follow in this the new dating given by Prof. Ormrod in 'The royal nursery: a household for the younger children of Edward III', *English Historical Review*, no. 120, 2005, p. 413, n. 83.

8. II Corinthians 2:14.

9. Wilkins (ed.), *Concilia Magnae*, Vol. II, p. 738. Trans. Horrox, *Black Death*. pp. 113–14.

10. *Fœdera, Conventiones, Literae* (ed. Rymer), Vol. V, 1708, p. 642. Trans. Horrox, *Black Death*, p. 250.

11. In addition there was a presentation to the nearby rectory of Bincombe by the king on 8th October 1348, though no induction was made until 4th November.

12. The twenty-day figure is an average figure arrived at through a careful study of episcopal registers: Wood, Ferrel and DeWitte-Aviña, 'Temporal dynamics'.

13. The abnormal mortality at Cadland manor across the Solent reported in January and June 1348 cannot be attributed to the plague.

14. Hampshire Record Office, *Reg. Edyngdon*, 21M65 A1/9 fo.17; trans. Horrox, *Black Death*, p. 116.

15. *Knighton's Chronicle* (ed. Martin), pp. 98–9. The precise extent of the mortality is unclear from this passage.

16. *Eulogium* (ed. Haydon), p. 213. Trans. Horrox, *Black Death*. p. 62.

17. HRO, *Reg. Edyngdon*; trans. Horrox, *Black Death*, p. 116.

18. The following account, and later references to Thornbury, is taken from Franklin, 'Thornbury manor'.

19. Sheppardine, Westend and Cowhill nearest the river, Oldbury, Kington, Woolford and Sibland scattered around Thornbury borough, and Morton, Buckover, Whitfield and Falfield on either side of the Bristol–Gloucester road.

20. The early infection of Thornbury, and the fact that the hamlets on the estuary were hit first, strongly suggests that it was infected by water, not along the roads out of Bristol.

21. The pestilence had passed through by the court of 3rd May 1349, by which time about two thirds of the tenantry had died. We may assume, given the emergence of the disease nearby, that the epidemic was well underway in Mells by the late autumn of 1348.

22. John Smith was already in old age by 1348 and so his death that year is not altogether surprising. However, one of his sons – Thomas – also

died that year. It is possible that both were early victims of the pestilence, just entering the West Wiltshire Downs.

23. *Register of Ralph of Shrewsbury* (ed. Holmes), Vol. X, p. 555. Trans. Horrox, *Black Death*, p. 113.

24. Jonah 3:10.

4. *Colonial Ireland*

1. Surviving fragment of a carol from the first half of the fourteenth century, from *Medieval English Lyrics* (ed. Davies), p. 99.

2. Friar John Clyn states that the plague was present in Dublin in the beginning of August. Given the numbers flocking to St Mullins, we must assume that the disease was evident in New Ross and/or Waterford by September.

3. *Annals of Ireland* (ed. Butler), p. 36. Trans. Horrox, *Black Death*. p. 84.

4. ibid., p. 35. Trans. Horrox, *Black Death*. p. 82.

5. In the period 1301–3 Dublin imported an average of approximately 1,260 tuns of wine per annum; in the period 1346–66 the city imported an average of approximately 180 tuns per annum.

6. Clyn states that the plague was present in Dublin in the beginning of August. At the latest, therefore, the disease must have come to Dalkey in July.

7. This is my supposition: Clyn states that the disease entered Howth, Dalkey and Drogheda at the same time. Dalkey was often the first stop on the way to Drogheda. It was also south of Howth and landing there was marginally easier. Dalkey would, therefore, seem the most obvious point at which ships from Bordeaux would dock first if plying the eastern Irish seaboard, especially if they had sick hands who needed to be taken on land.

8. Knowles, *Religious Orders, Vol. II: The End of the Middle Ages* (1957), p. 116.

9. *Annals of Ireland* (ed. Butler), p. 36. Trans. Horrox, *Black Death*. p. 84.

10. The Nenagh chronicler states that the pestilence first broke out in Drogheda, then spreading to Dublin and the surrounding area.

11. *Annals of Ireland* (ed. Butler), pp. 36–7. Trans. Horrox, *Black Death*. pp. 82–4.

12. *Annals of Ireland* (ed. Butler), p. 38; my translation.

13. Average per annum crown revenue 1278–99 – £6,300; 1368–84 – £2,512.

14. *Strassburg Urkundenbuch*; trans. Horrox, *Black Death*. p. 220.

15. In addition, the popular response to the pope's mandate was conditioned by a widespread and longstanding distrust of the papacy's motives in protecting the Jews. There was a suspicion that the papacy benefited

from its proximity to Jewish moneylenders, especially during the Avignon exile, which in itself was deeply unpopular. For a later English voice on this, see Langland, *Piers Plowman*, Passus XXI, ll. 422, p. 358.

16. Simonsohm (ed.), *Apostolic See and the Jews*, no. 373, p. 397. Trans. Horrox, *Black Death*. p. 221.

17. According to Clyn, twenty-five and twenty-three brothers respectively. I do not expect that these houses were substantially larger than the one destroyed at Dundalk by the Scots, in which case this level of mortality will have comprised the larger part of the previous complement of friars.

18. According to jurors at a 1351 inquisition (Kelly, *Black Death in Ireland*, p. 128).

19. i.e. the continuator of Ralph Higden's *Polychronicon*.

20. Dominican houses were almost always smaller than the Franciscan equivalents. For a town like Kilkenny, eight Dominican friars seems a likely number for a full friary.

21. *Annals of Ireland* (ed. Butler), p. 37. Trans. Horrox, *Black Death*, p. 84.

22. Lucien Febvre on the Roman frontier: 'elle se double d'une frontière morale'.

23. *Annals of Ireland* (ed. Butler), p. 38; my translation.

24. Ibid., p. 37; my translation.

5. *London Succumbs*

1. William FitzStephen's 'Description of London', in the translation by Stow, *Survey of London* (1603), p. 473. FitzStephen, the biographer of Thomas Becket, wrote this description c.1173. The work was nevertheless well-known in the fourteenth century, as can be seen from the rough-and-ready transcription made in a Londoner's common-place book c.1360–88. The emendations made to the text in this version suggest that contemporaries felt that much of the description was still accurate.

2. Ackroyd, *London*, pp. 59 and 338.

3. *London Assize of Nuisance* (eds. Chew and Kellaway), p. 102.

4. Boccaccio, *Decameron*, p. 6.

5. Wilkins (ed.), *Concilia*, Vol. II, p. 738. Trans. Horrox, *Black Death*, p. 114.

6. *Chronicon Galfridi le Baker* (ed. Thompson), p. 100. Trans. Horrox, *Black Death*, p. 81.

7. Hampshire Record Office, *Reg. Edyngdon*, 21M65 A1/9 fo.17; trans. Horrox, *Black Death*, p. 116.

8. 'Fama, malum qua non aliud velocius ullum: / mobilitate viget virisque adquirit eundo' (*Aeneid*, Bk IV, ll. 174–5).

9. Mandates for prayers, sermons, masses and processions were included

in the prior of Christchurch's letter, sent to the bishop of London for distribution on 28th September 1348, for which see above on page 54 and 101.

10. Parets, *Journal of the Plague Year*, p. 44.

11. *Chron. Johannis de Reading* (ed. Tait), pp. 108. Trans. Horrox, *Black Death*, p. 74.

12. Among the merchants and officials of the city the toll was equally severe. Thomas Marins, the chamberlain of the Grocers' Company, died on 25th April and was replaced by Thomas Walden, who was also the (evidently unsuccessful) apothecary of Westminster Abbey throughout the crisis. The Company of Goldsmiths lost four wardens. Both the Company of Hatters and the Company of Cutlers had to replace all of their wardens in the plague year. Likewise, William Raven, who was elected and sworn in as weigher at the Small Balance on 1st July 1349, was dead within a week and a new weigher had to be elected in his place. Six of the eight men enrolled as supervisors of shearmen had been struck out of the records by the year's end as they were either dead or had fled. Richard de Basynstock, an alderman and sheriff in 1348, died in 1349, whilst the deputy coroner – John de Foxton – is not mentioned in official records after August 1348. (This post, like that of sheriff, was officially a crown nomination – although in London the city, sometimes successfully, claimed the right to appoint its own sheriffs.) Indeed, it is not quite clear which aldermen acted as sheriff for the period 1348–9 and we must assume that the appointments changed hands at least once during the year.

13. 'Anno Domini 1349, regnante magna pestilentia consecratum fuit hoc Cœmiterium, in quo et infra septa presentis monasterii, sepulta fuerunt mortuorum corpora plusquam quinquaginta millia, præter alia multa abhinc usque ad presens, quorum animabus propitietur Deus. Amen.' Stow, *Survay*, p.384.

14. Stow's estimate is close to that given in the papal bull of 1351 establishing Manny's college of the Annunciation, which mentions a figure of 60,000 burials.

15. *Robertus de Avesbury* (ed. Thompson), p. 407. Trans. Horrox, *Black Death*, pp. 64–5.

16. *1348:* October – 2, November – 3; *1349:* January – 18, February – 42, March – 41, May – 120, June – 31, July – 51, October – 18, November – 27, December – 7; *1350:* January – 4, February – 19, March – 6, April – 6, May – 1, June – 3, July – 2, October – 2, November – 3. (*Calendar of Wills Proved and Enrolled in the Court of Husting*, Pt 1).

17. The number of wills enrolled in the key months of March, April and May – roughly reflecting deaths in February, March and April – is almost

exactly equivalent to two a day. If Robert of Avesbury is correct in believing that 200 people were buried in the new cemetery in Smithfield between 2nd February and 12th April, then this would mean that for every death involving a will there were roughly one hundred who were buried at Smithfield, almost all of whom would not have made a will. If a ratio of 100:1 is extrapolated from this and applied to the number of deaths involving wills in 1349 which are additional to the mean average from the three previous years (i.e. 334 additional deaths), a total nominal mortality rate of 33,400 is returned. It should be remembered that the ratio is calculated for the period February to April only and involves only the cemetery at West Smithfield: it will almost certainly underestimate mortality therefore. Moreover, although the calculation is unscientific it still sits neatly within the range decided upon by other historians, who have used similarly unreliable methods of computation: 15,000–30,000 (Shrewsbury), over 40,000 (Camden – at Smithfield only), 50,000 (Stow – at Smithfield only), 20,000–30,000 (Ziegler). If London's population was indeed 80,000–100,000, then the mortality suggested was between a third and a half of the total populace of London. (Ziegler, *Black Death*, p. 164; Shrewsbury, *Bubonic Plague in the British Isles*, pp. 82–4).

18. On 8th April, 1349. *Calendar of the Close Rolls*, Edward III, Vol. IX: 1349–54, pp. 65–6.

19. Barnes, *History of that Most Victorious Monarch Edward III*, p. 436.

20. *Register of William Edington* (ed. Hockey), Pt 1, p. 86.

6. Winter Crawl

1. 'Sir Gawain and the Green Knight', in *The Poems of the Pearl Manuscript* (eds. Andrew and Waldron), Fit II, l. 502, p. 226.

2. *Chronicon Galfridi le Baker* (ed. Thompson), p. 99. Trans. Horrox, *Black Death*, p. 81.

3. There is no surviving evidence for the assertion that Edward was involved in the decision but given the funding required, the probable use of royal masons and the fact that the work was being executed around – and because of – the king's father's tomb, it is unthinkable that Edward was not involved in the decision. The glazing in the great east window would seem to confirm that.

4. I agree here with Christopher Wilson's dating (Wilson, 'Origins of the perpendicular style', p. 135), not least because the abbey's resumption of building in 1351 – despite their financial problems – suggests that they had no choice but to build, a choice that would most obviously be forced by a lack of a roof.

5. *Eulogium* (ed. Haydon), Vol. III, p. 213. Trans. Horrox, *Black Death*. pp. 63–4.

6. Hugh de Rissingdone.

7. Twenty-three out of twenty-six.

8. There is a correlation between the number of priests instituted and the number of wills proved in the city, so this at least shows a similar mortality of priests and the privileged. Ten out of twenty-four of the cathedral canons perished, although many of these may have been absentees.

9. Furthermore, to the north-west at Mells – infected in the late autumn of 1348 – the mortality rate was also around two thirds.

10. Mandate issued from Edington's manor at Esher on 17th November 1348. (Gasquet, *Black Death*, p. 126.)

11. James, 'The Black Death: a turning point for Winchester?', p. 36.

12. Hudson and Tingey, *Records of the City of Norwich*, p. 208.

13. The balance of probabilities lies in favour of infection via London, as Great Yarmouth seems to have been struck some time after Norwich.

14. Gasquet, *Black Death*, p. 118.

15. It was Thorold Rogers (J. Thorold Rogers, *Six Centuries of Work and Wages*, Vol. I, London, 1884. p. 221) who first ascribed the survival of Christchurch to the priory's proprietary water supply, although for a monastery it was hardly unique in enjoying this. Nonetheless, we may suspect that it permitted the priory to institute the kind of precautions that other religious houses were unwilling – or simply too slow – to adopt.

7. *Spring and Death*

1. Gerard Manley Hopkins, 'Spring and Death', in W. Gardner and N. MacKenzie (eds.), *The Poems of Gerard Manley Hopkins*, 4th edn (Oxford: Oxford University Press, 1970), p. 14.

2. This description of the city's timekeeping and market schedule is based on an account made in the late fifteenth century; the routine of the middle of the fourteenth century will not have been that different. Holy Trinity was a priory church but as it was not the conventual church it was staffed by regular clergy. The order of doorkeeper was the lowliest of the minor orders and conferred responsibilities similar to those undertaken by a sacristan or verger: it was they who had the responsibility of opening up the church and ringing the bells.

3. Langland, *Piers Plowman*, Passus IX, l. 40, p. 163. Langland describes them as 'wyckede wayes' and 'brugges tobrokene by the heye wayes', giving

a clear inference of the earthly journey to God, made straight by charitable giving. Truth is here an ambiguous figure, representing the corrupted papal office, that whilst not demonic has nonetheless perverted the truths of the church for its own financial ends. Thus Langland, whilst not denying the benefit of such endowments, is clear that they are tainted by self-interest and are thus not pure acts of charity.

4. Harrison, *Bridges of Medieval England,* p. 198.

5. The exceedingly complex arrangements for the maintenance of London Bridge are a case in point.

6. Russell (*British Medieval Population*, p. 246) gives a figure of 6,000 for the population of Oxford. Salter (*Mediæval Oxford*, p. 109) suggests a pre-plague student population of around 1,500. Both these figures are probably conservative estimates, so it is possibly accurate to accept that the ratio between the two was similar.

7. 'Merton College', *History of the County of Oxfordshire: Vol. 3: The University of Oxford* (1954), p.105. The chancellors were John de Northwode and William de Hawkesworth.

8. *Knighton's Chronicle* (trans. and ed. Martin), pp. 98–9.

9. Russell (*British Medieval Population*, p. 246) estimates the pre-plague population as 4,800, whereas Thompson (in Billson, *Mediæval Leicester*, p. 143) puts it at 6,000. As elsewhere in his estimates of urban population, it is safe to assume that Russell has underestimated and I take, therefore, Thompson's figure. On mortality, Britnell ('Black Death in English towns', p. 199) comes to a lower figure than my rough calculation would suggest, based on a population distribution within Leicester from 200 years later. I think this to be unnecessarily complicated and in any case, the churches of St Nicholas, All Saints and St Mary de Castro will have served not insubstantial parishes in the mid-fourteenth century, given their proximity to the river and the old heart of the town.

10. Anon., 'Lenten is come with love to toune', in *Medieval English Lyrics* (ed. Davies), ll. 1–12, pp. 84–6.

11. John de Rilla.

12. William Carnek.

13. Robo ('Black Death in the hundred of Farnham', pp. 561–2) suggests that there was an early outbreak due to the calculations he makes on defaults of rent. I am inclined to distrust his assumptions but nonetheless it is possible there was an outbreak, given Farnham's position on the main London–Winchester road. I have, therefore, allowed for both possibilities.

14. *Historia Roffensis*; trans. Horrox, *Black Death*. p. 70. Although the author has been named as William Dene, this attribution is uncertain.

15. ibid., p.73.

16. *Duchy of Lancaster court rolls*; trans. Horrox, *Black Death*, p. 276.

17. Rees, 'Black Death in Wales', p. 118.

18. *Chron. Johannis de Reading* (ed. Tait), p. 109. Trans. Horrox, *Black Death*. p. 74.

19. At Cuxham, Robert Oldman, the bailiff, died at the end of March 1349. He was succeeded by his son John, who died in April. Thomas Green was the next bailiff – he died in June. A fourth bailiff died in July and the fifth had died or fled within a year.

20. There have been a number of efforts to estimate a general death rate from the proportions of smaller populations – be they beneficed clerics, tied tenants, nobles or landless labourers. Inevitably, any attempt to draw broader conclusions from these local and particular studies has always been heavily hedged with caveats; such is the variable quality and coverage of record keeping in fourteenth-century England that it will never be possible to come to an empirically satisfactory estimate of mortality. Nonetheless, anecdotal evidence, looking from place to place – monastery, village, family and town – gives a broadly consistent impression of the extraordinary scale of the deaths, which in very many cases exceeds 50 per cent of the population. The villages of this southern central region of England, which are reasonably well-documented, provide a good sample. Indeed, the numbing repetition of high death rates is impressive in its own way. On the other side of Oxford from Iffley at Kidlington, six out of fourteen villein yardlanders perished (43 per cent), but at Islip two miles away eleven out of seventeen villein tenants died (65 per cent), whilst at Woodeaton just a mile and a half to the south again, only two tenants remained in the village. A little to the west, at Crawley, a third of the tenants died but in the hamlet of Hailey – only a mile away – the proportion was two thirds. Beyond Witney, in Stanton Wyard, over half the villeins died, as did their lord – John Wyard. At neighbouring South Leigh, seven out of the thirteen (54 per cent) tenants died and in the manor of Witney itself the estimate is 66 per cent, including John Hickes, who came into his property on the death of his father during the plague, only to fall victim himself. (Perhaps the plague was introduced on the return of the two men who were paid 1s. 6d. in that year to drive eleven pigs to London.) In northeast Oxfordshire the death toll was much the same. At Steeple Barton all thirty-two villein tenements (yardlands) were lying fallow and uncultivated, as every one of the tenants had died. The land had reverted to the lord – John St John – who was also killed, passing the whole holding to his granddaughter Margaret, which suggests that the generation in between had been struck down too. The small village of Hethe lost twenty-one of its twenty-seven tenants (78 per cent).

21. For some reason the abbot decided not to follow this course of action at Woodeaton, where he came to a new agreement with the two remaining tenants which made it worth their while to stay and keep the community going.

22. When Abbot Upton was restored in 1344, the bishop of Lincoln – who was the patron of Eynsham Abbey – placed two other monks in charge of the spiritual and temporal affairs of the abbey, acting as trustees. When one died and another fell ill as a result of the pestilence, two monks were sent by the community to John Gynewell, the bishop of Lincoln, to give him the news. On 13th May 1349, the bishop placed these two monks in charge. However, the two brothers themselves died before they returned to Eynsham and so the bishop was forced to rescind the suspension of the abbot, who was allowed to exercise his full powers until the bishop's next visitation. Upton resigned in 1351 with a generous allowance, which suggests that the bishop in the end paid him off in order to get him out of the abbacy.

23. *Historia Roffensis*; trans. Horrox, *Black Death*, p. 72.

24. 'Parishes: Padworth', *History of the County of Berkshire*, Vol. III (1923), p. 413.

25. 'Social and economic history', ibid., Vol. II (1907), p. 184.

26. 'The market town of Bicester', *History of the County of Oxfordshire*, Vol. VI (1959), p. 32.

27. Gasquet, *Black Death*, p. 116.

28. *Knighton's Chronicle* (trans. and ed. Martin), pp. 100–101.

29. 'Social and economic history', *History of the County of Rutland*, Vol. I (1908), p. 218.

30. The mortality at the little Benedictine priory of Henwood in Warwickshire, on the outskirts of modern-day Solihull, was perhaps representative: twelve of the fifteen nuns were dead by August, including the prioress.

31. Walsingham, *Gesta* (ed. Riley), Vol. II, p. 369. Trans. Horrox, *Black Death*, p. 252.

32. Previous ordinances had limited the full number to one hundred, which would mean the death of forty-seven monks would be a mortality rate of roughly half. Toms (*Story of St Albans*, p. 50) claims that the mortality represented over three quarters of the strength of the house. I have suggested a death rate between the two, as both a higher or a lower figure is possible.

33. Walsingham, *Gesta* (ed. Riley), Vol. II, p. 370. Trans. Horrox, *Black Death*, p. 252.

34. The Petition was made on Sunday, 15th November 1349.

35. Bransford died at his manor of Hartlebury on Thursday, 6th August 1349.

36. T. Nash, *Collections from the History of Worcestershire*, Vol. I (London: 1781), p. 227; trans. Horrox, *Black Death*, p. 268.

37. *Chronicon Galfridi le Baker* (ed. Thompson), pp. 99–100. Trans. Horrox, *Black Death*, p. 81.

8. *Cadwallader's Curse, Plantagenet Pride*

1. The first words of Merlin's prophecy to Vortigern, given by the pool at Dinas Emrys. From Geoffrey of Monmouth's 'Prophecies of Merlin', incorporated within his *Historia Regum Britanniae* (*History of the Kings of Britain*), completed in 1136. (Geoffrey of Monmouth, *Kings of Britain* (trans. Thorpe), vii. 3, p. 171.)

2. Cf. Gerald of Wales's journey in the opposite direction, from Basingwerk Abbey to Chester (Gerald of Wales, *Journey through Wales* (trans. Thorpe), Bk II, Ch. 10, pp. 195–8).

3. According to Geoffrey of Monmouth's account; cf. Geoffrey of Monmouth, *Kings of Britain* (trans. Thorpe), v. 8, p. 133.

4. Goldcliff had been complaining of poverty as far back as 1290.

5. 'Holding [them] to the point of maximum diminishment.' R. R. Davies, *Lordship and Society*, p. 193.

6. At Longdon in Worcestershire, divided from Herefordshire by the Malvern Hills, Andrew Eyloff the reeve died on 14th April 1349, the Tuesday after Easter.

7. While it was normally the case that many in the lower orders would never progress to priesthood, many more deacons did make the full journey, not least because a good number had already been assigned a benefice. All the deacons ordained by the bishop the following September, for instance, eventually became priests.

8. Many hundreds from Hereford, at this time a small border town, must have died. The mortality in the countryside around is hard to gauge, although if it was anything like that seen in the manors of the bishop of Worcestershire – where the death rate amongst tenants ranged from 17 to 80 per cent, averaging overall 46 per cent – it did not differ from more central parts of England, either in the number of deaths or in the degree of variation from place to place.

9. The rector of Quatt died on Wednesday, 29th April 1349.

10. In Salop archdeaconry it took longer than in any other place in the diocese of Coventry and Lichfield to appoint a new priest on the death of an incumbent, owing to the poor roads and distance from the centre of diocesan administration at Coventry.

11. Through his wife, Harleigh had owned a quarter part of the manor of Yokelton, in the borderlands of Stafford's marcher lordship. Here rents

from the freemen fell from £8 to £1 10s. 0d. (£1.50) and both mills fell into disuse 'for lack of grinding, . . . because of the pestilence'.

12. It claimed the lives, for instance, of forty-three tenants in the Prince of Wales's manor of Drakelow before 24th June 1349, by which time the pestilence was only just starting to make an impression on Shropshire to the south.

13. A bovate (10–18 acres) here was shared by six tenants, three of whom disappeared during these months.

14. From £240 to £166.

15. It is notable that the receipts from the lordship of Pembroke were un-affected in 1349 (it was valued at £320 in that year, compared with £247 in 1323) – which may indicate that the epidemic did not penetrate this far west into the principality until at least after the harvest. It may well be, therefore, that Geoffrey le Baker was correct when he alleged that the native Welsh did not contract the disease until 1350 – given that it would have been the new year before the disease established itself among the mountain communities.

16. R. R. Davies, *Conquest, Coexistence and Change*, p. 353.

17. Cf. Gerald of Wales's description of poetic soothsayers (Gerald of Wales, *Description of Wales* (ed. Thorpe), Bk I, Ch. 16, pp. 246–51).

18. William of Newburgh in c.1190: 'It is quite clear that everything this man wrote about Arthur and his successors, or indeed about his pre-decessors Vortigern onwards, was made up, partly by himself and partly by others, either from an inordinate love of lying, or for the sake of pleasing the Britons' (William of Newburgh, *Historia Rerum Anglicarum*, quoted in Lewis Thorpe's introduction to Geoffrey of Monmouth, *Kings of Britain* (trans. Thorpe), p. 17).

19. Geoffrey of Monmouth, *Kings of Britain* (trans. Thorpe), xii. 15, p. 281.

20. 'Cadwallader shall summon Conanus and shall make an alliance with Albany [Scotland]. Then the foreigners shall be slaughtered and the rivers will run with blood. The mountains of the Armorica [Brittany] shall erupt and Armorica itself shall be crowned with Brutus' diadem. Kambria [Wales] shall be filled with joy and the Cornish oaks shall flourish. The island shall be called by the name of Brutus and the title given to it by the foreigners shall be done away with.'

21. Geoffrey of Monmouth, *Kings of Britain* (trans. Thorpe), pp. 175, 281–4.

22. *Calendar of the Close Rolls*, Edward III, Vol. IX: 1349–54, p. 1.

23. ibid., p. 66.

24. ibid.

9. Uses and Abuses

1. Francis Bacon, 'Of Adversity', *Essays I–XX*, no. 5, 2nd edn, ed. A. F. Watt (London: University Tutorial Press, 1908), p. 24.

2. Lincoln's common clerk wrote in the Blickling Homilies 'that in 1349 there was that great pestilence in Lincoln which spread all over parts of the world beginning on Palm Sunday [5th April] in the year aforesaid until the Feast of the Nativity of St John the Baptist [24th June] next following, when it ceased, God be praised who reigns for ever and ever, Amen' (Hill, *Mediæval Lincoln*, p. 242).

3. The vigil of the feast of the Ascension. Although a sure diagnosis of plague is impossible, especially as the man was already 'infirm and paralysed' (*Historia Roffensis*; trans. Horrox, *Black Death*, p. 71), the correspondence of his death with that of three of his chief clerks may not be coincidental: Henry Edwinstowe (disappeared after May 1348), Thomas Cottingham (died by April 1350) and John Morton (died by December 1349) – all Chancery clerks of the first grade. There were only twelve senior clerks and it must be supposed that at least one of these men died of plague. Perhaps they also made contact with the chancellor, Ufford, when infected.

4. *Historia Roffensis*; trans. Horrox, *Black Death*, p. 71.

5. Indeed, it may have been present in an early infection at nearby Crowland Abbey: see Ch. 6, p. 114.

6. The Jubilee celebrations were to start at Christmas in 1349 and the Jubilee proper was declared for the year 1350. Avignon could be reached – at a push – within a month; Rome might take two.

7. The order was made on 1st October 1348.

8. A number of other English bishops had secured papal permission for looser rules governing confession and so Lisle, on 26 March, had a copy despatched to Ely for proclamation. A similar indulgence had been sent to Lincoln on Sunday, 1st March 1349, and to York on Monday, 23rd March 1349. It is probable that this was a standard form replicated whenever a request from a diocese arrived at the papal curia. No sooner had this 'indulgence' been sent off than Lisle received reports that the plague had finally arrived in the diocese. Avignon itself had only recently been brought low by the pestilence and offered sad evidence to the bishop of how virulent the disease could be.

9. Aberth, 'Black Death in the diocese of Ely', p. 284.

10. Gonville was rector from 1343 to 1351.

11. Plague killed fourteen of the villein tenants by Easter (12th April) and seventeen more by Whitsun (31st May).

12. At Landbeach, between the two, the plague was present between May and June, just as in Soham; here too it killed at least half the population. It was the same at Oakington, five miles west of Landbeach, where seventeen of the thirty-five tenants on the largest manor in the village died.

13. King's Hall (1337); Clare Hall (1326 and 1346); Pembroke Hall (1347).

14. 'Hospitals: St John the Evangelist, Cambridge', *History of the County of Cambridgeshire*, Vol. II (1948), p. 305.

15. A Franciscan chronicler in Lynn claimed that the pestilence arrived around Easter; the evidence from Hunstanton, just to the north of Lynn on the eastern shore of the Wash, seems to bear this out: eleven tenants had died by 23rd April, within two weeks of Easter.

16. He made two collations to positions in South Elmham on 29th April 1349.

17. He was there on 11th June.

18. By Hugh atte Mille of Honingham.

19. As many as forty monks. At Redgrave, one of the cluster of villages that included Rickinghall, Botesdale and Thelnetham, 169 tenants had died during these months – 54 per cent of the previous number.

20. Swanton was replaced on 10th July by John Heders, so it is likely that he died towards the end of the previous month. He had been ill for some time.

21. Just beyond the stone cloister only recently completed by the second generation of Ramsey masons.

22. Given as Ralph de Swantone.

23. John Gaddesden (see p. 195 and following) treated one of Edward I's sons for smallpox by wrapping the boy in scarlet and laying him in a bed with red bed hangings.

24. R. Hoeniger, *Der schwarze Tod* (Berlin: 1882), App. 3, p. 156; trans. Horrox, *Black Death*, p. 163.

25. Edict of the Fourth Lateran Council of 1215 (as quoted in Dohar, *Black Death and Pastoral Leadership*, p. 3).

26. Chaucer, *The Canterbury Tales*, 'General Prologue', ll. 422–4, in *Riverside Chaucer* (ed. Benson), p. 30.

27. Abingdon, Donnington, Hungerford, Newbury, Reading, Wallingford, Windsor.

28. Indeed, this must suggest that the relatively small numbers in hospitals elsewhere may well hide the scale of their operations, although very few approached the size of St Leonard's.

29. These details are taken from a visitation of 1364, so are not exactly contemporary. However, they refer to the customary activities of the hospital so it is safe to assume that their obligations had not changed from 1349.

30. Boccaccio, *Decameron*, pp. 5–6.

31. Gaddesden was probably born in the 1280s so would have been in his sixties by the time the plague struck. It is as likely, therefore, that old age was the cause of the doctor's death as was plague. Either way, he did not live long enough to offer an opinion on the disease.

32. Luke 4:23.

33. *Registrum Zouche*; trans. Horrox, *Black Death*, p. 269.

34. See Ch. 2, p. 46–7.

35. Melton Mowbray: 30th April 1349.

36. Thompson, 'Registers of John Gynewell', p. 313.

37. During June there were only two days when Gynewell did not make an appointment: 18th and 26th June.

38. Thompson ('Registers of John Gynewell') posits that the rate across the diocese was 40.17 per cent, although this discounts multiple institutions to the same benefice as well as resignations, which accounted for 201 of the 1,025 vacancies in this year. Given the rate of mortality elsewhere, there is good reason to suppose that many of the resignations were as a result of the plague, as some rectors would presumably resign from their cure once they knew they had the disease, knowing that their condition was terminal. None of this makes any difference to the assertion that the turnover was over 50 per cent, however, as whether by resignation or death the number of vacancies less the number of repeated institutions (i.e. 1,025 − 74 = 951) is more than half the total number of benefices to which the bishop had power to appoint (i.e. 1,857).

39. Sempringham was the mother house of the Gilbertines, England's only indigenous religious order. There were several other foundations in Lincolnshire, some of which were exceedingly poor. The Gilbertines were characterized by their distinctive 'double' monasteries, in which there were both monks and nuns, living separately but praying together – divided by a partition – in the same church. The format of the 'double' monastery was by no means new, however: it had been popular in the early days of Christianity in England, most famously at St Hild's abbey of Whitby, and was to be repeated by the Brigittines at Syon.

40. Thompson, 'Registers of John Gynewell', p. 318.

41. Thomas Sibthorpe – a royal clerk who had made sufficient money to be able to pay for a chantry in the church at Newark, not far away.

42. It should be noted that Gynewell was a famous pluralist and that this abuse did not necessarily predicate, therefore, a lack of pastoral consideration in the offender.

43. Presumably because he had acted as guarantor for the Master, Loth' Nicholyn. It might well be that the trouble had something to do with the coining of the gold noble, which began in 1343–4.

44. The death of the Keeper of the King's Exchange, John Horton, around May 1349, may well be connected to this failure of supervision: the King's Exchange was also housed in the Tower.

45. The Exchequer's quick action in 1349 did not stop the abuse of the Mint, however. In 1350 Nicholyn's successor as Master of the Mint, Philip Neyre, was incarcerated in the Fleet prison for theft of money and money-producing instruments; he subsequently escaped and the authorities frantically attempted to seize as much of his property in London as they could in an effort to recoup their loss.

46. 'How Death Comes', by an anonymous poet, in *Medieval English Lyrics* (ed. Davies), ll. 15–20, p. 75.

47. More precisely, the Office of the Dead followed the pre-Benedictine rite of the Lucernarium, in which Vespers formed the final service of the day. The addition of Compline into the Divine Office was not reflected in the Office of the Dead, even though that office in its final form post-dates the advent of Compline.

48. Psalm 130 in the Anglican usage.

49. Ps. 130:1–8 (*NIV*).

50. It should be noted that the Seven Trumpet sequence of the Book of Revelation (Rev. 8:2–11:19) is a free adaptation of the Ten Plagues visited on Egypt (Ex. 7–10).

51. Chaucer, *The Legend of Good Women*, ll. 36–9, in *Riverside Chaucer* (ed. Benson), p. 589.

52. Including the *Anonimalle Chronicle*, *Eulogium*, Thomas Walsingham's *Historia Anglicana*, the *Historia Roffensis*, John of Reading's *Chronica*, and John Clyn's *Annals*.

53. Boccaccio, *Decameron*, p. 10.

54. See Ch. 5, p. 103.

55. Burton, *Chronica Monasterii de Melsa* (ed. Bond), Vol. III, p. 72. Trans. Horrox, *Black Death*, p. 69.

56. Cf. Ralph Shrewsbury's injunction, Ch. 6, p. 120–1.

57. There are many instances in the clerical registers where clerical appointments lagged some way behind the arrival of the disease in the parish. Not every one of these delays can be explained away as a result of diocesan inefficiency; the efforts made by so many in the episcopate attest to the fact that haste was more common than delay.

58. Only Clyn makes direct reference to people avoiding funerals. On the Continent, the connection was made: Louis Heyligen, in his letter from Avignon, states that mixing with people should be avoided (see Ch. 2, p. 33).

59. *Historia Roffensis*; trans. Horrox, *Black Death*, p. 70.

60. That 'no one who can reap or work to the value of 1d. per day shall give lodging to any stranger or suspect, to harvest the lord's grain in the fields' ('Social and economic history', *History of the County of Hertfordshire*, Vol. IV (1914), p. 190). There is also evidence of villagers attempting to control wages within set limits locally – a clear indication of the importance of reasonably priced labour to villagers themselves (i.e. Poos, 'Social context', p. 36).

61. See Ch. 5, pp. 103–4.

62. It is worth noting that Henry Knighton specifically stated that it was not until 'the following autumn' that wages increased. It is noticeable that Knighton then goes on to exaggerate the new rates of pay: it seems much comment relied on this exaggeration, even at the time (*Knighton's Chronicle* (trans. and ed. Martin), pp. 100–101).

63. *Historia Roffensis*; trans. Horrox, *Black Death*, p. 70.

64. According to Robert of Avesbury, who worked in London as a clerk in the court of the archbishop of Canterbury at Lambeth Palace, the pestilence ceased in London by Pentecost, which in 1349 fell on the last day of May.

65. He received Richard FitzRalph on Monday, 1st June, the day after Whit Sunday: see Ch. 10, pp. 219–20.

66. The extent of Thoresby's pluralism should be noted: he possessed no fewer than twenty-one benefices, all of which were sub-contracted out to vicars. The income from these parishes supplemented that of the archbishopric, which was – compared to some other English bishoprics – not great.

67. Indeed, Edward II's government had sought to control prices during the Great Famine of 1315–18.

68. *Statutes of the Realm* (eds. Luders et al.), Vol. I, p. 307. Trans. Horrox, *Black Death*, p. 289. My italics.

69. *Statutes of the Realm* (eds. Luders et al.), Vol. I, p. 308. Trans. Horrox, *Black Death*, p. 289.

70. The version of the Ordinance enrolled in the Statutes of the Realm has an additional paragraph addressed to Edington, ordering its proclamation in all the parishes in his diocese. It is likely that this was the instruction that Edington had had drawn up as a template for sending to all the other dioceses.

71. The mandate is dated (Wednesday) 1st July 1349.

72. *Registrum Hamonis Hethe Diocesis Roffensis* (ed. Johnson), Vol. II, p. 884. Trans. Horrox, *Black Death*, p. 290.

10. *Northern March*

1. The chapter was normally held after chapter Mass, which at this time was celebrated around 8am.

2. 29th December 1170.

3. The present fifteenth-century chapter house was built on the plan of the previous building.

4. The oft-repeated suggestion (for example, in Bradwardine's entry by Gordon Leff in the *Oxford Dictionary of National Biography*) that there was a dearth of candidates to choose from is incorrect: of the eligible clergy available at the time of the previous election, all – Ufford excepted – were still alive.

5. FitzRalph argued, rather weakly, that his principal reason for travelling to the curia was to settle some outstanding debts owed by his archdiocese to the papacy.

6. Given that Bradwardine was consecrated in Avignon on Sunday, 19th July, only six weeks after his election, it seems unlikely that he stayed in London long enough to attend the council meeting that decided upon the Ordinance of Labourers on 18th June. The journey to Avignon took a month at the very least and the new archbishop will have had some waiting to do at the other end before being received by the pope.

7. On Friday, 19th June, the day after the Ordinance of Labourers was issued.

8. On average there were only three clerical institutions each year in the archdeaconry of Stafford; by 17th May 1349 this number had already been met.

9. On 18th May 1349.

10. Wake is variously described as having died on 30th May and 31st May: the confusion may have been caused by his death during the night, although this is speculation. In any case, I have chosen the date given in his Inquisition Post Mortem.

11. 5th April 1349: this is the opinion of the city's common clerk, recording the fact some time later. The date seems a little early but is just within the range of possibility.

12. For example, Thornbury, see pp. 160–1.

13. The sub-dean, precentor, treasurer, three archdeacons and fourteen prebendaries all died, although not all were resident in Lincoln. It is worth noting that Thomas Bradwardine had lately been the dean but after his promotion the post was temporarily vacant. The deanery was a popular and important sinecure: William Bateman and John Ufford had also been holders of the position.

14. Egbert, bishop of York 732–66, was elevated to archbishop in 735.

15. Thompson, 'Pestilences of the fourteenth century', p. 104.

16. Thomas Stubbs, writing in the 1370s, claims that it appeared around Ascension Day, 21st May 1349. It is worth noting that John Ufford had died the day before, on Wednesday, 20th May. Thus, if he had indeed been a victim of the disease, he had caught the tail of the epidemic as it disappeared from London and the south-east, just as it was beginning to devour victims in the Northern capital.

17. A few days after Ascension (21st May 1349).

18. Thursday, 18th June 1349 ('The medieval church', *History of the County of Staffordshire*, Vol. III (1970), p. 40).

19. It is unclear precisely where the year starts in this series. However, for the purposes of comparison this has little bearing on the figures.

20. His successor, Thomas Brembre, was appointed in 1349.

21. 'Social and economic history', *History of the County of Yorkshire*, Vol. III (1913), p. 441.

22. Roger Northburgh, the infirm bishop of Coventry and Lichfield, also appointed a suffragan – the Franciscan Thomas of Brakenberg, bishop of Leighlin, from 20th March 1349. Brakenberg ensured that the diocesan administration continued to operate efficiently, so that most parishes received a new vicar within twenty days of the death of the previous incumbent. Indeed, in the archdeaconry of Stafford, the pace of institution during the hectic plague year was marginally quicker than during the other years of Bishop Roger's pontificate (during 1349 the median period from death to institution was eighteen days as opposed to nineteen days for the period 1322–58). Considering the distances that had to be covered, sometimes on foot, this was not an unimpressive feat of organization. Only a very few villages were waiting for their new priest for as much as half a year, although I doubt this was due to administrative incompetence, merely an efficient shuffling of candidates into those most populous and remunerative cures, leaving a few parishes to be filled once candidates made themselves available. This, I believe, is the most likely explanation for the long – albeit small – 'tail' in institutions found by Wood, Ferrel and DeWitte-Aviña, 'Temporal dynamics', p. 440.

23. The measured distance between the locations mentioned in his register, as the crow flies, comes to 339 miles. We should allow an additional 50 per cent for deviations, round-trips and the twisting roads. His pace was fairly constant: he travelled, on average, every other day, covering about twenty miles (i.e. thirteen miles measured directly).

24. He stayed at the Augustinian abbey of Wellow, in the middle of the town, as the guest of the abbot, John Holton.

25. From Michaelmas 1347 to Easter 1348 over 3,000 sacks of wool were exported from both Boston (Lincoln's satellite port on the mouth of

the Witham) and Kingston-upon-Hull; however, there were no wool exports made from Grimsby.

26. Louth Abbey, to the south, was not infected until July and Meaux Abbey, across the Humber, was not infected until August. It is likely that the disease was not yet showing itself in Grimsby, therefore.

27. It is possible that in the town's hinterland – relatively isolated and fore-warned – there was a somewhat lower death rate (there was a mortality among the priests of 'only' 35 per cent). As Lincoln, York, Hull and Grimsby were all infected before the disease spread into the country-side, some villagers may well have been able to avoid contact with outsiders in the period of the epidemic's spread.

28. The bishop arrived at Louth, after a detour, on 9th July 1349. The distance from Stow Park to Newark is twenty-nine miles as the crow flies.

29. Walter of Louth died on 13th July and Richard de Lincoln was installed on 22nd July. There is no explicit explanation why he would return to Louth: it can have been no other than the intermediate death of the abbot.

30. *Chronicon Abbatiae de Parco Lude* (ed. Venables), p. 38. Trans. Horrox, *Black Death*, pp. 66–7.

31. Gen. 7:5 and 9.

32. He arrived on 5th August; he had previously left on 13th May.

33. In direct distances, he had gone 575 miles, travelling on forty-one days, achieving an average of fourteen miles per day on the road.

34. Yet still he was not finished. On 7th August he set out once again, travel-ling through Huntingdonshire, Northamptonshire, north Bedfordshire and north Buckinghamshire and arriving via Banbury at Thame in south Oxfordshire on Saturday, 29th August 1349. He was back in Lyddington within two weeks. Even then his marathon was not complete, as he made a tour of south Lincolnshire, stopping only at the end of November – again in Lyddington – until March next year.

35. The mandate would have been coeval with the archbishop's receipt of the petition from the Liberty itself. We may imagine, therefore, that the disease had been in Beverley for at least a couple of weeks.

36. William de Wolfreton.

37. Aylmer and Cant (eds.), *History of York Minster*, p. 160. The will had been made out the year before, on 15th June 1348.

38. It seems that the Minster staff began 'setting-out' works in 1350, perhaps just to fulfil the terms of Sampson's will, as work would not begin on the new choir for some time yet.

39. 12th August 1349.

40. It took several storms to wipe out Ravenser, at least one of which was in 1349, probably coinciding with the surge that had caused such damage at Sempringham on 6th June.

41. One of those present, John Dowson, remembered fifty-three years later (1402) that it was a summer's day.

42. See p. 19.

43. The time of vespers varied between monasteries but was usually in the late afternoon. The 'Magnificat' comes early in the liturgy.

44. Luke 1:52.

45. Burton also claims that they were 'both masculine and feminine', perhaps indicating an inaccuracy that has crept into the story over time.

46. Burton, *Chronica Monasterii de Melsa* (ed. Bond), Vol. III, p. 72. Trans. Horrox, *Black Death*, pp. 68–70.

47. Burton wrote the chronicle some time between c.1388 and 1396.

48. The relationship between cosmology and medicine was explicitly made by Geoffrey of Meaux in his plague treatise, for which see below on p. 229.

49. Geoffrey of Meaux's preface suggests that he was writing after the outbreak of plague but before its retreat, or at least by implication its conclusion in the British Isles.

50. Bodleian Library MS Digby 176 fos. 26–9; trans. Horrox, *Black Death*, p. 167.

51. Commissioned by Philip VI to identify the causes and possible remedies of the plague, the Paris scholars reported back in October 1348 that the pestilential vapours originated in a direct transfer of gases within the atmosphere during the 1345 conjunction. They argued that Jupiter, whose qualities were hot and wet, attracted vapours with similar malevolent qualities from the earth and Mars, a process given increased force by Aquarius, whose qualities were hot and wet too. These noxious gases were further intensified by maleficent Mars, then spread around the earth by winds generated through the strong repelling forces caused by the proximity of Mars with Jupiter, mixing with the air and causing its corruption.

52. Given on 24th April 1348: see p. 34. Jacme d'Agramont's discussion is wide-ranging but his conclusions, where the issues correspond, are similar.

53. R. Hoeniger, *Der schwarze Tod* (Berlin: 1882), App. 3, p. 156; trans. Horrox, *Black Death*, p. 163.

54. Although Boccaccio, insightful as ever, separates the two causes quite deliberately: 'Some say that it descended upon the human race through the influence of the heavenly bodies, others that it was a punishment signifying God's righteous anger at our iniquitous way of life' (Boccaccio, *Decameron*, p. 5).

55. The identity of the Dominican friar is unknown, although given that Blofield was from Norfolk, not far from Norwich itself, it is more than likely that his correspondent was an old friend from home.

56. The left shoulder was significant, for it was the shoulder on which Christ was said to have borne the cross on the way to Calvary.

57. Normally, the northern leg of the journey could be made by boat as well – along the River Seine, via Paris and the River Yonne to Auxerre, leaving just a relatively short overland trip to Chalon-sur-Saône. However, given the fact that a Franco-Castilian fleet had been harassing English ships in the Seine since the spring, it seems likely that FitzRalph and Bradwardine opted for the overland route from Calais. By whatever means they reached the Rhône, the last leg of their journey down the river was by no means free of risk. The river was famously dangerous. Madame de Sévigné commented in 1671 on the 'raging Rhône', so different from the 'gentle Loire', and on hearing of a near accident under the bridge at Avignon she exclaimed: 'That Rhône terrifies everybody!' (Madame de Sévigné, *Selected Letters*, trans. and ed. L. Tancock (Harmondsworth: Penguin, 1982), pp. 71 and 76).

58. Richard FitzRalph only five years earlier, Thomas Bradwardine thirteen.

59. The city wall was rebuilt, as it appears today, between 1349 and 1368.

60. 1342–52. His extensions to the work undertaken by Benedict XII were largely complete by 1349.

61. Following the death, from plague, of Michael Mentmore, for which see p. 157. Also in Avignon were lawyers acting on behalf of the earl of Salisbury and his steward, Sir Thomas Holland, who were arguing over which one of them was rightly married to Joan, daughter of Margaret, countess of Kent and sister of Thomas Wake of Liddel. It is remarkable that this dispute continued to be debated despite the pestilence – a sign, perhaps, that the noble litigants were confident enough of their survival to persist with the time, money and effort required to resolve their argument. Sir Thomas eventually won through when, on 13th November 1349 the pope issued a bull declaring Salisbury's marriage void. Shortly after Sir Thomas Holland's death eleven years later Joan (who would become known as the 'Fair Maid of Kent') married Edward, Prince of Wales.

62. It is likely that the sermon was given before Clement issued bulls, on 18th August 1349, to the metropolitans of England, Ireland and Scotland concerning the Jubilee indulgence.

63. Most likely the chapel but sermons could also be heard in audience, in one of the several rooms used for consistories.

64. Matt. 8:25.

65. Forwarded to Durham cathedral priory in March 1349 and to the bishop of Carlisle on 28th April 1349.

66. *Statutes of the Realm* (eds. Luders et al.), Vol. I, p. 307. Trans. Horrox, *Black Death*, p. 287.

67. The halmote was the bishop's seigneurial court, held at ten set locations in the palatinate, to which tenants from surrounding villages came. The estate was not divided up into manorial units as in the South but townships.

68. i.e. the Ordinance of Labourers.

69. PRO Durham 3/12, transcribed by R. Britnell; trans. Horrox, *Black Death*, p. 284.

70. Certainly there was no mention of it in the Inquisition Post Mortem taken at Kirbymoorside, a manor of Thomas Wake, nine miles north of Barton-le-Street, on 1st July 1349.

71. Persons – i.e. those not in religious orders.

72. Thompson, 'Pestilences of the fourteenth century', p. 119.

73. His will was proved on 14th September 1349. Gasquet, *Black Death*, p. 180.

74. Paying = pleasure; *Medieval English Lyrics* (ed. Davies), ll. 61–2 pp. 109–10.

75. The peak period for clerical institutions in the archdeaconry of Chester, which included Cheshire and south Lancashire, was 10th August 1349. Usually this would correspond to a peak in deaths that came approximately twenty days before. However, because of its distance from Lichfield, this was one of the slower parts of the diocese to have replacements appointed, so the peak in clerical deaths may well have occurred up to a month before. If the assumption is made that south Lancashire was infected somewhat later than Cheshire, it is reasonable to posit that the plague was established in south Lancashire by the end of July, peaking by the middle of August.

76. The oft-quoted figures given in the archdeacon of Richmond's claim from the dean of Amounderness are extremely unreliable. However, even if they are reduced to a third of their stated numbers (see following note) they still indicate a death toll running into the thousands.

77. The archdeacon of Richmond estimated the deaths at 3,000, of which 400 made wills to the value of £13.33 (20 marks). A local jury then revised this figure down to £4. It would seem reasonable, therefore, to think that perhaps a third or so of the archdeacon's exaggerated figure would be correct.

78. In 1349, 257 fewer reaping and binding works were performed at Stockton than in 1348, equivalent to a quarter of all autumn works, a fall attributed directly to the pestilence.

79. The four ploughmen of Coatham Mundeville, ten miles inland of Stockton and not four miles out of Darlington, were dead by the end of September.

80. The same was true of the two Heworth hamlets – Over and Nether –

the former losing 36 per cent of its tenants whilst the latter lost 72 per cent.

81. Southwick, Fulwell and Monk Wearmouth; East and West Rainton, Moorsley, North and South Pittington.

82. Britnell, 'Feudal reaction', p. 31.

83. It is worth noting that a year before, on 25th October 1348, Edward had despatched Bishop Kirkby to collect the body of Princess Joan from Bordeaux. Her remains were returned but there is no record of when his journey began or when he returned to his diocese.

84. The epidemic was present in Dijon and the area around Chalon-sur-Saône during August 1349.

85. Robo, 'Black Death in the hundred of Farnham', p. 565.

86. *Registrum Hamonis Hethe* (ed. Johnson), pp. 894–5. Trans. Horrox, *Black Death*, pp. 117–8.

87. Tuesday, 29th September 1349.

88. *Robertus de Avesbury* (ed. Thompson), pp. 407–8. Trans. Horrox, *Black Death*, pp. 153–4.

89. There is no explicit record of an action being taken but Thomas Walsingham, writing in the 1390s, records that 'it was said that [the flagellants were practising] ill advisedly, in that they did not have permission from the apostolic see.' Clearly something was done about them.

11. *Barbarians*

1. Themistius, Oration 10. Delivered to Valens before the Senate of Constantinople in 370. Heather, Peter and John Matthews, *The Goths in the Fourth Century* (Liverpool: Liverpool University Press, 1991).

2. See Ch. 4, pp. 88–9.

3. 'nacionem Hibernicam aut Scoticam que unius sunt lingue notabiliter attegit sive lesit', from Walsh, *Richard FitzRalph*, p. 294 and n.

4. It was also somewhat disingenuous, especially given his by now well-publicized views on the equality of Gaelic- and Anglo-Irish barbarity. Moreover, FitzRalph would probably have been aware that apart from some parts of Galloway, Scots Gaelic was not spoken south of the Forth–Clyde line.

5. 12th August 1348.

6. By the time the official papers arrived in Armagh, plague was spreading down the eastern shore of the colony, making it all but impossible for the archbishop to bring the colonists and their native enemies together.

7. At Rokeby, on the Tees in Richmondshire.

8. *Chronicon de Lanercost*, p. 351. Trans. *ODNB*: Rokeby.

9. Limerick, it seems, was still free of disease. A friar died of plague there on 1st November and it must be doubted whether this small port had a population large enough to sustain the epidemic for four months.

10. Kelly, *Black Death in Ireland*, p. 36.

11. In July 1349.

12. *Annals of the Four Masters*, Vol. 3, pp. 594–5.

13. The passage starts: 'One thousand three hundred and fifty years until tonight since J.C. Amen was born and in the second year after the coming of the plague into Ireland that was written.' Quoted elsewhere (i.e. Kelly, *Black Death in Ireland*, p. 60; Henry and Marsh-Micheli, 'Manuscripts and illuminations', p. 796), this passage has been dated as Christmas Eve 1350. This, I believe, is a mistake. The Mac Aodhagáin family were hereditary scribes (*brehons*), attached to ruling families in Connacht, Ormond and later northern Thomond. There is no evidence – and it is highly improbable – that the plague lasted a full year in any of these places, all of which showed infection at some point in 1349. Moreover, as the plague arrived in Ireland in the summer of 1348, a dating of Christmas Eve 1349 would tally with Aodh's assertion that he was writing 'in the *second* year after the coming of the plague into Ireland' (my italics). A more likely explanation for the unusual dating he uses can be found in Aodh's careful wording, in which he seems to take the date of the Nativity as the beginning of the New Year.

14. Kelly, *Black Death in Ireland*, p. 60.

15. For instance, the 'ring fort' – a dwelling bounded by a ditch. Stone had long been used in churches and on ecclesiastical sites, and latterly in fortifications; otherwise buildings were more rudimentary.

16. As reported by Froissart, *Chronicles* (ed. and trans. Brereton), p. 410.

17. Raymond, viscount of Perelhos and Roda in Roussillon (from Watt, 'Approaches to the history of fourteenth-century Ireland', in Cosgrove, *New History of Ireland*, p. 309).

18. Sir John Carew, deputy justiciar 3rd October–19th December (in Rokeby's absence), had spent his few weeks in the post defending Dublin against attacks from the O'Byrnes of Wicklow.

19. Kelly, *Black Death in Ireland*, p. 72.

20. *Calendar of the Close Rolls*, Edward III, Vol. IX: 1349–54, p. 92.

21. In 1344 Edward had appointed Ralph d'Ufford as justiciar, sending him with a considerable army with which to enforce the royal will. D'Ufford had used the soldiers well but was dead within two years,

by which time Edward was once again completely absorbed in the preparations for his Continental campaign. No more happened until peacemaking powers were conferred on FitzRalph in August 1348.

22. Guy de Nesle.

23. He now attempted to activate this alliance, although in the event Count Louis was found wanting.

24. This was the second instalment of the three-year tax granted by parliament in April 1348. For details, see Ch. 2 note x, p. 28.

25. It is possible that the keeper of Westminster Palace, John Sench, who was also responsible for the Fleet Prison, was another casualty (*Calendar of the Fine Rolls*, Edward III, Vol. VI: 1347–1356, p. 179).

26. Amusingly, the steward of the chamber who ordered the seizure, Philip de Weston, was himself later arraigned for fraud (ibid., p. 249).

27. I am grateful to Dr Jeremy Ashby, Assistant Curator at the Tower of London, for this point.

28. On Wednesday, 26th August 1349.

29. Edward had already taken the precaution of asking the pope to appoint his nominee and Clement obliged a little over a fortnight after the monks had made their choice, on 7th October 1349. It showed swift action on the part of Edward, as this was only forty-two days since Bradwardine's death. A messenger must have been sent almost immediately.

30. *Registrum Trillek* (ed. Parry), p. 148, from Dohar, *Black Death*, p. 60. Becket's body had been translated to the Trinity Chapel in Canterbury Cathedral in 1220.

31. See Ch. 3, p. 67.

32. It is not entirely clear whether de Pavia intended a sting or simply lost his courage, although the sequence of events – and the balance of chronicle reports – suggests that it was the latter.

33. He was sixty-seven in 1348.

34. Nicholson, *Scotland*, p. 156.

35. There is evidence of Balliol issuing mandates from the islet of Hestan and from the castles of Caerlaverock and Buittle.

36. In Edward III's first foreign treaty, at Northampton. It was here that Edward first recognized Balliol as king of Scots.

37. In 1370: there is no reason to think that it was substantially different in 1349–50.

38. *Chronicon Galfridi le Baker* (ed. Thompson), p. 100. Trans. Horrox, *Black Death*, p. 81.

39. In his approach to Bannockburn, Edward II was said to have taken only six days to complete the journey from the Tweed to Falkirk, forty miles further than Edinburgh, and that with all the machinery and baggage of war.

40. Including one marked on the English Gough map that ran from Perth direct to Aberdeen.

41. Fordun's chronicle (c.1350–63) provides the earliest surviving Scottish account of the pestilence. He may well have had family connections in Perthshire, so his account could well have been informed by information from here as well.

42. Fordun, *Chronica Gestis Scotorum*, Vol. I, pp. 368–9. Trans. Horrox, *Black Death*, p. 84.

43. In Scotland feudalism had overlaid previous landholding structures – mainly an ancient kin-based system of food rents – and the money rent economy reflected this. It was the development of this cash economy that had brought about the substitution of food rents by money rents, so much so that leases across Scotland were by the mid-fourteenth century paid for in coin.

44. Prof. Benedictow claims that Norway had a pre-plague population of around 350,000, the vast majority of which was rural. It is reasonable to assume that at least a third of Scotland's population was distributed through the Highlands.

45. Norway was infected via merchant traffic from London, if contemporary Norse annals are to be believed.

46. Benedictow, *The Black Death*, p. 154.

47. The complete lack of hard information makes it impossible to give dates to the progress of the plague through Scotland, although political events provide some clue as to the course of the epidemic. A petition to allow the marriage of John Macdonald, the lord of the Isles, to Robert Stewart's eldest daughter, Margaret, was sent to Avignon around April (it was heard by the papal court on 14th June 1350): this might suggest that plague had not yet established itself fully north of the Forth–Clyde line, which was Macdonald's powerbase. Certainly the plague was clearly still raging in the summer of 1350, as the pope was persuaded to grant the same Jubilee indulgence to the earls of Ross and Mar that he had refused to Edward and the English, although the epidemic plague did not prevent the abbot of Dunfermline from making the journey to Rome that year (he may well have caught the disease on his return, however, as the pope had to appoint a successor in 1351). However, Sir William Douglas travelled to Scotland to lobby for the terms of a proposed treaty later in 1350, in December – a journey he may well have delayed until the epidemic had left the Lowlands. It seems likely, therefore, that pestilence arrived over the border (and possibly in Edinburgh) in very late 1349 or early 1350, established itself there during the spring and moved gradually north through the year, perhaps ending in the northern Highlands and islands

in late 1350 or early 1351. Such a pattern would accord with how the epidemic would be expected to move, given the experience in England and elsewhere.

12. *Resurgam*

1. Langland, *Piers Plowman* (ed. Pearsall), Passus XII, l. 110, p. 366; my translation.
2. It is difficult to judge precisely when this was. Although the letter has been dated to 28th December 1349, this would have been impossible had the action at Calais happened, as Jonathan Sumption believes to be the case – after a full assessment of the sources – on the morning of 2nd January 1350 (Sumption, *Trial by Fire*, p. 61).
3. Wilkins (ed.), *Concilia*, Vol. II, p. 752. Trans. Horrox, *Black Death*, p.118.
4. Nicholas Worlingworth was an associate of Adam Walpol, who had been implicated in the fraud at the royal mint, for which see Ch. 9, p. 206.
5. On 8th September 1350, just before Joanna Bret died.
6. Fratres Cruciferi or Crossed Friars, an early twelfth-century Flemish foundation.
7. There were, of course, other beneficiaries in London other than the friars, although their accumulation of wealth in the period stands out. The Priory and Hospital of St Mary Spital, for instance, took advantage of the depression in land prices during the plague to purchase five houses and shops and a hundred acres in Shoreditch and Hackney in 1349. Around 1351 they purchased a further sixty acres in Hackney, via a trust as a mechanism to get round the Statute of Mortmain (1279).
8. *Calendar of the Fine Rolls*, Edward III, Vol. VI: 1347–1356, p. 181; the order was repeated on 12th April and sent to other towns across England.
9. This was to be judged under the rules that governed the alienation of land and property to religious institutions.
10. *Calendar of the Patent Rolls*, Edward III, Vol. VIII: 1348–50, p. 459.
11. Hill, *Mediæval Lincoln*, p. 298.
12. In 1350 William Brigge, a Salisbury dyer, took over a tenement in Fisherton, one of the many villages around the city where dying racks were laid out. Although the property had previously been owned by two Salisbury drapers, there is no reason to think that Brigge did not use the whole plot, producing the same in total as the two had done before.
13. It is a crude measure but worth noting nonetheless that between September 1349 and September 1350 the household of Lady Elizabeth de Burgh, which numbered about 250, consumed more than 83,000 herrings, every one of which was sourced from Yarmouth.

14. The following year the port was one of three along the Lincolnshire coast (Barton and Boston being the others) that shipped provisions, including corn, pigs and beef, to the English garrisons of Gascony, Brittany and Calais.

15. On 20th September 1349. He was instructed to desist from drawing the stipend as soon as the parish was again able to support him. Aberth, 'Black Death in the diocese of Ely', p. 285.

16. The foundation deed was signed on 15th January 1350.

17. Elsewhere the mendicants were expanding too during 1349–51: in Leicester (Franciscans), Ipswich and Dunwich (both Dominicans) while the Crutched Friars in Oxford bought a new site, although this was short-lived.

18. It was pulled down sometime between 1350 and 1400.

19. Rent received by St John's Hospital in the city fell from £30 per annum from before the Great Death to £11 in 1349–50.

20. *Historia Roffensis*; trans. Horrox, *Black Death*, pp. 73–4.

21. ibid., pp. 72–3.

22. Hugh Despenser, who held lands in the Vale of Glamorgan, died on 8 February 1349 (although it remains unclear where, the date of his death suggests that he most probably caught the disease in London). Despenser had served Edward III with valour in the French campaigns. Nonetheless, it was to Edward's father that Despenser linked himself in death: the design of Hugh's tomb in Tewkesbury Abbey was clearly influenced by that of Edward II's at Gloucester.

23. The figure comes from Russell's generous sample from the Inquisitions Post Mortem, where of 505 nobles in possession of their inheritance at the time of the Great Death only 138 appear to have perished (Russell, *British Medieval Population*, pp. 215–18).

24. If one counts the two deaths of the archbishops of Canterbury (John Ufford and Thomas Bradwardine) that could be attributable to pestilence, the other being Wulstan de Bransford, bishop of Worcester.

25. i.e. as many as ten of the thirty-four dioceses in Ireland lost their bishop in the pestilence. Probably Ferns, Killala, Waterford, and possibly Clonmacnoise, Derry, Dublin, Meath, Tuam and Waterford – a second time (the remainder being: Ardagh, Ardfert, Armagh, Cashel, Cork, Clogher, Clonfert, Cloyne, Connor, Down, Dromore, Elphin, Emly, Kildare, Kilfenora, Killaloe, Kilmacduagh, Limerick, Lismore, Mayo, Ossory, Raphoe, Ross). The bishop of Leighlin, William St Leger, died at Avignon at the beginning of May 1348, most probably from the pestilence; I have not counted St Leger as a plague death in Ireland as a result. None of the four Welsh bishops (Bangor, Llandaff, St Asaph and St David's) died and there is no record of any of the twelve Scottish bishops (Aberdeen,

Brechin, Dornoch, Dunblane, Dunkeld, Fortrose, Glasgow, Iona-Hy, Kirkwall, Lismore, St Andrews, Whithorn) dying, although records here are even poorer than in Ireland. A possible explanation for a comparatively higher mortality among the Irish bishops may reveal why the lesser clergy suffered so terribly in England. For in the greater part, the Irish bishops ran tiny bishoprics, many of which were inherited. Theirs was a personal and pastoral episcopacy, far removed from the kind of prelacy practised by the grand magnate-bishops who presided over the larger English dioceses, who had in some cases a whole number of palaces in which to hide. Like the Irish bishops, this was not a privilege enjoyed by the lesser clergy in England, who were tied to their parish or religious house; they, like the parishioners they ministered to, could only hope and pray that they might be spared.

26. It is an impression given added weight by the mortality of abbots in the most reclusive closed monastic orders. It is likely that at least seventeen heads (twelve of monks, five of nuns) of the 104 Cistercian foundations in England died during the Pestilence (Bindon, Byland, Catesby (nuns), Cookhill (nuns), Kirkstall, Louth Park, Meaux, Sawtry, Sewardsley (nuns), Robertsbridge, Roche, Stoneleigh, Thame, Vale Royal, Waverley, Whistones (nuns), Wintney (nuns)). Even if some have been missed, it seems unlikely that no more than 20 per cent of the heads of Cistercian houses died. It is also worth noting that there is no record of a Carthusian prior dying during the plague years, out of three houses (Witham, Hinton, Beauvale) extant at the time.

27. *Knighton's Chronicle* (trans. and ed. Martin), pp. 100–101.

28. Indeed, in Kent it was this, not the mortality – which had already passed by harvest time – which meant that much of the harvest was simply left in the fields to rot.

29. *Historia Roffensis*; trans. Horrox, *Black Death*, p. 73.

30. Much of this estate had just been valued on Thomas's death. Margaret had died on 29th September 1349, so the escheator was forced to repeat the whole process again, although a backlog of cases delayed the second valuation until the New Year.

31. On the death of any great lord (i.e. those who held land directly from the king), the king's escheator in each county was required to conduct an Inquisition Post Mortem to establish the extent, value and condition of their possessions.

32. Customary rents fell from £6 5s. 5d. (£6.27) to £4 5s. 5d. (£4.27); rents from farmers fell from 35s. (£1.75) to 16s. 4d. (£0.82).

33. It was now worth 6s. 8d. (approx. £0.33).

34. From £8 to 50s. (£2.50) (*Inquisitions Post Mortem*, 23 Edward III Pt 1, no. 88, quoted in Gasquet, *Black Death*, p. 159).

35. It had been worth £20 but was now valued at just 20s. (i.e. £1.00).

36. PRO Ministers' Accounts, SC 6/801/4; trans. Horrox, *Black Death*, p. 283.

37. John de Vere.

38. The fine had been 2s. and he reduced it to 6d. Suffolk Record Office (Ipswich branch), HA68:484:135; trans. Horrox, *Black Death*, p. 286.

39. The cartulary states that Walter had been required to work for five days per week between Michaelmas (29th September) and Martinmas (11th November), and four days per week between Martinmas and the feast of St John the Baptist (Midsummer, or 24th June) – all of which comes to 158 days. In addition, Walter was required to carry services as far as Eynsham if it was necessary.

40. PRO Durham 3/12; trans. Horrox, *Black Death*, p. 328.

41. Dene, *Historia Roffensis*. Trans. Horrox, *Black Death*, pp. 72–3.

42. Langland, *Piers Plowman* (ed. Pearsall), Prologue, ll. 81–4; my translation. The A text of *Plowman*, which includes these lines of the Prologue, was completed by 1370.

43. *Knighton's Chronicle* (trans. and ed. Martin), pp. 102–3.

44. Ch. 9, pp. 216–7.

45. Bishop Bateman, for instance, was permitted (by a bull issued on 13th October) to lower the minimum canonical age for ordination to twenty-one in the case of sixty potential ordinands, while John Thoresby, the new chancellor and bishop of Worcester, gained the pope's approval to ordain illegitimates (something that had for a long time been proscribed by the English church), so long as they were of good character. Archbishop Zouche of York received permission (issued on 12th October 1349 and published on 4th January 1350) to hold an additional four ordinations in 1350 so that he could get men through the system quickly, a task that he delegated (once again) to his suffragan, Hugh, archbishop of Damascus.

46. Some monastic patrons simply appointed one of their own, as did Barnwell Priory to their parish of Waterbeach, in Cambridgeshire, in 1349; it was not until 1390 that a secular priest was presented here again – although it must be admitted that it was not that unusual for Augustinian canons to serve their own parishes.

47. John Thoresby charged the prior of Llanthony, in his letter of appointment making the prior his vicar-general in the diocese of February 1350, 'to appoint a remedy for the want of rectors and parish chaplains, owing to loss of so many priests in so many churches' and condemned those priests who 'made no personal residence, not celebrating zealously nor ministering to their parishioners', and admonished all the clergy not to take excessive payments for burials

or masses for the dead. Thoresby did not actually go to Worcester until 1351: clearly the demands of the chancellorship kept him from visiting his new diocese until then ('Ecclesiastical History', *History of the County of Worcestershire*, Vol. II (1906), pp. 32–3). Two months later William Edington issued a similar letter to all the clergy in his diocese, instructing them to remain resident in their churches. Simon Islip had also sent out several letters to the same effect.

48. On 28th May 1350.

49. *Registrum Simonis de Sudbiria* (ed. Fowler), Vol. I, pp. 190–91. Trans. Horrox, *Black Death*, pp. 307–8.

50. 'Memorials: 1350', *Memorials of London and London Life* (trans. and ed. Riley), pp. 251–2.

51. *Calendar of the Patent Rolls*, Edward III, Vol. VIII: 1348–50, p. 594.

52. *Knighton's Chronicle* (trans. and ed. Martin), pp. 102–3.

53. *Statutes of the Realm* (eds. Luders et al.), Vol. I, p. 307. Trans. Horrox, *Black Death*, p. 288.

54. *Historia Roffensis*; trans. Horrox, *Black Death*, p. 73.

55. *Statutes of the Realm* (eds. Luders et al.), Vol. I, p. 311. Trans. Horrox, *Black Death*, p. 313.

56. In Farnham, Surrey, recorded wages slipped back slightly from their peak in 1349–50 (from 3–4*d*. per day for a labourer in 1349–50 to 2–3*d*. per day for a labourer in 1350–51).

57. Passed as a reconfirmation of the Statute of Westminster of 1335.

58. John Malwayn administered the customs from 20th July 1350 for three years, following the collapse of the Chiriton company.

59. Burton, *Chronica* (ed. Bond), Vol. III, p. 37. Trans. Horrox, *Black Death*, p.68.

60. The house of Llanthony Secunda, for instance, had to lobby Trillek for the revenues of an additional church to be appropriated to them to offset the financial losses they were suffering as a result of the plague (granted in 1351). Buildwas had in 1350 to contend, in addition to falling rents, with a raid of thieving Welshmen from Powys who stole some of the abbey's treasures, including chalices, jewels, vestments and books.

61. York, Borthwick Institute of Historical Research, Reg. 10 fo.145; trans. Horrox, *Black Death*, p. 300.

62. Franklin, 'Thornbury manor', p. 361.

63. St Mary Graces was further endowed in 1353 with properties nominally owned by John Corey, and again in 1358 and 1367.

13. *Reorder and Reaction*

1. Carney, 'Literature in Irish', p. 690.
2. At Loughmoran, Lady Elizabeth de Burgh's bailiff had let the demesne to the steward of the manor; at her manor of Palmerstown the tenants were remitted a third of their rents, although the large number of entry fines flattered the manor accounts into showing an income similar to the one produced before the plague. However, at Callan half the tenements were still vacant in 1350: even though this vacant land was farmed out, the income generated was nonetheless much reduced. At Lisronagh much of the customary land was still in the steward's hands, untilled, in 1351–2, and rents from those tenements that were still let had halved.
3. Admissions in Colchester were about 50 per cent higher in the 1350s than they had been in the 1340s, i.e. from around fifteen per annum in the 1340s to around twenty-two per annum in the 1350s. More people were given burghal rights to Colchester during 1353–4 than at any other time during the remainder of the century.
4. Williamson, 'Plague in Cambridge', p. 51.
5. For example, Walter Burley and John Maudith had both died; John Baconthorpe, Simon Bredon and Richard Kilvington had left the university before the Great Death came.
6. *Chron. Johannis de Reading* (ed. Tait), p. 10. Trans. Horrox, *Black Death*, p. 75.
7. 'Ecclesiastical history', *History of the County of Durham*, Vol. II (1907), p. 20.
8. Zouche had died in 1352.
9. Dohar, *Black Death and Pastoral Leadership*, p. 77.
10. Sumption, *Trial by Fire*, p. 133.
11. In some places the drop was unspectacular: Haverford, in west Pembroke, had been worth £161 in 1325 but in 1355 was valued at £153 – a decline of only 5 per cent. However, Maelienydd, in Powys, saw its value fall considerably after the pestilence, a drop that continued through the following decade – in 1360 it was worth 26 per cent less than it had been three years earlier.
12. In the lordship of Narberth, in Pembroke, revenue doubled from £47 in 1360 to £94 in 1366. Yet this was by no means a universal experience: income from the duke of Lancaster's lordship of Ogmore, to the west in Glamorgan, was in the 1360s down by a third on the level achieved before the Great Death.
13. For example, at Banstead in Surrey a quarter of all plots in the manor still had no replacement tenant in 1353, while the following year the vice-sheriff of Cumberland reported that 'the great part of the manor

lands attached to the king's castle at Carlisle' was still, in 1354, uncultivated, 'by reason of the mortal pestilence lately raging in those parts'
(Gasquet, *Black Death*, p. 183).

14. At Easington in 1355 for six years; at Urpeth in 1357.

15. 'Social and economic history', *History of the County of Durham*, Vol. II
(1907), p. 215.

16. This figure excludes the palatinates of Cheshire, Durham and Lancashire.
In Wiltshire deputies were appointed by the justices, who also sat
themselves, a practice that must have been common elsewhere. So the
actual number of people sitting on benches will have been far higher
than even 500. One way or other the enforcement of the Statute of
Labourers must have involved a significant proportion of the landed
class.

17. As in Caldecott.

18. I have rounded Prof. Ormrod's estimates for these years, which come
to just over £109,748 (from Ormrod, *Reign of Edward III*, p. 189).

19. Gasquet, *Black Death*, p. 181.

20. *Knighton's Chronicle* (trans. and ed. Martin), pp. 118–19.

14. *Flowering amidst Failure*

1. *Major Latin Works of John Gower* (ed. Stockton), pp. 98–9.

2. See Ch. 2, pp. 31–2.

3. Bowsky, *Black Death*, p. 137.

4. France, 'History of the Plague in Lancashire', p. 27.

5. Fordun, *Chronica Gestis Scotorum*, Vol. I, pp. 380–81. Trans. Horrox, *Black
Death*, p. 88.

6. Jillings, *Scotland's Black Death*, p. 34.

7. Newton, *Thaxted in the Fourteenth Century*, p. 25.

8. *Knighton's Chronicle* (trans. and ed. Martin), pp. 184–5.

9. This is my very free translation of the poor Leonine verse inscribed on
the inside north wall of the tower, from the transcription by Sherlock
(*Medieval Drawings and Writings*, pp. 5–6), with his interpolations:

M.C.T[er] x penta miseranda ferox violenta
[discessit pestis] supersat plebs pessima testis in fine q^{e}vent[us] [erat]
valid[us]
[. . . h]oc anno maurus in orbe tonat ^{MCCC}LXI

In the modern calendar the year was actually 1362, so I have substituted
this to avoid confusion. The fact that the author thinks that the plague

left Ashwell in 1350, rather than in 1349 as it should correctly be, suggests that he was remembering an event that was by this point quite distant. Alternatively he was carrying on from the second graffito on the wall, which states: 'In 1349 there was a plague and [in 13]50' (ibid., p. 5). This is undoubtedly later, as all the local manorial evidence makes it plain that the plague had left by 1350; it may, however, record a local murrain or some other epidemic. Either way, it seems likely that the inscription was made sometime in the 1360s, most probably during the building works to secure the tower.

10. It is worth noting that Thomas de la Mare crenellated St Alban's in 1357.

11. The precise chronology of the rebuilding of Winchester Cathedral is contested. My hypothesis is that Edington built the west front, without the gable and possibly without tracery in the great west window, probably in the 1360s, after he had completed Edington church around 1360 and his resignation as chancellor in 1363 but substantially before his death in 1366. Wykeham may have had the porch added early in his episcopacy for weather-proofing reasons (possibly in the early 1370s, when Wykeham's register mentions building work being undertaken). There is something of a pastiche about the triple porch, with references both to other parts of Winchester and to the work of masons elsewhere. It may not be far-fetched to imagine this to be the best attempt by a capable mason to sort out the mess of the west end as it had been left on – or shortly after – Edington's death. Then, when Wykeham turned his mind to the nave's completion late in his episcopacy (just as Edington had done), he commissioned William Wynford to do the work. Wynford raised the height of the aisles but was forced to incorporate Edington's west front as best he could, for to start again would have been prohibitively expensive. I would speculate that the tracery to the west window is by Wynford (notice the tear-drop motif common to this window and his clerestory windows, absent in Edington's aisle windows).

12. Langland, *Piers Plowman* (ed. Pearsall), Passus IX, l. 64, p. 164.

13. 'Memorials: 1351', *Memorials of London and London Life* (ed. Riley), pp. 266–9.

14. Baldwin, 'Sumptuary legislation', p. 34.

15. *Eulogium* (ed. Haydon), Vol. III, p. 231. Trans. Horrox, *Black Death*. p. 133.

16. *Chron. Johannis de Reading* (ed. Tait), pp. 167–8. Trans. Horrox, *Black Death*, p. 134.

17. *Eulogium* (ed. Haydon), Vol. III, pp. 214. Trans. Horrox, *Black Death*. p. 64.

18. It is striking is that the recording of women's occupations tended to be

most rigorous in those surveys of growing and successful towns, and least good in small and declining towns.

19. The Malmesbury monk provides a further, intriguing, assertion that female survivors of the pestilence remained barren for many years and that the proportion of deaths in childbirth – both women and children – increased. This is the single source that mentions this phenomenon and it is difficult to see how it can be substantiated, or even explained.

20. *A Fourteenth-Century Chronicle from the Grey Friars at Lynn* (ed. Gransden), p. 275, trans. Horrox, *Black Death*, p. 86, and *Chronicon Abbatie de Parco Lude* (ed. Venables and trans. Maddison), pp. 40–41.

21. Child mortality was already exceptionally high: life expectancy in late-medieval Essex at birth was about thirty-three, but for those who reached twelve it was about forty – a stark difference that amply displays what challenging years filled this first decade of life.

22. Bowsky, *Black Death*, pp. 225–6.

23. K. Sudhoff, 'Festschriften aus den ersten 150 Jahren nach der Epidemie des "schwarzen Todes" 1348: III', *Archiv für Geschichte der Medizin V*, 1912, pp. 62–9; trans. Horrox, *Black Death*, p. 186.

24. *A Little Book of Pestilence* (Manchester: 1911); trans. Horrox, *Black Death*, p. 177.

25. An appeal to better (and cleaner) times of old was a common refrain in injunctions such as these, although in this instance it may well have been a reference to William FitzStephen's comment, made two centuries before, that London enjoyed sweet air.

26. *Memorials of London and London Life*, p. 295. I have slightly modified the word order in this passage.

27. Rosser, *Medieval Westminster*. p. 69.

28. The growing debt of Haltemprice Priory, which owned the advowson of the village, suggests that the income they received from Wharram was less than the cost of providing a vicar.

29. *The Anonimalle Chronicle*, (ed. Galbraith), p. 77. Trans. Horrox, *Black Death*, p. 88.

30. The following heads of religious houses died during the 1369 epidemic: Augustinian (2) – Grimsby (Lincolnshire), Stonely (Huntingdonshire); Benedictine (4) – St Sepulchre, Canterbury (Kent), Colchester (Essex), Monk Sherborne (Hampshire), Vale Royal (Cheshire); Cistercian (1) – Fountains (Yorkshire); hospitals (2) – Fordingbridge (Hampshire); Little Maldon (Essex); also the dean of Chichester Cathedral in Sussex.

31. Johnston, *Galar Y Beirdd/Poets' Grief*, pp. 50–55.

32. Langland, *Piers Plowman* (ed. Pearsall), Prologue, l. 19, p. 28.

33. ibid., Passus X, ll. 269–72, p. 192.

34. Gower, *Confessio Amantis* (ed. Peck), 'Prologue', ll. 26–31; my translation.

35. Chaucer, *Book of the Duchess*, in *Riverside Chaucer* (ed. Benson), ll. 475–9, p. 336; my translation.

36. Other than the extraordinary figure of £667 registered for the Jubilee Year of 1350–51, receipts of shrine donations at Canterbury peaked in 1376–7 at £550, perhaps coinciding with the death of Edward, Prince of Wales, who was buried there; their previous peak was in 1319–20 at £500.

37. Chaucer, *Canterbury Tales*, 'Pardoner's Tale', in *Riverside Chaucer* (ed. Benson), VI (C), ll. 675–9, p. 199.

38. ibid., ll. 686–9, p. 199.

39. Cottle, *Triumph of English*, p. 20.

40. 'Medieval agriculture', *History of the County of Staffordshire*, Vol. VI (1979), p. 38.

41. It was for this reason that the receipts from feudal dues in manors across the South and East of England either rose in the thirty years after the Great Death or stayed static – representing a per capita rise on these reduced village populations. At Wheathampstead in Hertfordshire, perquisites of the manor court were 9 per cent higher in the period 1371–81 than they had been in between 1340 and 1347, when the village was double the size. At Meopham in Kent, fines had more than doubled over a similar period. Thus, by ramping up the receipts from feudal fines and fees, landlords were able to recover some of the losses they sustained in lower rents and higher labour costs.

42. *The Anonimalle Chronicle*, (ed. Galbraith), p. 77. Trans. Horrox, *Black Death*, p. 88.

43. A very loose translation of the epitaph, as printed in Blair, 'John Smith of Brightwell Baldwin', p. 431.

44. They reached £15,359 14s. 9 1/4d. (i.e. approximately £15,359.74).

45. £2,000 per annum to £500 per annum.

46. Bower, *Scotichronicon*, Vol. 7, Bk XIV, pp. 366–7.

47. A £1,878 17s. 1 1/4d (i.e. £1,878.86) surplus on revenues of £14,584 9s. 9 3/4d. (i.e. £14,584.49).

48. 1380–84: 56,400 hides exported per annum on average; 1385–9: 48,300 hides exported per annum on average.

49. Fordun, *Chronica Gestis Scotorum*, Vol. I, p. 42; trans. Vol. IV, p. 38.

50. For instance, at Caldicot, where the pestilence of 1361–2 had been particularly severe, there was rapid commutation of services and extensive leasing of demesne land. It was a sensible move on the part of the estate officials, as by 1366 profits from leasing exceeded the loss from still-vacant tenements: by 1367 demesne was let for £6 13s. 0d. and in 1369 demesne was let for £7 10s. 0d.; all demesne land farmed out in subsequent years for £8.

51. R. R. Davies, *Conquest, Coexistence and Change*, p. 437.

52. ibid., p. 435.
53. Watt, 'Anglo-Irish colony under strain', p. 373.
54. £14,733 in the period 1363–4, for instance.
55. Watt, 'Anglo-Irish colony under strain', p. 387.
56. Kelly, *Black Death in Ireland*, pp. 120, 141.
57. Watt, 'Anglo-Irish colony under strain', p. 373.
58. *Concilia* (ed. Wilkins), Vol. III, p. 100. Trans. Horrox, *Black Death*, p. 120.
59. W. Lyndewood, *Provinciale seu constitutiones Angliae* (Oxford: 1679), Appendix, pp. 58–9; trans. Horrox, *Black Death*, p. 311.
60. Gild in St Mary, Hatfield (1363); Fraternity of the Holy Trinity in Chelmsford (c.1368); Fraternity of the Holy Trinity, Rayleigh (c.1369); Gild of the Holy Trinity in All Saints, Maldon (1377); Fraternity of the Assumption of the Virgin, St Peter's Maldon (1379); Fraternity of Corpus Christi, founded by Adam, Simon and John Chaumpeneye and associates (1379).
61. *Sermons of Thomas Brinton* (ed. Devlin), Vol. I, no. 48, p. 216. Trans. Horrox, *Black Death*, p. 141.
62. Gasquet, *Old English Bible*, pp. 61, 63, 65–7, 75–6.
63. David Knowles, *Religious Orders in England*, Vol. II (1955), p. 59.
64. Walsingham, *Historia Anglicana* (ed. Riley), Vol. I, p. 89.
65. France, 'History of the Plague in Lancashire', p. 27.
66. Walsingham, *Historia Anglicana* (ed. Riley), Vol. I, p. 90.
67. Walter Bower, 1385–1449, writing 1441–5.
68. 'The later Middle Ages: City government and the Commonalty', *History of the County of Yorkshire: The City of York* (1961), p. 81.
69. Dobson (ed.), *Peasants' Revolt*, p. 203.

Epilogue

1. A (liberal) translation of a fragment of a fifteenth-century wall painting in Acle church in Norfolk. Coulton, 'A medieval inscription in Acle church'.

Appendix 2.
The Spread of the Black Death in the British Isles: Mapping the Epidemic

1. Carpentier, 'Autour de la peste noire', pp. 1062–92.

Select Bibliography

Many books and articles have informed this book. This bibliography is restricted to those works on which the text relies.

It is right that I point to a number of books and authors to whom I am especially indebted. *The Black Death*, by Rosemary Horrox, is an invaluable compendium of the key sources relating to the period. Where possible, I have used her translations, which are the best available. My treatment of the Hundred Years War follows almost entirely the definitive work of Jonathan Sumption. In addition, I have made use of a number of unpublished papers, theses and dissertations, namely those of Paula Arthur, Carolyn Fenwick, P. A. Franklin, Lori Gates, Eileen and Arthur Gooder, Philip Lindley, Marilyn Livingstone, Simon Pawley, Andrew Prescott, A. Saul, R. M. Smith and Christopher Wilson. All these volumes are given their full reference below.

Printed Primary Sources

Adami Murimuthensis Chronica sui temporis, nunc primum per decem annos aucta (MCCCIII–MCCCXLVI), cum eorundem continuatione (ad MCCCLXXX) a quodam anonymo, ad fidem codicum manuscriptorum edidit et recensuit, ed. T. Hog (London: English Historical Society, 1846)

Annála Connacht. The Annals of Connacht – A.D. 1224–1544, trans. and ed. A. Martin Freeman (Dublin: Dublin Institute for Advanced Studies, 1944)

Annála Rioghachta Eireann. Annals of the Kingdom of Ireland by the Four Masters from the Earliest Period to the Year 1616, trans. and ed. J. O'Donovan, 7 vols. (Dublin: Hodges & Smith, 1851)

Annála Uladh. Annals of Ulster: From the Earliest Times to the Year 1541, trans. and ed. W. M. Hennessey, 2nd edn (Blackrock: Edmund Burke, 1988)

Annales Monastici, ed. Henry Richards Luard, Rolls Series No. 36, 5 vols. (London: Longman, Green, Longman, Roberts, and Green, 1864–9), Vol. III. *Annales Prioratus de Dunstaplia (A.D. 1–1297); Annales Moasterii de Bermundeseia (A.D. 1042–1432)* (1866)

Annals of Clonmacnoise, being Annals of Ireland from the Earliest Period to A.D. 1408, trans. Conell Mageoghagan and ed. Rev. D. Murphy (Dublin: Royal Society of Antiquaries of Ireland, 1896)

The Anonimalle Chronicle, 1333–1381, from a Manuscript Written at St Mary's Abbey, York, ed. V. H. Galbraith, 1st edn reprinted with minor corrections (Manchester: Manchester University Press, 1970)

Boccaccio, Giovanni, *The Decameron*, trans. G. McWilliam (London: Penguin, 1995)

Bower, Walter, *Scotichronicon*, eds. D. E. R. Watt et al., 9 vols. (Aberdeen: Aberdeen University Press, 1998)

The Brut or the Chronicles of England, ed. F. W. D. Brie, Early English Text Society Publications Original Series Nos. 131 and 136, 2 vols. (London: Kegan, Paul, Trubner and Co., 1906–8)

Burton, Thomas, *Chronica Monasterii de Melsa*, etc., ed. Edward A. Bond, Rolls Series No. 43, 3 vols. (London: Longmans, Green, Reader, and Dyer, 1866–8)

Calendar of Charter Rolls, etc., ed. Sir H. C. Maxwell Lyte et al., Rolls Series No. 142 (London, 1903–27)

Calendar of Coroners' Rolls of the City of London, A.D. 1300–1378, ed. by R. R. Sharpe (London: Richard Clay & Sons, 1913)

Calendar of Entries in the Papal Registers Relating to Great Britain and Ireland: Papal Letters, 20 vols. (London: Her Majesty's Stationery Office, 1893–2005), *Vol. III. 1342–1362* and *Vol. IV. 1362–1404*

Calendar of Inquisitions Miscellaneous, eds. Sir H. C. Maxwell Lyte et al., 1308–1388, Vols. II–IV, Rolls Series No. 155 (London: Her Majesty's Stationery Office, 1916–57)

Calendar of Inquisitions Post Mortem, eds. Sir H. C. Maxwell Lyte et al., Edward III and Richard II, Vols. VII–XVI, Rolls Series No. 154 (London: Her Majesty's Stationery Office, 1909–74)

A Calendar of the Cartularies of Adam Fraunceys and John Pyel, ed. Stephen O'Connor, Camden Society, 5th ser., Vol. II (London: University College London, 1993)

Calendar of the Close Rolls, eds. Sir H. C. Maxwell Lyte et al., Edward III and Richard II, Rolls Series Nos. 133–134 (London: Her Majesty's Stationery Office, 1896–1927)

Calendar of the Fine Rolls, ed. Sir H. C. Maxwell Lyte, Edward III and Richard II, Vols. IV–XI, Rolls Series No. 149 (London: Her Majesty's Stationery Office, 1913–29)

Calendar of Letter-Books Preserved Among the Archives of the City of London, ed. R. R. Sharpe, 12 vols. (London: J. E. Francis, 1899–1912), *Letter-Book F, circa A.D. 1337–1352, Letter-Book G, circa A.D. 1352–1374* and *Letter-Book H, circa A.D. 1375–1399*

Calendar of Letters from the Mayor and Corporation of the City of London, circa A.D. 1350–70, etc., ed. R. R. Sharpe (London: J. C. Francis, 1885)

Calendar of the Patent Rolls, eds. Sir H. C. Maxwell Lyte et. al., Edward III and Richard II, Rolls Series Nos. 162–172 (London: Her Majesty's Stationery Office, 1891–1909)

Calendar of Plea and Memoranda Rolls, ed. A. H. Thomas, 6 vols. (Cambridge: Cambridge University Press, 1926–61), *A.D. 1323–1364* (1926) and *A.D. 1364–1381* (1929)

A Calendar of the Register of Bishop Wolstan de Bransford, Bishop of Worcester, 1339–49, ed. Roy Martin Haines, Worcestershire Historical Society Publications No. 4 (London: Her Majesty's Stationery Office, 1966)

Calendar of Wills Proved and Enrolled in the Court of Husting, London, A.D. 1258–A.D. 1688, ed. R. R. Sharpe, 2 vols. (London: Corporation of London, 1889–90)

Capgrave, John, *The Chronicle of England*, ed. Rev. Francis Charles Hingeston, Rolls Series No. 1 (London, 1858)

Chapters of the Augustinian Canons, ed. Rev. H. E. Salter (Oxford: Canterbury and York Society, 1922)

Chronica Johannis de Reading et Anonymi Cantuariensis, 1346–1367, ed. J. Tait, Historical Series, Vol. XX (Manchester: Victoria University Publications, 1914)

The Chronicle of Adam Usk, 1377–1421, trans. and ed. C. Given-Wilson (Oxford: Clarendon Press, 1997)

The Chronicle of Froissart, trans. Sir John Bourchier, Lord Berners and ed. W. P. Ker, 6 vols. (London: 1901–3)

The Chronicle of Lanercost: 1272–1346, trans. Herbert Maxwell (Cribyn: Llanerch Press, 2001)

Chronicon Abbatiae de Parco Lude. The Chronicle of Louth Park Abbey, etc., ed. E. Venables, trans. A. R. Maddison, Lincolnshire Record Society Publications No. 1 (Horncastle: Lincolnshire Record Society, 1891)

Chronicon Galfridi le Baker de Swynebroke, ed. E. M. Thompson (Oxford: Clarendon Press, 1889)

Clyn, John, *The Annals of Ireland*, ed. R. Butler, Irish Archæological Society Publications No. 12 (Dublin: Irish Archæological Society, 1849)

The Complete Works of John Gower, ed. G. C. Macaulay, 4 vols. (Oxford: Clarendon Press, 1899–1902)

De Orygynale Cronykil of Scotland, etc., ed. D. Laing, Historians of Scotland Vols. II, III and IX, 3 vols. (Edinburgh: Edmonston & Douglas, 1872–9)

English Historical Documents, 1327–1485, ed. A. R. Myers, English Historical Documents, Vol. IV (London: Eyre & Spottiswoode, 1969)

Eulogium (historiarum sive temporis): Chronicon ab orbe condito usque ad annum Domini MCCCLXVI, a monacho quodam Malmesburiensi exaratum, ed. Frank

Scott Haydon, Rolls Series No. 9, 2 vols. (London: Longman, Brown, Green, Longmans, and Roberts, 1858–63)

Fœdera, conventiones, literae, et cujuscunque generis Acta publica, inter Reges Angliæ, et alios quosvis Imperatores, Reges, Pontifices, Principes, vel Communitates, etc., ed. Thomas Rymer, 20 vols. (London: 1704–32)

Fordun, John, *Chronicle of the Scottish Nation,* trans. F. J. H. Skene and ed. W. F. Skene (Edinburgh: Edmonston & Douglas, 1872)

A Fourteenth-Century Chronicle from the Grey Friars at Lynn, ed. A. Gransden, *English Historical Review,* no. 72, 1957

Froissart, Geoffrey, *Chronicles,* selected, ed. and trans. Geoffrey Brereton (Harmondsworth: Penguin Books, 1978)

Geoffrey of Monmouth, *The History of the Kings of Britain,* trans. Lewis Thorpe (Harmondsworth: Penguin Books, 1966)

Gerald of Wales, *The Journey through Wales and The Description of Wales,* trans. Lewis Thorpe (Harmondsworth: Penguin Books, 1978)

Gower, John, *Confessio Amantis,* ed. R. Peck (Toronto: University of Toronto Press, 1980)

Historical Papers and Letters from the Northern Registers, ed. J. Raine, Rolls Series No. 61 (London: Longman & Co., 1873)

Horrox, Rosemary (trans. and ed.), *The Black Death* (Manchester: Manchester University Press, 1994)

Johannis de Fordun, *Chronica Gentis Scotorum,* ed. W. F. Skene and trans. (Vol. IV) F. J. H. Skene, Historians of Scotland Vols. I and IV (Edinburgh: Edmonston & Douglas, 1871)

Johnston, Dafydd, *Galar Y Beirdd: Marwnadau Plant / Poets' Grief: Medieval Welsh Elegies for Children* (Cardiff: TAFOL, 1993)

Knighton's Chronicle, 1337–1396, trans. and ed. G. H. Martin (Oxford: Clarendon Press, 1995)

Langland, William, *Piers Plowman: The C Text,* ed. D. Pearsall (Exeter: University of Exeter Press, 1994)

Langland, William, *Piers the Ploughman,* trans. J. F. Goodridge (Harmondsworth: Penguin Books, 1959)

London Assize of Nuisance 1301–1431: A Calendar, ed. Helena M. Chew and William Kellaway (London: London Record Society, 1973)

London Possessory Assizes. A Calendar, ed. Helena A. Chew, London Record Society Publications, Vol. I (London: London Record Society, 1965)

The Major Latin Works of John Gower. The 'Voice of One Crying' and the 'Tripartite Chronicle', etc., ed. Eric W. Stockton (Seattle: University of Washington Press, 1962)

Medieval English Lyrics. A Critical Anthology, ed. R. L. Davies (London: Faber and Faber, 1963)

Memorials of London and London Life, in the XIIIth, XIVth, and XVth Centuries.

Being a Series of Extracts, Local, Social, and Political, from the Early Archives of the City of London. A.D. 1276–1419, trans. and ed. Henry Thomas Riley (London: Longmans & Co., 1868)

Missale ad usum insignis et præclaræ ecclesiæ Sarum, ed. Francis Dickinson (Burntisland: E Prelo of Pitsligo, 1861–83)

Munimenta Gildhallae Londoniensis: Liber Albus, Liber Custumarum et Liber Horn, ed. Henry Thomas Riley, 4 vols. (London: Longman, 1859–62)

Le Neve, John, Fasti Ecclesiae Anglicanae 1300–1541. Vol VI. Northern province (York, Carlisle and Durham), compiled by B. Jones (London: University of London Institute of Historical Research, 1963).

Parets, Miquel, A Journal of the Plague Year: Diary of the Barcelona Tanner 1651, trans. and ed. James S. Amelang (Oxford: Oxford University Press, 1991)

Petrarch, Francesco, Canzoniere, trans. J. G. Nichols (Manchester: Fyfield Books, 2002)

The Poems of Laurence Minot 1333–1352, ed. Thomas Beaumont James and John Simons (Exeter: University of Exeter Press, 1989)

The Poems of the Pearl Manuscript, ed. Malcolm Andrew and Ronald Waldron, 5th edn (Exeter: University of Exeter Press, 2007)

Polychronicon Ranulphi Higden, Monachi Cestrensis, etc., ed. C. Babington and J. R. Lumby, Rolls Series 41, 9 vols. (London: 1865–86)

The Records of the City of Norwich, ed. Rev. William Hudson and J. C. Tingey, 2 vols. (Norwich and London: Jarrold & Sons, 1906–10)

Regiment de Preservacio a Epidemia o Pestilencia e Mortaldats: Epistola de Maestre Jacme d'Agramont als honrats e discrets, etc. 1348, trans. M. L. Duran-Reynolds and C. E. A. Winslow, Bulletin of the History of Medicine, vol. 23, no. 1, 1949

The Register of John de Grandisson, Bishop of Exeter, A.D. 1327–1369, ed. Rev. F. C. Hingeston-Randolph, 3 vols. (London: George Bell & Sons, 1894–9)

The Register of Ralph of Shrewsbury, Bishop of Bath and Wells, 1329–1363, etc., ed. T. S. Holmes, Somerset Record Society Publications Nos. 9–10, 2 vols. (London: Somerset Record Society, 1896)

Register of the Freemen of the City of York. Vol. I 1272–1558, ed. F. Collins, Publications of the Surtees Society Vol. 96 (Durham: Surtees Society, 1897)

The Register of William Edington, Bishop of Winchester 1346–66, ed. S. F. Hockey, Hampshire Record Series Nos. 7–8, 2 vols. (Winchester: Hampshire Record Office, 1986–7)

Registrum Hamonis Hethe, Diocesis Roffensis, ed. Charles Johnson, 3 vols. (London: Canterbury and York Society, 1914–48)

Registrum Johannis de Trillek, Episcopi Herefordensis, A.D. MCCCXLIV–MCCCLXI, transcribed and ed. Joseph Henry Parry, Canterbury and York Society

Publications Vol. VIII, Nos. 25 and 29, 2 vols. (London: Canterbury and York Society, 1912)

Registrum Simonis de Sudbiria Diocesis Londoniensis AD 1362–1375, ed. R. C. Fowler, Canterbury and York Society Publications, several parts (Oxford: Oxford University Press, 1916–38)

The Riverside Chaucer, ed. Larry D. Benson, 3rd edn (Oxford: Oxford University Press, 1987)

Robertus de Avesbury, *De Gestis Mirabilibus Regis Edwardi Tertii*, ed. Edward Maunde Thompson, Rolls Series No. 93 (London: Her Majesty's Stationery Office, 1889)

Scottish Historical Documents, ed. Gordon Donaldson (Edinburgh: Scottish Academic Press, 1970)

Select Cases from the Coroners' Rolls A.D. 1265–1413, etc., ed. C. S. Gross, Publications of the Selden Society No. 9 (London: Bernard Quaritch, 1896)

Select Cases in the Court of the King's Bench under Edward III, Vol. VI, ed. G. O. Sayles, Selden Society Vol. 82 (London: Bernard Quaritch, 1958–65)

The Sermons of Thomas Brinton, ed. Sister Mary Aquinas Devlin, Camden Society 3rd ser., Nos. 85–6, 2 vols. (London: Offices of the Royal Historical Society, 1954)

Simonsohm, Shlomo (ed.), *The Apostolic See and the Jews. Documents: 492–1404*, Studies and Texts No. 94, Vol. I (Toronto: Pontifical Institute of Medieval Studies, 1988)

Sir Gawain and the Green Knight, trans. Simon Armitage (London: Faber, 2007)

Sir Gawain and the Green Knight, trans. Brian Stone, 2nd edn (Harmondsworth: Penguin Books, 1974)

Statutes of the Realm. From Original Records, etc. 1101–1713, ed. A. Luders et al., 12 vols. (London: 1810–28)

Walsingham, Thomas, *Chronicon Angliæ, ab anno domini 1328 usque ad annum 1388*, etc., ed. Sir Edward Maunde Thompson, Rolls Series No. 64 (London: Longman, 1874)

Walsingham, Thomas, *Gesta abbatum monasterii Sancti Albani*, etc., ed. Henry Thomas Riley, Rolls Series No. 28, 3 vols. (London: Longmans, Green, Reader, and Dyer, 1867–9)

Walsingham, Thomas, *Historia Anglicana*, ed. H. T. Riley, Rolls Series No. 28, 2 vols. (London: Longman, Green, Longman, Roberts, and Green, 1862–4)

Walsingham, Thomas, *The St Albans Chronicle: The Chronica Maiora of Thomas Walsingham. Vol. I. 1376–1394*, ed. John Taylor, Wendy R. Childs and Leslie Watkiss (Oxford: Clarendon Press, 2003)

Wilkins, D. (ed.), *Concilia Magnae Britanniae et Hiberniae*, etc., 4 vols. (London: 1737)

'The Will of William Edington', *Wiltshire Notes and Queries*, vol. 3 (March 1900), pp. 214–21

Wynnere and Wastoure, ed. Stephanie Trigg, Early English Text Society Publications No. 297 (Oxford: Oxford University Press, 1990)

Unpublished Papers, Theses and Dissertations

Arthur, P., 'Black Death and mortality – a reassessment' (unpublished paper, 2007)

Fenwick, Carolyn Christine, 'The English poll taxes of 1377, 1379 and 1381: a critical examination of the returns' (unpublished doctoral thesis, University of London, 1983)

Franklin, P. A., 'Thornbury manor in the age of the Black Death: peasant society, landholding and agriculture in Gloucestershire, 1328–1352' (unpublished doctoral thesis, University of Birmingham, 1982)

Gates, L. A., 'A Glastonbury estate complex in Wiltshire: survival and prosperity in the medieval manor, 1280–1380' (unpublished doctoral thesis, University of Toronto, 1991)

Gooder, Eileen and Arthur Gooder, 'Coventry at the Black Death and afterwards' (unpublished paper, 1965)

Lindley, Philip Graham, 'The monastic cathedral at Ely, c.1320 to c.1350: art and patronage in medieval East Anglia' (unpublished doctoral thesis, University of Cambridge, 1985)

Livingstone, Marilyn, 'Sir John Pulteney's landed estates: the acquisition and management of land by a London merchant' (unpublished MA dissertation, University of London, 1990)

Pawley, Simon, 'Lincolnshire coastal villages and the sea 1300–1600: economy and society' (unpublished doctoral thesis, University of Leicester, 1984)

Prescott, Andrew John, 'Judicial records of the rising of 1381' (unpublished doctoral thesis, London University, 1984)

Saul, A., 'Great Yarmouth in the fourteenth century: a study in trade, politics and society' (unpublished doctoral thesis, University of Oxford, 1975)

Smith, R. M., 'English peasant life-cycles and socio-economic networks: a quantitative geographical case study' (unpublished doctoral thesis, Cambridge University, 1975)

Wilson, Christopher, 'The origins of the perpendicular style and its development to circa 1360' (unpublished doctoral thesis, London University, 1979)

Secondary Sources

Aberth, John, 'The Black Death in the diocese of Ely: the evidence of the bishop's register', *The Journal of Medieval History*, vol. 21, no. 3 (September 1995), pp. 257–87

Achtman, M., et al., 'Microevolution and history of the plague bacillus, *Yersinia pestis*', *Proceedings of the National Academy of Sciences of USA*, vol. 101, issue 51 (21 December 2004), pp. 17837–42

Achtman, M., K. Zurth, G. Morell, et al., '*Yersinia pestis*, the cause of the plague, is a recently emerged clone of *Y. pseudotuberculosis*', *Proceedings of the National Academy of Sciences of USA*, vol. 96 (1999), pp. 14043–8

Ackroyd, Peter, *London: The Biography* (London: Chatto & Windus, 2000)

Alcock, N. W., 'The medieval peasant at home: England, 1250–1550', *International Medieval Research*, vol. 12 (2003), pp. 449–68

Allan, J. P. and S. R. Blaylock, 'The west front I: the structural history of the west front', in Kelly, Francis (ed.), *Medieval Art and Architecture at Exeter Cathedral*, pp. 94–115

Allen, Martin, 'The volume of the English currency, 1158–1470', *Economic History Review*, vol. 54, no. 4 (November 2001), pp. 595–611

Allison, K. J., 'The Lost Villages of Norfolk', *Norfolk Archaeology*, vol. 31, pt 1 (1955), pp. 116–62

Andersen, M., 'The Fear of Black Death', *UNISA Medieval Studies*, vol. 5 (1995), pp. 36–50

Ariès, Philippe, *The Hour of Our Death*, trans. Helen Weaver (London: Allen Lane, 1981)

Arthur, P., 'Per pestilentiam: the Bishop of Winchester's pipe roll for 1348–9', *The Hatcher Review*, vol. 5, no. 46 (1998), pp. 50–57

Ashford, L. J., *History of the Borough of High Wycombe* (London: Routledge & Kegan Paul, 1960)

Aston, T. H. (ed.), *Social Relations and Ideas: Essays in Honour of R. H. Hilton* (Cambridge: Cambridge University Press, 1983)

Aston, T. H. and C. H. E. Philpin (eds.), *The Brenner Debate: Agrarian Class Structure and Economic Development in Pre-Industrial Europe* (Cambridge: Cambridge University Press, 1985)

Austin, David, 'Barnard Castle, Co. Durham. First interim report: excavations in the town ward, 1974–6', *Journal of the British Archaeological Association*, vol. 132 (1979), pp. 50–72

—, 'Barnard Castle, Co. Durham. Second interim report: excavations in the inner ward, 1976–8', *Journal of the British Archaeological Association*, vol. 133 (1980), pp. 74–85

Aylmer, G. E. and R. Cant (eds.), *A History of York Minster* (Oxford: Clarendon Press, 1977)

Badham, Sally, 'Monumental brasses and the Black Death: a reappraisal', *The Antiquaries Journal*, vol. 80 (2000), pp. 207–47

Baker, Timothy, *Medieval London* (London: Cassell, 1970)

Bailey, Mark D., 'Blowing up bubbles: some new demographic evidence for the fifteenth century?', *Journal of Medieval History*, vol. 15, no. 4 (December 1989), pp. 347–58

—, 'Coastal fishing off south east Suffolk in the century after the Black Death', *Proceedings of the Suffolk Institute of Archaeology and History*, vol. 37, no. 2 (1990), pp. 102–14

—, 'Peasant welfare in England: 1290–1348', *Economic History Review*, vol. 51, no. 2 (May 1998), pp. 223–51

—, *The Bailiff's Minute Book of Dunwich, 1404–1430* (Woodbridge: Boydell Press, 1992)

Baillie, Mike, *New Light on the Black Death. The Cosmic Connection* (Stroud: Tempus, 2006)

Baldwin, Frances Elizabeth, *Sumptuary Legislation and Personal Regulation in England*, Johns Hopkins University Studies in Historical and Political Science Series 44, No. 1 (Baltimore: The Johns Hopkins Press, 1926)

Ballard, A., 'The manors of Witney, Brightwell, and Downton', in Vinogradoff (ed.), *Oxford Studies in Social and Legal History, Vol. V* (1916), pp. 181–220

Barbé, L. A., 'The Plague in Scotland', *Chambers' Journal*, 7th ser., vol. 4 (1914), pp. 234–7

Barnes, Sir Joshua, *The History of That Most Victorious Monarch Edward IIId King of England and France*, etc. (Cambridge: John Hayes, 1688)

Barrow, G. W. S., *Scotland and Its Neighbours in the Middle Ages* (London: The Hambledon Press, 1992)

Bartsocas, Christos S., 'Two fourteenth-century Greek descriptions of the "Black Death"', *Journal of History of Medicine and Allied Sciences*, vol. 21, no. 4 (1966), pp. 394–400

Bean, J. M. W., 'The Black Death: the crisis and its social and economic consequences', in Williman (ed.), *Black Death*, pp. 23–38

—, 'Plague, population and economic decline in England in the later Middle Ages', *Economic History Review*, 2nd Ser., vol. 15, no. 3 (1963), pp. 423–37

Beardwood, Alice, *Alien Merchants in England 1350 to 1377: Their Legal and Economic Position* (Cambridge, Mass.: The Medieval Academy of America, 1931)

Beattie, Cordelia, 'The problem of women's work identities in post-Black Death England', in Bothwell, Goldberg and Ormrod (eds.), *Problem of Labour in Fourteenth-Century England*, pp. 1–19

Beidler, Peter G. 'The plague and Chaucer's Pardoner', *Chaucer Review*, vol. 16, no. 3 (Winter 1982), pp. 257–69

Bell, R. D. and M. W. Beresford et al., *Wharram: A Study of Settlement on the Yorkshire Wolds, Vol. III – Wharram Percy: The Church of St Martin*, Society for Medieval Archaeology Monograph Series No. 11 (London: Society for Medieval Archaeology, 1987)

Benedictow, Ole, *The Black Death, 1346–1353: The Complete History* (Woodbridge: Boydell Press, 2004)

Bennett, Judith M., 'Medieval peasant marriage: an examination of marriage license fines in *Liber Gersumarum*', in Raftis (ed.), *Pathways to Medieval Peasants*, pp. 193–246

Bennett, Michael, 'The impact of the Black Death on English legal history', *Australian Journal of Law and Society*, vol. 11 (1995), pp. 191–203

—, 'Richard II, Henry Yevele and a new royal mansion on the Thames', *Antiquaries Journal*, vol. 82 (2002), pp. 343–9

Beresford, M. W., *Lost Villages of England* (London: Lutterworth Press, 1954)

Beresford, Maurice and John Hurst, *Wharram Percy: Deserted Medieval Village* (London: B. T. Batsford/English Heritage, 1990)

— (eds.), *Deserted Medieval Villages: Studies* (London: Lutterworth Press, 1971)

Bernardo, Aldo S., 'The plague as meaning in Boccacio's "Decameron"', in Williman (ed.), *Black Death*, pp. 39–64

Beveridge, W. H., 'Wages in the Winchester manors', *Economic History Review*, vol. 7, no. 1 (November 1936), pp. 22–43

—, 'Westminster wages in the manorial era', *Economic History Review*, 2nd Ser., vol. 8, no. 1 (1955–6), pp. 18–35

Biddick, K., 'Medieval English peasants and market involvement', *Journal of Economic History*, vol. 45 (1985), pp. 823–31

Billson, Charles James, *Mediæval Leicester* (Leicester: Edgar Backus, 1920)

Binski, Paul, 'John the Smith's grave', in L'Engle, Susan and Gerald B. Guest (eds.), *Tributes to Jonathan J. G. Alexander: The Making and Meaning of Illuminated Medieval & Renaissance Manuscripts, Art & Architecture* (London: Harvey Miller, 2006), pp. 386–93

—, *Medieval Death: Ritual and Representation* (London: British Museum Press, 1996)

Biraben, Jean Noël, *Les Hommes et la peste en France et dans les pays européens et méditerranéens*, 2 vols. (Paris: Mouton, 1975–6)

Blair, John, 'John Smith of Brightwell Baldwin', *Monumental Brass Society Bulletin*, no. 81 (May 1999), p. 431

Blake, Norman (ed.), *The Cambridge History of the English Language*, 6 vols. (Cambridge: Cambridge University Press, 1992–2001), *Vol. II: 1066–1476* (1992)

Blashill, Thomas, *Sutton-in-Holderness. The Manor, the Berewic, and the Village Community* (Hull: William Andrews & Co., 1896)

Bleukx, Koenraad, 'Was the Black Death (1348–9) a real plague epidemic? England as a case study', in Verbeke, W., et al. (eds.), *Serta Devota in Memoriam Guillelmi Lourdaux* (Louvain: Leuven University Press, 1995), pp. 65–113

Bois, Guy, *The Crisis of Feudalism: Economy and Society in Eastern Normandy c.1300–1550* (Cambridge: Cambridge University Press, 1984)

Bolton, Jim, 'The world upside down', in Ormrod and Lindley (eds.), *Black Death in England*, pp. 17–78

Bonser, Wilfrid, 'Epidemics during the Anglo-Saxon period', *Journal of the British Archaeological Association*, 3rd ser., vol. 9 (1944), pp. 48–71

Borsch, Stuart J., *The Black Death in Egypt and England: A Comparative Study* (Austin, Texas: University of Texas Press, 2005)

Bothwell, James, P. J. P. Goldberg and W. M. Ormrod, *The Problem of Labour in Fourteenth-Century England* (Woodbridge: York Medieval Press, 2000)

Boucher, Charles E., 'The Black Death in Bristol', *Transactions of the Bristol and Gloucestershire Archaeological Society*, vol. 9, no. 60 (1938), pp. 31–46

Bowsky, William M., 'The impact of the Black Death upon Sienese government and society', *Speculum*, vol. 39, no.1 (1964), pp. 1–34

— (ed.), *The Black Death: A Turning Point in History?* (Huntington, NY / London: Holt, Reinhart and Winston, 1978)

Boyle, J. R., *The Lost Towns of the Humber*, etc. (Hull: A. Brown & Sons, 1889)

Brady, Karl and Connie Kelleher, 'Swords, plague and pestilence', *Archaeology Ireland*, vol. 14, no. 3 (Autumn 2000), pp. 8–11

Bray, R. S., *Armies of Pestilence: The Effects of Pandemics on History* (Cambridge: The Lutterworth Press, 1996)

Bridbury, A. R., 'The Black Death', *Economic History Review*, 2nd ser., vol. 26 (1973), pp. 557–92

—, Review of *Plague, Population and the English Economy: 1348–1530* by John Hatcher, *Population Studies*, vol. 31 (1977), pp. 606–7

Briggs, Chris, 'Credit and the peasant household economy in England before the Black Death: evidence from a Cambridgeshire manor', *International Medieval Research*, vol. 12 (2003), pp. 231–48

Britnell, R. H., 'The Black Death in English towns', *Urban History*, vol. 21 (1994), pp. 195–210

—, *The Commercialisation of English Society, 1000–1500* (Cambridge: Cambridge University Press, 1993)

—, 'Feudal reaction after the Black Death in the palatinate of Durham', *Past and Present*, vol. 128 (1990), pp. 28–47

—, 'Forstall, forestalling and the Statute of Forestallers', *English Historical Review*, vol. 102, no. 402 (January 1987), pp. 89–102

—, *The Winchester Pipe Rolls and Medieval English Society* (Woodbridge: The Boydell Press, 2003)

Britton, C. E., *A Meteorological Chronology to A.D. 1450*, Meteorological Office Geophysical Memoirs No. 70 (London: Meteorological Office, 1937)

Brooke, C. N. L., 'Earliest times to 1485', in Matthews, W. R. and W. M. Atkins (eds.), *A History of St Paul's Cathedral* (London: Baker, 1964), pp. 1–99

Brooke, Christopher, *A History of Gonville and Caius College Cambridge* (Woodbridge: The Boydell Press, 1985)

Brown, Andrew, 'Review of *The Black Death and Pastoral Leadership: The Diocese of Hereford in the Fourteenth Century* William J. Dohar', *English Historical Review*, vol. 112, no. 447 (June 1997), pp. 718–19

Burne, A. H., *The Battlefields of England*, new edn (London: Penguin Books, 2002)

Burns, J. H. (ed.), *The Cambridge History of Medieval Political Thought, c.350–c.1450* (Cambridge: Cambridge University Press, 1988)

Butcher, A. F., 'English urban society and the revolt of 1381', in Hilton and Aston (eds.), *English Rising of 1381*, pp. 84–111

Campbell, Anna Montgomery, *The Black Death and Men of Learning*, History of Science Society Publications No. 1 (New York: Columbia University Press, 1992)

Campbell, B. M. S., 'Agricultural progress in medieval England: some evidence from eastern Norfolk', *Economic History Review*, 2nd ser., vol. 36 (February 1983), pp. 26–46

—, 'Arable productivity in medieval England: some evidence from Norfolk', *Journal of Economic History*, vol. 43, no. 2 (June 1983), pp. 379–404

—, 'Matching supply to demand: crop production and disposal by English demesnes in the century of the Black Death', *Journal of Economic History*, vol. 57, no. 4 (1997), pp. 827–58

—, 'Population pressure, inheritance, and the land market in a fourteenth-century peasant community', in Smith (ed.), *Land, Kinship and Life-Cycle*, pp. 87–135

—, 'A unique estate and a unique source: the Winchester Pipe Rolls in perspective', in Britnell (ed.), *Winchester Pipe Rolls and Medieval English Society*, pp. 21–43

—, *Before the Black Death: Studies in the 'Crisis' of the Early Fourteenth Century* (Manchester: Manchester University Press, 1991)

Campbell, B. M. S., K. C. Bartley and J. P. Power, 'The demesne-farming systems of post-Black Death England: a classification', *Agricultural History Review*, vol. 44, no. 2 (1996), pp. 131–79

Canning, J. P., 'Introduction: politics, institutions and ideas, c.1150–c.1450', in Burns (ed.), *Cambridge History of Medieval Political Thought*, pp. 341–66

Carleton Williams, E., 'Mural painting of the three living and the three dead in England', *Journal of the British Archaeological Association*, 3rd ser., vol. 7 (1942), pp. 31–40

Carney, James, 'Literature in Irish, 1169–1534', in Cosgrove (ed.), *New History of Ireland*, pp. 688–707

Carpentier, Elisabeth, 'Autour de la peste noire: épidémies dans l'histoire du XIVe siècle', *Annales: Economies, Sociétés, Civilisations*, vol. 17 (1962), pp. 1062–92

Cartwright, Frederick and Michael Biddiss, *Disease and History: The Influence of Disease in Shaping the Great Events of History*, 2nd edn (Stroud: Sutton, 2000)

Chadwyck Healey, Charles E. H., *The History of the Part of West Somerset Comprising the Parishes of Luccombe, Selworthy, Stoke Pero, Porlock, Culbone and Oare* (London: Henry Sotheran & Co., 1901)

Chanteau, Suzanne, et al., 'Development and testing of a rapid diagnostic test for bubonic and pneumonic plague', *The Lancet*, vol. 361 (18th January 2003), pp. 211–16

Childs, Wendy and Timothy O'Neill, 'Overseas trade', in Cosgrove (ed.), *New History of Ireland*, pp. 492–524

Christakos, George and Ricardo A. Olea, 'New space–time perspectives on the propagation characteristics of the Black Death epidemic and its relation to bubonic plague', *Stochastic Environmental Research and Risk Assessment*, vol. 19 (2005), pp. 307–14

Christakos, George, Ricardo A. Olea, Marc L. Serre and Hwa-Lung Yu, *Interdisciplinary Public Health Reasoning and Epidemic Modelling: The Case of the Black Death* (New York: Springer, 2005)

Christakos, George, Ricardo A. Olea and Hwa-Lung Yu, 'Recent results on the spaciotemporal modelling and comparative analysis of Black Death and bubonic plague modelling', *Public Health*, vol. 121 (2007), pp. 700–20

Christie, A. B., *Infectious Diseases: Epidemiology and Clinical Practice*, 3rd edn (Edinburgh and London: E. & S. Livingstone, 1969)

Clark, Elaine, 'Debt litigation in a late medieval English vill', in Raftis (ed.), *Pathways to Medieval Peasants*, pp. 247–79

—, 'Medieval labor law and the English courts', *American Journal of Legal History*, vol. 27 (1983), pp. 330–53

—, 'Social welfare and mutual aid in the medieval countryside', *Journal of British Studies*, vol. 33 (1994), pp. 381–406

Cohn, Samuel K., *The Black Death Transformed: Disease and Culture in Early Renaissance Europe* (London: Arnold, 2002)

—, 'Review of *Scotland's Black Death* by Karen Jillings', *Scottish Economic and Social History*, vol. 23, pt 1 (2003), pp. 48–50

Collins, Frances and J. Oliver, 'Lomer: a study of a deserted medieval village', *Proceedings of the Hampshire Field Club & Archaeological Society*, vol. 28 (1971), pp. 67–76

Colvin, H. M. (ed.), *A History of the King's Works: The Middle Ages*, 2 vols (London: Her Majesty's Stationery Office, 1963)

Connell, C. W., 'Western views of the origin of the "Tartars": an example of the influence of myth in the second half of the thirteenth century', *The Journal of Medieval and Renaissance Studies*, vol. 3, no. 1 (Spring 1973), pp. 115–37

Cook, G. C. (ed.), *Manson's Tropical Diseases* (London: W. B. Saunders, 1996)

Cook, G. H., *Old S. Paul's Cathedral: A Lost Glory of London* (London: Phoenix House, 1955)

Cosgrove, Art (ed.), *A New History of Ireland, Vol. II: Medieval Ireland, 1169–1534* (Oxford: Clarendon Press, 1987)

Cottle, B., *The Triumph of English 1350–1400* (London: Blandford Press, 1969)

Coulton, G. G., *The Black Death* (London: Ernest Benn, 1929)

—, 'A medieval inscription in Acle church', *Norfolk and Norwich Archaeological Society*, vol. 20, pt 2, pp. 141–8

Courtenay, William J., 'The effect of the Black Death on English higher education', *Speculum*, vol. 55, no. 4 (1980), pp. 696–714

Cowley, F. G., *The Monastic Order in South Wales, 1066–1349* (Cardiff: University of Wales Press, 1977)

Creighton, Charles, *A History of Epidemics in Britain From A.D. 664 to the Extinction of the Plague*, 2 vols. (Cambridge: Cambridge University Press, 1891)

Crook, J. M., 'Winchester Cathedral and the Black Death', *The Hatcher Review*, vol. 5, no. 46 (1998), pp. 43–9

— (ed.), *Winchester Cathedral: Nine Hundred Years 1093–1993* (Chichester: Phillimore, 1993)

Crook, J. M. and Y. Kusaba, 'The perpendicular remodelling of the nave: problems and interpretations', in Crook (ed.), *Winchester Cathedral*, pp. 215–30

Cullum, P. H., 'Boy/man into clerk/priest: the making of the late-medieval clergy', in McDonald and Ormrod (eds.), *Rites of Passage*, pp. 51–65

Davies, J. Silvester, *A History of Southampton*, etc. (Southampton: Gilbert & Co., 1883)

Davies, R. A., 'The effect of the Black Death on the parish priests of the medieval diocese of Coventry and Lichfield', *Historical Research*, vol. 62, no. 147 (February 1989), pp. 85–90

Davies, R. R., *Conquest, Coexistence and Change: Wales 1063–1415* (Oxford: Clarendon Press/University of Wales Press, 1987)

—, *Lordship and Society in the March of Wales, 1282–1400* (Oxford: Clarendon Press, 1978)

Davis, David E., 'The scarcity of rats and the Black Death: an ecological history', *Journal of Interdisciplinary History*, vol. 16 (1986), pp. 455–70

Davis, Paul S. and Susan Lloyd-Fern, *Lost Churches of Wales and the Marches* (Stroud: Alan Sutton, 1990)

Deaux, George, *The Black Death, 1347* (London: Hamish Hamilton, 1969)

Derbes, Vincent J., 'De Mussis and the Great Plague of 1348: a forgotten episode of bacteriological warfare', *Journal of the American Medical Association*, vol. 196, no. 1 (1966), pp. 179–82

Derksen, John, 'Review of *After the Black Death: A Social History of Early Modern Europe*, 2nd edn, by George Huppert', *Near East School of Theology Theological Review*, vol. 23, no. 2 (November 2002), pp. 152–3

Devlin, Sister Mary Aquinas, 'Bishop Thomas Brunton and his sermons', *Speculum*, vol. 14, no. 3 (July 1939), pp. 324–44

—, 'The chronology of bishop Brunton's sermons', *Proceedings of the Modern Language Association*, vol. 51, no. 1 (March 1936), pp. 300–302

DeWitte, Sharon N. and James W. Wood, 'Selectivity of Black Death mortality with respect to pre-existing health', *Proceedings of the National Academy of Sciences*, vol. 105, no. 5 (January 2008), pp. 1436–41

Dickinson, Philip G. M., 'Little Wratting Church', *Proceedings of the Suffolk Institute of Archaeology*, vol. 27, pt 1 (1956), pp. 34–6

Dickson, Gary, 'The flagellants of 1260 and the crusades', *Journal of Medieval History*, vol. 15, no. 3 (September 1989), pp. 227–68

Ditchburn, David and Alastair J. Macdonald, 'Medieval Scotland, 1100–1560', in Houston, R. A. and W. W. J. Knox (eds.), *The New Penguin History of Scotland* (London: Allen Lane, 2001), pp. 96–181

Dobson, R. B. (ed.), *The Peasants' Revolt of 1381*, 2nd edn (London: Macmillan, 1983)

Dodd, J. Phillip, 'The population of Frodsham manor, 1349–50', *Transactions of the Historic Society of Lancashire and Cheshire*, vol. 131 (1981–2), pp. 21–33

Dodds, Ben, 'Durham Priory tithes and the Black Death between the Tyne and the Tees', *Northern History*, vol. 39, no. 1 (March 2002), pp. 5–24

Dohar, William J., *The Black Death and Pastoral Leadership: The Diocese of Hereford in the Fourteenth Century* (Philadelphia: University of Pennsylvania Press, 1995)

Dols, Michael W., 'Al-Manbiji's "Report of the Plague": a treatise on the plague of 1362–64 in the Middle East', in Williman (ed.), *Black Death*, pp. 65–75

—, *The Black Death in the Middle East* (Princeton, NJ: Princeton University Press, 1977)

Donaldson, A. M., A. K. G. Jones and D. J. Rackham, 'Barnard Castle, Co. Durham. A dinner in the great hall: report on the contents of a fifteenth-century drain', *Journal of the British Archaeological Association*, vol. 133 (1980), pp. 86–96

Down, Kevin, 'Colonial society and economy in the high Middle Ages', in Cosgrove (ed.), *New History of Ireland*, pp. 439–91

Drancourt, Michel, et al., 'Detection of 400-yr-old *Yersinia pestis* DNA in human dental pulp: an approach to the diagnosis of ancient septicaemia', *Proceedings of the National Academy of Sciences*, vol. 95 (1998), pp. 12637–40

Drancourt, Michel, Linda Houhamdi and Didier Raoult, '*Yersinia pestis* as a telluric, human ectoparasite-borne organism', *Lancet Infectious Diseases*, vol. 6 (2006), pp. 234–41

Draper, Peter and Richard K. Morris, 'The development of the east end of Winchester Cathedral from the 13th to the 16th centuries', in Crook (ed.), *Winchester Cathedral*, pp. 177–92

Douthwaite, William Ralph, *Gray's Inn, Its History and Associations*, etc. (London: Reeves and Turner, 1886)

Duffy, Eamon, *The Stripping of the Altars: Traditional Religion in England c.1400–c.1580* (New Haven, Conn./London: Yale University Press, 1992)

Duffy, Mark, *Royal Tombs of Medieval England* (Stroud: Tempus, 2003)

Duncan, C. J. and S. Scott, 'What caused the Black Death', *Postgraduate Medical Journal*, vol. 81, no. 955 (May 2005), pp. 315–20

Duncan, Kirsty, 'The possible influence of climate on the bubonic plague in Scotland', *Scottish Geographical Magazine*, vol. 108, no. 1 (April 1992), pp. 29–34

Duncan, S. R., S. Scott and C. J. Duncan, 'Time series analysis of oscillations in a population model: the effects of plague, pestilence and famine', *Journal of Theoretical Biology*, vol. 158, no. 3 (7th October 1992), pp. 293–312

Dunn, Alison, 'Review of *English Law in the Age of the Black Death, 1348–1381* by Robert C. Palmer', *The Modern Law Review*, vol. 59, no. 1 (January 1996), pp. 149–53

Dyer, Christopher C., 'The English medieval village community and its decline', *Journal of British Studies*, vol. 33, no. 4 (1994), pp. 407–29

—, *Lords and Peasants in a Changing Society: The Estates of the Bishopric of Worcester, 680–1540* (Cambridge: Cambridge University Press, 1980)

—, *Making a Living in the Middle Ages: The People of Britain 850–1520* (London: Penguin, 2003)

—, 'The rising of 1381 in Suffolk', *Proceedings of the Suffolk Institute of Archaeology and History*, vol. 36 (1988), pp. 277–87

—, 'The social and economic background to the rural revolt of 1381', in Hilton and Aston (eds.), *English Rising of 1381*, pp. 9–42

—, *Standards of Living in the Later Middle Ages: Social Change in England c.1200–1520* (Cambridge: Cambridge University Press, 1989)

—, 'Work ethics in the fourteenth century', in Bothwell, Goldberg and Ormrod (eds.), *Problem of Labour in Fourteenth-Century England*, pp. 21–41

Eames, Elizabeth, *English Medieval Tiles* (London: British Museum Publications, 1985)

Ecclestone, Martin, 'Mortality of rural landless men before the Black Death: the Glastonbury head-tax lists', *Local Population Studies*, vol. 63 (Autumn 1999), pp. 6–29

Edwards, C. M. Hay, *A History of Clifford's Inn*, etc. (London: Thomas Werner Laurie, 1912)

Ell, S. R., 'Interhuman transmission of medieval plague', *Bulletin of the History of Medicine*, vol. 54 (1980), pp. 497–510

Elliott-Binns, L. E., *Medieval Cornwall* (London: Methuen & Co., 1955)

Fairbrother, J. R, *Faccombe Netherton: Excavations of a Saxon and Medieval Manorial Complex*, British Museum Occasional Paper No. 74 (London: British Museum, 1990)

Faith, Rosamond Jane, 'The 'Great Rumour' of 1377 and peasant ideology', in Hilton and Aston (eds.), *English Rising of 1381*, pp. 43–73

Farmer, D. L., 'Prices and wages', in Hallam, H. E. (ed.), *The Agrarian History of England and Wales, Vol. II: 1042–1350* (Cambridge: Cambridge University Press, 1988), pp. 716–817

—, 'Prices and wages, 1350–1500', in Miller, E. (ed.), *The Agrarian History of England and Wales, Vol. III: 1350–1500* (Cambridge: Cambridge University Press, 1991), pp. 431–525

Fawcett, Richard, *Scottish Medieval Churches: Architecture and Furnishings* (Stroud: Tempus, 2002)

Finberg, H. P. R. (ed.), *The Agrarian History of England and Wales*, 8 vols. (Cambridge: Cambridge University Press, 1967–2000), *Vol. II, 1042–1350*, ed. H. E. Hallam (1988) and *Vol. III, 1348–1500*, ed. E. Miller (1991)

Fisher, John L., 'The Black Death in Essex', *Essex Review*, vol. 52 (1943), pp. 13–20

Fishwick, Henry, *A History of Lancashire* (London: Elliot Stock, 1894)

Fletcher, J. M. J., 'The Black Death in Dorset, 1348–1349', *Proceedings of Dorset Natural History Antiquarian Field Club*, vol. 43 (1922), pp. 1–14

Foa, Anna, *The Jews of Europe after the Black Death*, trans. Andrea Glover (Berkeley, Calif.: University of California Press, 2000)

Fowler, Kenneth, *The King's Lieutenant: Henry of Grosmont, First Duke of Lancaster, 1310–61* (London: Elek, 1969)

Fletcher, H. L. V., *Herefordshire* (London: Robert Hale, 1948)

France, R. Sharpe, 'A History of the Plague in Lancashire', *Transactions of the Historic Society of Lancashire and Cheshire*, vol. 90 (1938), pp. 1–175

French, Roger, 'Introduction: the "long fifteenth century" of medical history', in French, Roger, et al. (eds.), *Medicine from the Black Death to the French Disease* (Aldershot: Ashgate, 1998), pp. 1–5

Fryde, E. B., 'Some business transactions of York merchants John Goldbeter,

William Acastre and partners, 1336–1349', *Borthwick Papers No. 29* (York: St Anthony's Press, 1966), pp. 3–21

Gani, R. 'Epidemiologic determinants for modelling pneumonic plague outbreaks', *Emerging Infectious Diseases*, vol. 10 (2004), pp. 608–14

Gardiner, Dorothy, *Historic Haven: The Story of Sandwich* (Derby: Pilgrim Press, 1954)

Gasquet, Francis Aidan, *The Great Pestilence, A.D. 1348–9, Now Commonly Known as the Black Death* (London: Simpkin, Marshall & Co., 1893), 2nd edn, *The Black Death of 1348 and 1349* (London: George Bell & Sons, 1908)

—, *The Old English Bible, and other essays*, etc., 2nd edn (London: George Bell & Sons, 1908)

Gibb, Andrew, *Glasgow: The Making of a City* (London: Croom Helm, 1983)

Gilbert, M. T. P., et al., 'Absence of *Yersinia pestis*-specific DNA in human teeth from five European excavations of putative plague victims', *Microbiology*, vol. 150 (2004), pp. 341–54

Gillett, Edward, *A History of Grimsby* (London: Oxford University Press for the University of Hull, 1970)

Goldberg, Jeremy, 'Introduction', in Ormrod and Lindley (eds.), *The Black Death in England*, pp. 1–15

Goldberg, P. J. P., 'Female labour, service and marriage in the late medieval urban north', *Northern History*, vol. 22 (1986), pp. 18–38

—, 'Urban identity and the poll taxes of 1377, 1379, and 1381', *Economic History Review*, 2nd ser., vol. 43 (1990), pp. 194–216

—, *Women, Work and Life-Cycle in a Medieval Economy: Women in York and Yorkshire c.1300–1520* (Oxford: Clarendon Press, 1992)

Gottfried, Robert S., *The Black Death: Natural and Human Disaster in Medieval Europe* (New York/London: Free Press/Collier Macmillan, 1983)

—, *Doctors and Medicine in Medieval England, 1340–1530* (Princeton, NJ/Guildford: Princeton University Press, 1986)

—, 'Plague, public health, and medicine in late medieval England', in Bulst, N. and R. Delort (eds.), *Maladies et société*, (Paris: Editions du Centre National de la Recherche Scientifique, 1989), pp. 336–65

Grainger, Ian, Duncan Hawkins, Lynne Cowal and Richard Mikulski, *The Black Death cemetery, East Smithfield, London*, MoLAS Monograph No. 43 (London: Museum of London Archaeology Service, 2008)

Green, B. and R. M. R. Young, *Norwich – The Growth of a City. An Exhibition at the Castle Museum, Norwich, 6th July–29th September, 1963* (Norwich: Norwich Museums Committee, 1963)

Green, Valentine, *The History and Antiquities of the City and Suburbs of Worcester*, 2 vols. (London: G. Nicol, 1796)

Grimwood, C. G. and S. A. Kay, *History of Sudbury, Suffolk* (Sudbury: The Authors, 1952)

Gwynn, Aubrey, 'The Black Death in Ireland', *Studies: An Irish Quarterly Review of Letters, Philosophy and Science*, vol. 24 (1935), pp. 25–42

Gwynn, Aubrey and R. Neville Hadcock, *Medieval Religious Houses: Ireland* (London: Longmans, 1970)

Haddock, David D. and Lynne Kiesling, 'The Black Death and property rights', *The Journal of Legal Studies*, vol. 31, no. 2, pt 2 (June 2002), pp. S545–S588

Haines, Charles Reginald, *Dover Priory: A History of the Priory of St Mary the Virgin, and St Martin of the New Work*, etc. (Cambridge: Cambridge University Press, 1930)

Harding, Vanessa, 'Burial choice and burial location in late medieval London', in Basset, Steven (ed.), *Death in Towns* (Leicester: Leicester University Press, 1992), pp. 119–35

Hargreaves, P., 'Seignorial reaction and peasant responses: Worcester Priory and its peasants after the Black Death', *Midland History*, vol. 24 (1999), pp. 53–78

Harper-Bill, Christopher, 'The English church and English religion after the Black Death', in Ormrod and Lindley (eds.), *Black Death in England*, pp. 79–124

Harris, James C., 'The plague of Ashdod', *Archives of General Psychiatry*, vol. 63 (March 2006), pp. 244–5

Harrison, David, *The Bridges of Medieval England: Transport and Society, 400–1800* (Oxford: Clarendon Press, 2004)

Harriss, G. L., *King, Parliament and Public Finance in Medieval England to 1369* (Oxford: Clarendon Press, 1975)

Hart, Evelyn, 'The Creative Years: 1220–1535', in Shortt, Hugh (ed.), *City of Salisbury* (London: Phoenix House, 1957), pp. 28–53

Harvey, Barbara, 'Introduction', in Campbell, Bruce M. S. (ed.), *Before the Black Death*, pp. 1–24

Harvey, Barbara and Jim Oeppen, 'Patterns of morbidity in late medieval England: a sample from Westminster Abbey, c.1320–c.1420', *Economic History Review*, 2nd ser., vol. 54, no. 2 (May 2001), pp. 215–39

Harvey, John H., *English Mediaeval Architects: A Biographical Dictionary down to 1550*, etc., rev. edn (Gloucester: Alan Sutton, 1984)

—, *The Mediæval Architect* (London: Wayland (Publishers), 1972)

—, *The Perpendicular Style, 1330–1485* (London: B. T. Batsford, 1978)

Harvey, P. D. A. (ed.), *Manorial Records of Cuxham, Oxfordshire, circa 1200–1359*, Royal Commission on Historical Manuscripts Joint Publication No. 23 and Oxfordshire Record Society Publications No. 50 (London: Her Majesty's Stationery Office, 1976)

— (ed.), *The Peasant Land Market in Medieval England* (Oxford: Clarendon, 1984)

Hatcher J., 'England in the aftermath of the Black Death', *Past and Present*, vol. 144 (1994), pp. 3–35

—, *Plague, Population and the English Economy, 1348–1530* (London: Macmillan Education, 1977)

—, *Rural Economy and Society in the Duchy of Cornwall, 1300–1500* (Cambridge: Cambridge University Press, 1970)

Hawkins, Duncan, 'The Black Death and the new London cemeteries of 1348', *Antiquity*, vol. 64 (1990), pp. 637–42

Hay-Edwards, C. M., *A History of Clifford's Inn* (London: Thomas Werner Laurie, 1912)

Hecker, J. F. C., *The Epidemics of the Middle Ages*, trans. B. G. Babington, 3rd edn (London: Trübner & Co., 1859)

Henneman, J. B., 'The Black Death and royal taxation in France, 1347–1351', *Speculum*, vol. 43 (1968), pp. 309–49

Henry, Françoise and Geneviève Marsh-Micheli, 'Manuscripts and illuminations, 1169–1603', in Cosgrove (ed.), *New History of Ireland*, pp. 780–815

Herbert, Florentia C., 'The history of Wrockwardine: the lords of the manor', *Transactions of the Shropshire Archaeology and Natural History Society*, 4th ser., vol. 1 (1911), pp. 191–231

Herlihy, David, *The Black Death and the Transformation of the West* (Cambridge, Mass./London: Harvard University Press, 1997)

Hill, Sir (I. W.) Francis, *Mediæval Lincoln* (Cambridge: Cambridge University Press, 1948)

Hilton, R. H., *The Decline of Serfdom in Medieval England* (London: Macmillan, 1969)

—, 'Introduction', in Hilton and Aston (eds.), *English Rising of 1381*, pp. 1–8

—, 'Peasant movements in England before 1381', *Economic History Review*, 2nd ser., vol. 2 (1949–50), pp. 117–136

Hilton, R. H. and T. H. Aston (eds.), *The English Rising of 1381* (Cambridge: Cambridge University Press, 1987)

Hinton, David A., *Gold and Gilt, Pots and Pins: Possessions and People in Medieval Britain* (Oxford: Oxford University Press, 2005)

Hirshleifer, Jack, 'Disaster and Recovery: The Black Death in Western Europe', *The International Library of Critical Writings in Economics*, vol. 178, no. 1 (2004), pp. 3–33

Hirst, L. Fabian, *The Conquest of Plague: A Study of the Evolution of Epidemiology* (Oxford: Clarendon Press, 1953)

Hockey, S. F., *Insula Vecta: The Isle of Wight in the Middle Ages* (Chichester: Phillimore, 1982)

Hollingsworth, T. H., *Historical Demography* (Cambridge: Cambridge University Press, 1969)

Holmes, G. A., *The Estates of the Higher Nobility in Fourteenth-Century England* (Cambridge: Cambridge University Press, 1957)

Holt, Richard A., 'Gloucester in the century after the Black Death', *Transactions of the Bristol and Gloucestershire Archaeological Society*, vol. 103 (1985), pp. 149–61

Holt, Richard and Gervase Rosser (eds.), *The Medieval Town: A Reader in English Urban History 1200–1540* (London: Longman, 1990)

Honeybourne, Marjorie, 'The reconstructed map of London under Richard II', *London Topographical Record*, vol. 22 (1965), pp. 29–76

—, *A Sketch Map of London under Richard II*, London Topographical Society Publication No. 93 (London: London Topographical Society, 1960)

Hope, Valerie, *My Lord Mayor: Eight Hundred Years in London's Mayoralty* (London: Weidenfeld & Nicolson in association with the Corporation of London, 1989)

Hope, W. H., *The History of the London Charterhouse from Its Foundation until the Suppression of the Monastery* (London: Society for the Propagation of Christian Knowledge, 1925)

Howell, Cicely, *Land, Family and Inheritance in Transition: Kibworth Harcourt 1280–1700* (Cambridge: Cambridge University Press, 1983)

Hurst, J. G., 'The changing medieval village in England', in Raftis (ed.), *Pathways to Medieval Peasants*, pp. 27–64

Hyatte, Reginalde, 'Boccaccio's *Decameron* and de Ferrière's *Songe de Pestilence*', *The Explicator*, vol. 53, no. 1 (Fall 1994), pp. 3–5

Inglesby, Thomas V., et al., 'Plague as a biological weapon', *Medical and Public Health Management: Journal of the American Medical Association*, vol. 283, no. 17 (3rd May 2000), pp. 2281–90

James, Tom Beaumont, 'The Black Death: a turning point for Winchester?', *The Hatcher Review*, vol. 5, no. 46 (1998), pp. 32–42

—, 'The Black Death in Berkshire and Wiltshire', *The Hatcher Review*, vol. 5, no. 46 (1998), pp. 11–20

—, 'The Black Death in Hampshire', *Hampshire Papers*, no. 18, (December 1999), pp. 1–28

—, 'Introduction & Conclusion: The Black Death in Wessex', *The Hatcher Review*, vol. 5, no. 46 (1998), pp. 4–10 and 58–62

—, *The Palaces of Medieval England, c.1050–1550: Royalty, Nobility, the Episcopate and Their Residences from Edward the Confessor to Henry VIII* (London: Seaby, 1990)

—, 'Years of Pestilence', *British Archaeology*, issue 61 (October 2001), pp. 8–13

Jessopp, A., 'The Black Death in East Anglia', in *Coming of the Friars*, pp. 166–261

—, *The Coming of the Friars and Other Historic Essays*, 5th edn (London: T. Fisher Unwin, 1922 (first published 1889))

Jillings, Karen, *Scotland's Black Death: The Foul Death of the English* (Stroud: Tempus, 2003)

Johnson, A. H. (ed.), *The History of the Worshipful Company of the Drapers of London*, etc., 5 vols. (Oxford: Clarendon Press, 1914–22)

Jones, E. D., 'Going round in circles: some new evidence for population in the later Middle Ages', *Journal of Medieval History*, vol. 15, no. 4 (December 1989), pp. 329–46

Jones, Peter Murray, 'Thomas Fayreford: an English fifteenth-century medical practitioner', in French, Roger, et al. (eds.), *Medicine from the Black Death to the French Disease* (Aldershot: Ashgate, 1998), pp. 156–83

Jordan, W. C., *The Great Famine: Northern Europe in the Early Fourteenth Century* (Princeton, NJ/Chichester: Princeton University Press, 1996)

Karlsson, Gunnar, 'Plague without rats: the case of fifteenth-century Iceland', *Journal of Medieval History*, vol. 22, no. 3 (September 1996), pp. 263–84

Keen, M. H., *England in the Later Middle Ages: A Political History* (London: Methuen & Co. Ltd, 1973)

Keene, D. J., *Survey of Medieval Winchester* (Oxford: Clarendon, 1985)

Keene, Derek, 'A new study of London before the Great Fire', *Urban History Yearbook* (Leicester: Leicester University Press, 1984), pp. 11–21

Keil, Ian, 'The chamberer of Glastonbury Abbey in the fourteenth century', *Proceedings of the Somerset Archaeological Society*, vol. 107 (1963), pp. 79–92

Kelly, Francis (ed.), *Medieval Art and Architecture at Exeter Cathedral*, British Archaeological Association Conference Transactions No. 11 (Leeds: British Archaeological Association, 1991)

Kelly, Maria, *The Great Dying: The Black Death in Dublin* (Stroud: Tempus, 2003)

—, *A History of the Black Death in Ireland*, 2nd edn (Stroud: Tempus, 2004)

Kennedy, Hugh, *Muslim Spain and Portugal: A Political History of al-Andalus* (London: Longman, 1996)

Kershaw, I., 'The Great Famine and agrarian crisis in England, 1315–1322', *Past and Present*, no. 59 (May 1973), pp. 3–50

Kieckhefer, Richard A., 'Radical tendencies in the flagellant movement of the mid-fourteenth century', *Journal of Medieval and Renaissance Studies*, vol. 4, no. 2 (Fall 1974), pp. 157–76

Kiple, F. F. (ed.), *Plague, Pox and Pestilence* (London: Weidenfeld & Nicolson, 1997)

Kitsikopoulos, Harry, 'The impact of the Black Death on peasant economy in England, 1350–1500', *Journal of Peasant Studies*, vol. 29, no. 2 (January 2002), pp. 71–90

—, 'Standards of living and capital formation in pre-plague England: a peasant budget model', *Economic History Review*, vol. 53 (2000), pp. 237–61

—, 'Technological change in medieval England: a critique of the neo-

Malthusian argument', *Proceedings of the American Philosophical Society*, vol. 144, no. 4 (December 2000), pp. 397–449

Kleineke, Hannes, 'Carleton's book: William FitzStephen's "Description of London" in a late fourteenth-century common-place book', *Historical Research*, vol. 74, no. 183 (2001), pp. 117–26

Knight, Charles Brunton, *A History of the City of York from A.D. 71 (foundation of Eboracum) – A.D. 1901* (York and London: Herald Printing Works, 1944)

Knowles, David, *The Religious Orders in England*, 3 vols. (Cambridge: Cambridge University Press, 1950–59)

Knowles, David and W. F. Grimes, *Charterhouse. The Medieval Foundation in the Light of Recent Discoveries.* (London: Longmans, Green & Co., 1954)

Knowles, John, 'The periodic plagues of the second half of the fourteenth century and their effects on the art of glass-painting', *Archaeological Journal*, vol. 79 (1922), pp. 343–52

Kyriacou, Demetrios N., et al., 'Clinical predictors of bioterrorism-related inhalational anthrax', *The Lancet*, vol. 364 (2004), pp. 449–52

Lambert, Henry Charles Miller, *History of Banstead in Surrey*, 2 vols. (Oxford: Oxford University Press, 1912, 1931)

Le Strange, Hamon, *Le Strange Records: A Chronicle of the Early Le Stranges . . . A.D. 1100–1310* (London: Longmans, Green & Co., 1916)

Lea, Frederic Simcox, *The Royal Hospital and Collegiate Church of Saint Katherine near the Tower*, etc. (London: Longmans, Green, and Co., 1878)

Lerner, Robert E., 'The Black Death and western European eschatological mentalities', in Williman (ed.), *Black Death*, pp. 77–105

Lethaby, W. R., *Westminster Abbey and the King's Craftsmen: A Study of Mediæval Building* (London: Duckworth & Co., 1906)

Levett, A. E., 'The Black Death on the estates of the see of Winchester', in Vinogradoff (ed.), *Oxford Studies in Social and Legal History, Vol. V* (1916), pp. 1–220

Lindley, Phillip G., 'The Black Death and English art: a debate and some assumptions', in Ormrod and Lindley (eds.), *Black Death in England*, pp. 125–46

—, 'The medieval sculpture of Winchester Cathedral', in Crook (ed.), *Winchester Cathedral*, pp. 109–10

Livi-Bacci, Massimo, 'The nutrition–mortality link in past times: a comment', *Journal of Interdisciplinary History*, vol. 14, no. 2 (Autumn 1983), pp. 293–8

Lloyd, T. H., 'Overseas trade and the English money supply in the fourteenth century', in Mayhew, N. J. (ed.), *Edwardian Monetary Affairs (1279–1344)*, pp. 96–124

Lock, R., 'The Black Death in Walsham-le-Willows', *Proceedings of the Suffolk Institute of Archaeology and History*, vol. 37, pt 4 (1992), pp. 316–37

Lomas, Richard A., 'The Black Death in County Durham', *Journal of Medieval History*, vol. 15, no. 2 (June 1989), pp. 127–40

Longman, William, *The History of the Life and Times of Edward the Third*, 2 vols. (London: Longmans, Green, and Co., 1869)

Lynch, Michael, *Scotland: A New History*, new ed. (London: Pimlico, 1992)

Mackinnon, James, *The History of Edward the Third, 1327–1377* (London: Longmans & Co., 1900)

Marks, Richard, *Image and Devotion in Late Medieval England* (Stroud: Sutton, 2004)

—, *Stained Glass in England during the Middle Ages* (London: Routledge, 1993)

Marr, John S. and James B. Kiracofe, 'Was the Huey Cocolizti a haemorrhagic fever?', *Medical History*, vol. 44, no. 3 (July 2000), pp. 341–62

Massingberd, W. O., 'The Black Death and the Lincolnshire clergy', *Lincoln Diocesan Magazine*, vol. 20, no. 219, September 1904, pp. 137–8

Mate, Mavis E., 'The agrarian economy after the Black Death: the manors of Canterbury Cathedral, 1348–91', *Economic History Review*, vol. 37, no. 3 (1984), pp. 341–54

—, *Daughters, Wives and Widows after the Black Death: Women in Sussex, 1350–1535* (Woodbridge: Boydell Press, 1998)

Matthew, H. C. G. and Brian Harrison (eds.), *Oxford Dictionary of National Biography*, new edn (Oxford: Oxford University Press, 2004)

Mayhew, N. J., 'Numismatic evidence and falling prices in the fourteenth century', *Economic History Review*, 2nd ser., vol. 27, no. 1 (1974), pp. 1–15

—, 'Population, money supply, and the velocity of circulation in England 1300–1700', *Economic History Review*, vol. 48, no. 2 (1995), pp. 238–57

— (ed.), *Edwardian Monetary Affairs (1279–1344): Proceedings of a Symposium Held in Oxford, August 1976*, British Archaeological Reports 36 (Oxford: British Archaeological Reports, 1977)

McDonald, Nicola and W. M. Ormrod (eds.), *Rites of Passage: Cultures of Transition in the Fourteenth Century* (Woodbridge: York Medieval Press, 2004)

McGarvie, M., 'Mells during the Black Death', *Somerset and Dorset Notes and Queries*, vol. 24 (2000), pp. 409–13

McNeill, W. H., *Plagues and Peoples* (Garden City, NY: Anchor Press, 1976)

Megson, Barbara E., *Such Goodly Company: A Glimpse of the Life of the Bowyers of London 1300–1600* (London: Worshipful Company of Bowyers, 1993)

—, 'Mortality among London citizens in the Black Death', *Medieval Prosopography*, vol. 19 (1998), pp. 125–33

Meiss, Millard, *Painting in Florence and Siena after the Black Death: The Arts, Religion and Society in the Mid-Fourteenth Century* (Princeton: Princeton University Press, 1951)

Milbourn, T. (rev. and ed.), *The Vintners' Company, Their Muniments, Plate, and Eminent Members, with Some Account of the Ward of Vintry* (London, 1888)

Miller, Edward and John Hatcher, *Medieval England: Rural Society and Economic Change, 1086–1348* (London: Longman, 1978)

—, *Medieval England: Towns, Commerce and Crafts, 1086–1348* (London: Longman, 1995)

Moalem, Sharon, 'Survival of the sickest', *New Scientist*, issue 2591 (17th February 2007), pp. 42–5

Moberly, G. H., *Life of William of Wykeham* (Winchester: Warren & Son, 1887)

Mogdridge, Jeremy, 'Anthrax and bioterrorism: are we prepared?', *The Lancet*, vol. 364 (2004), pp. 393–5

Moody, T. W., F. X. Martin and F. J. Burne (eds.), *A New History of Ireland, Vol. IX: Maps, Genealogies, Lists* (Oxford: Clarendon Press, 1984)

Moor, C., *Historical Notes Concerning the Deanery of Corringham, in the Archdeaconry of Stow, and the Diocese of Lincoln*, etc. (Gainsborough: C. Caldicott, 1897)

Morris, Christopher, 'The plague in Britain: Review of *A History of Bubonic Plague in the British Isles* by John F. D. Shrewsbury', *Historical Journal*, vol. 14, no. 1 (1971), pp. 205–15

Mortimer, Ian, *The Perfect King: The Life of Edward III, Father of the English Nation* (London: Jonathan Cape, 2006)

Mullan, John, 'The transfer of customary land on the estates of the bishop of Winchester between the Black Death and the plague of 1361', in Britnell (ed.), *Winchester Pipe Rolls and Medieval English*, pp. 81–107

Myers, A. R., *London in the Age of Chaucer* (Norman: University of Oklahoma Press, 1972)

Newton, K. C., *Thaxted in the Fourteenth Century. An Account of the Manor and Borough*, Essex Record Office Publications No. 33 (Chelmsford: Essex County Council, 1960)

Nicholls, Kenneth W., 'Gaelic society and economy in the high Middle Ages', in Cosgrove (ed.), *New History of Ireland*, pp. 397–438

—, *Gaelic and Gaelicised Ireland in the Middle Ages* (Dublin: Gill & Macmillan, 1972)

Nicholson, R., *Scotland: The Later Middle Ages* (Edinburgh: Oliver & Boyd, 1974)

Nightingale, Pamela, *A Medieval Mercantile Community: The Grocers' Company and the Politics and Trade of London, 1000–1485* (New Haven, Conn. / London: Yale University Press, 1995)

Nilson, Ben, *Cathedral Shrines of Medieval England* (Woodbridge: Boydell, 1998)

Nohl, Johannes, *Der schwarze Tod. The Black Death: A Chronicle of the Plague Compiled . . . from Contemporary Sources*, trans. C. H. Clarke (London: George Allen & Unwin, 1926)

Norman, Philip, 'Sir John Pulteney and his two residences in London', *Archaelogia*, vol. 57, pt 2 (1901), pp. 257–84

Norris, John, 'East or West? The geographic origin of the Black Death', *Bulletin of History of Medicine*, vol. 51, no. 1 (Spring 1977), pp. 1–24

Norton, Christopher, David Park and Paul Binski, *Dominican Painting in East Anglia: The Thornham Parva Retable and the Musée de Cluny Frontal* (Woodbridge: The Boydell Press, 1987)

O'Connor, Stephen, 'Finance, diplomacy and politics: royal service by two London merchants in the reign of Edward III', *Institute of Historical Research* (Oxford: Blackwell, 1994), pp. 18–39

Odgers, W. Blake (ed.), *Six Lectures on the Inns of Court and of Chancery*, etc. (London: Macmillan & Co., 1912)

Olea, Ricardo A. and George Christakos, 'Duration of urban mortality for the fourteenth-century Black Death epidemic', *Human Biology*, vol. 77, no. 3 (June 2005), pp. 291–303

Oman, Charles, *The Great Revolt of 1381*, 2nd edn (Oxford: Clarendon Press, 1969)

Orme, Nicholas, 'Mortality in fourteenth-century Exeter', *Medical History*, vol. 132, no. 2 (April 1988), pp. 195–203

Orme, Nicholas and Margaret Webster, *The English Hospital 1070–1570* (New Haven, Conn./London: Yale University Press, 1995)

Ormrod, Mark, 'The royal nursery: a household for the younger children of Edward III', *English Historical Review*, vol. 120 (2005), pp. 398–415

Ormrod, Mark and Philip Lindley (eds.), *The Black Death in England* (Stamford: Paul Watkins, 1996)

Ormrod, W. M., 'Coming to kingship: boy kings and the passage to power in fourteenth-century England', in McDonald and Ormrod (eds.), *Rites of Passage*, pp. 31–49

—, 'Edward III and the recovery of royal authority in England, 1340-1360', *History*, vol. 72 (1987), pp. 4–19

—, 'The English government and the Black Death of 1348–49', in Ormrod (ed.), *England in the Fourteenth Century*, pp. 175–88

—, 'An experiment in taxation: the English Parish Subsidy of 1371', *Speculum*, vol. 63 (1988), pp. 59–82

—, 'The Peasants' Revolt and the Government of England', *The Journal of British Studies*, vol. 29, no. 1 (January 1990), pp. 1–30

—, 'The personal religion of Edward III', *Speculum*, vol. 64, no. 4 (1989), pp. 849–77

—, 'The politics of pestilence: government in England after the Black Death', in Ormrod and Lindley (eds.), *Black Death in England*, pp. 147–79

—, 'The Protecolla Rolls and English government finance, 1353–1364', *English Historical Review*, vol. 102, no. 404 (July 1987), pp. 622–32

—, *The Reign of Edward III: Crown and Political Society in England 1327–1377*, updated edn (Stroud: Tempus, 2000)

— (ed.), *England in the Fourteenth Century: Proceedings of the 1985 Harlaxton Symposium* (Woodbridge: Boydell Press, 1986)

Owen, Hugh and John Brickdale Blakeway, *History of Shrewsbury*, 2 vols. (London: Harding, Lepard & Co., 1825)

Owst, Gerald R., *Literature and Pulpit in Medieval England: A Neglected Chapter in the History of English Letters* etc. (Cambridge: Cambridge University Press, 1933)

Packe, Michael, *King Edward III*, ed. L. C. B. Seaman (London: Routledge & Kegan Paul, 1983)

Page, F. M., *The Estates of Crowland Abbey: A Study of Manorial Organisation* (Cambridge: Cambridge University Press, 1934)

Page, Mark, 'The peasant land market on the estate of the Bishop of Winchester before the Black Death', in Britnell (ed.), *Winchester Pipe Rolls and Medieval English*, pp. 61–80

Palmer, Robert C., *English Law in the Age of the Black Death, 1348–1381: A Transformation of Governance and Law* (Chapel Hill, NC: University of Carolina Press, 1993)

Pantin, W. A., *The English Church in the Fourteenth Century*, etc. (Cambridge: Cambridge University Press, 1955)

Parsons, E. J. S. and F. M. Stenton, *The Map of Great Britain circa 1360, Known as the Gough Map. An Introduction to the Facsimile* etc. (Oxford: Oxford University Press, 1970)

Pearce, David, *London's Mansions: The Palatial Houses of the Nobility* (London: B. T. Batsford, 1986)

Pearson, Sarah, 'Houses, shops, and storage: building evidence from two Kentish ports', *International Medieval Research*, vol. 12 (2003), pp. 409–31

Pendrill, Charles, *London Life in the Fourteenth Century* (London: G. Allen & Unwin, 1925)

Pevsner, Nikolaus, *Hertfordshire*, 2nd edn, rev. Bridget Cherry (Harmondsworth: Penguin, 1977)

—, *Wiltshire*, 2nd edn, rev. Bridget Cherry (Harmondsworth: Penguin, 1975)

Phythian-Adams, Charles, *Desolation of a City: Coventry and the Urban Crisis of the Late Middle Ages* (Cambridge: Cambridge University Press, 1979)

Pickard, Ransom, *The Population and Epidemics of Exeter in Pre-Census Times* (Exeter: James Townsend & Sons, 1947)

Platt, Colin, *King Death: The Black Death and Its Aftermath in Late-Medieval England* (London: University College London Press, 1996)

Polzer, Joseph, 'Aspects of the fourteenth-century iconography of death and the plague', in Williman (ed.), *Black Death*, pp. 107–30

Poos, L. R., *A Rural Society after the Black Death: Essex 1350–1525* (Cambridge: Cambridge University Press, 1991)

—, 'The social context of the Statute of Labourers enforcement', *Law and History Review*, vol. 1 (1983), pp. 27–52

Poos, L. R. and R. M. Smith, '"Legal windows onto historical populations?" Recent research on demography and the manor court in medieval England', *Law and History Review*, vol. 2 (1984), pp. 128–52

—, '"Shades Still on the Window". A reply to Zvi Razi', *Law and History Review*, vol. 3 (1985), pp. 409–29

Post, John D., 'Climatic change and historical discontinuity: a review', *Journal of Interdisciplinary History*, vol. 14, no. 1 (Summer 1983), pp. 153–60

Postan, M. M., *Essays on Medieval Agriculture and General Problems of the Medieval Economy* (Cambridge: Cambridge University Press, 1973)

—, *The Medieval Economy and Society. An Economic History of Britain, 1100–1500* (London: Weidenfeld & Nicolson, 1972)

—, 'Some economic evidence of declining population in the later Middle Ages', *Economic History Review*, 2nd ser., vol. 2 (1949–50), pp. 221–89

Prestwich, M. C., 'Currency and the economy of early fourteenth-century England', in Mayhew (ed.), *Edwardian Monetary Affairs (1279–1344)*, pp. 45–58

Prestwich, Michael, *The Three Edwards: War and State in England, 1272–1377* (London: Weidenfeld & Nicolson, 1980)

Pusch, Carsten M., et al., 'Yersinial F1 antigen and the cause of the BD', *The Lancet Infectious Diseases*, vol. 4, no. 8 (August 2004), pp. 487–8

Putnam, B.H., *The Enforcement of the Statutes of Labourers During the First Decade after the Black Death, 1349–1359* (New York: Columbia College, 1908)

— 'The justices of labourers in the fourteenth century', *English Historical Review*, vol. 21, no. 83 (July 1906), pp. 517–38

—, 'The transformation of the keepers of the peace into the justices of the peace, 1327–1380', *Transactions of the Royal Historical Society*, 4th ser., vol. 12 (1929), pp. 19–48

—, 'Wage-laws for priests after the Black Death', *American Historical Review*, vol. 21 (1915–16), pp. 12–32

Quiney, Anthony, *Town Houses of Medieval Britain* (New Haven, Conn./London: Yale University Press, 2003)

Raftis, J. A., *The Estates of Ramsey Abbey: A Study in Economic Growth and Organization*, etc., Pontifical Institute of Mediæval Studies, Studies and Texts No. 3 (Toronto: Pontifical Institute of Mediæval Studies, 1957)

—, *Pathways to Medieval Peasants*, Papers in Mediæval Studies No. 2 (Toronto: Pontifical Institute of Mediæval Studies, 1981)

—, *Tenure and Mobility. Studies in the Social History of the Mediæval English*

Village, Pontifical Institute of Mediæval Studies, Studies and Texts No. 8 (Toronto: Pontifical Institute of Mediæval Studies, 1964)

—, *Warboys: Two Hundred Years in the Life of an English Medieval Village*, Pontifical Institute of Mediæval Studies, Studies and Texts No. 29 (Toronto: Pontifical Institute of Mediæval Studies, 1974)

Rahtz, P. A. and L. Watts, *Wharram: A Study of Settlement on the Yorkshire Wolds, Vol. IX – The North Manor Area and North-West Enclosure*, York University Archaeological Publications No. 11 (York: University of York, 2004)

Ranger, Terence and Paul Slack (eds.), *Epidemics and Ideas: Essays on the Historical Perception of Pestilence* (Cambridge: Cambridge University Press, 1992)

Ratsitorahina, Mahery, et al., 'Epidemiological and diagnostic aspects of the outbreak of pneumonic plague in Madagascar', *The Lancet*, vol. 355 (8 January 2000), pp. 111–13

Razi, Zvi, *Life, Marriage and Death in a Medieval Parish: Economy and Demography in Halesowen 1270–1400* (Cambridge: Cambridge University Press, 1991)

—, 'The Toronto School's reconstruction of medieval peasant society: a critical view', *Past and Present*, vol. 85, (November 1979), pp. 141–57

Razi, Zvi and Richard Smith (eds.), *Medieval Society and the Manor Court* (Oxford: Clarendon Press, 1996)

Rees, William, 'The Black Death in England and Wales as exhibited in manorial documents', *Proceedings of the Royal Society of Medicine*, vol. 16, pt 2, no. 34 (1923), pp. 27–45

—, 'The Black Death in Wales', *Transactions of the Royal Historical Society*, 4th ser., vol. 3 (1920), pp. 115–35

Riddle, John M., *Contraception and Abortion from the Ancient World to the Renaissance* (Cambridge, Mass./London: Harvard University Press, 1992)

—, 'Oral contraceptives and early-term abortificants during classical antiquity and the Middle Ages', *Past and Present*, vol. 132 (1991), pp. 3–32

Rigby, S. H., 'Gendering the Black Death: women in later medieval England', *Gender & History*, vol. 12, no. 3 (November 2000), pp. 745–54

—, *Medieval Grimsby: Growth and Decline* (Hull: The University of Hull Press, 1993)

Ritchie, Carson, 'The Black Death at St Edmund's Abbey', *Proceedings of the Suffolk Institute of Archaeology*, vol. 27, pt 1 (1956), pp. 47–50

Robo, Etienne, 'The Black Death in the hundred of Farnham', *English Historical Review*, vol. 44 (1929), pp. 560–72

Rogers, Alan, *The Medieval Buildings of Stamford*, Stamford Survey Group Report No. 1 (Nottingham: Department of Adult Education, University of Nottingham, 1970)

—, *The Making of Stamford* (Leicester: Leicester University Press, 1965)

Rogers, J. E. Thorold, 'England before and after the Black Death', *Fortnightly Review*, vol. 3, no. 14 (1865)

Rosser, Gervase, *Medieval Westminster* (Oxford: Clarendon Press, 1989)

Rushton, Neil S., 'Spatial aspects of the almonry site and the changing priorities of poor relief at Westminster Abbey', *Architectural History*, vol. 45 (2002), pp. 66–87

Russell, Josiah Cox, *British Medieval Population* (Albuquerque: University of New Mexico Press, 1948)

Russell, R. C., 'Effects of pestilence and plague, 1315–1385', *Comparative Studies in Society and History*, vol. 8, no. 4 (1966), 464–73

Salter, H. E., *Mediæval Oxford*, Oxford Historical Society Publications No. 100 (Oxford: Clarendon Press, 1936)

Saltmarsh, John, 'Plague and economic decline in England in the later Middle Ages', *Cambridge Historical Journal*, vol. 7 (1941), pp. 23–41

Saul, Nigel, *Richard II* (New Haven, Conn./London: Yale University Press, 1997)

Saunders, J. J., *The History of the Mongol Conquests* (London: Routledge & Kegan Paul, 1971)

Schevill, Ferdinand, *History of Florence, from the Founding of the City through the Renaissance* (London: G. Bell and sons, 1937)

Schofield, John, *Medieval London Houses* (New Haven, Conn./London: Yale University Press, 1995)

Schofield, John and Alan Vince, *Medieval Towns* (London: Leicester University Press, 1994)

Scott, Susan and Christopher J. Duncan, *Biology of Plagues: Evidence from Historical Populations* (Cambridge: Cambridge University Press, 2001)

—, *Return of the Black Death: the World's Greatest Serial Killer* (Chichester: Wiley, 2004)

Scrope, Sir Richard with Sir N. H. Nicholas, *The Scrope and Grosvenor Controversy, etc.*, 2 vols. (London: The Author, 1832)

Seebohm, Frederic, 'The Black Death and its place in English History', *Fortnightly Review*, vol. 2, 8 (1865), pp. 149–60

Sheppard, Francis, *London: A History* (Oxford: Oxford University Press, 1998)

Sherlock, David, *Medieval Drawings and Writings in Ashwell Church, Hertfordshire* (Ashwell: Ashwell Parish Church, 1978)

Shrewsbury, John F. D., *A History of Bubonic Plague in the British Isles* (Cambridge: Cambridge University Press, 1970)

Siraisi, Nancy, 'Introduction', in Williman (ed.), *Black Death*, pp. 9–22

Slack, Paul, 'The Black Death past and present, 2: some historical problems', *Transactions of the Royal Society of Tropical Medicine & Hygiene*, vol. 83, no. 4 (July–August 1989), pp. 461–3

—, 'Introduction', in Ranger and Slack (eds.), *Epidemics and Ideas*, pp. 1–20

Sloan, A. W., 'The Black Death in England', *South African Medical Journal*, vol. 59 (25 April 1981), pp. 646–50

Sloane, Barney and Gordon Malcolm, *Excavations at the Priory of the Order of the Hospital of St John of Jerusalem, Clerkenwell, London*, MOLAS Monograph No. 20 (London: Museum of London Archaeology Service, 2004)

Smith, R. M. (ed.), *Land, Kinship and Life-Cycle* (Cambridge: Cambridge University Press, 1984)

Smythe, Robert, *Historical Account of Charter-house*, etc. (London, 1808)

Stamper, P. A. and R. A. Croft, *Wharram: A Study of Settlement on the Yorkshire Wolds, Vol. VIII – The South Manor Area*, York University Archaeological Publications No. 10 (York: University of York, 2000)

Staples, Andy, 'The medieval farming year' (1999), http://www.witheridge-historical-archive.com/medieval-year.htm

Steinhoff, Judith, 'Artistic working relationships after the Black Death: a Sienese compagnia, c.1350–1363(?)', *Renaissance Studies*, vol. 14, no. 1 (March 2000), pp. 1–45

Stenton, F. M., 'Road system of medieval England', *Economic History Review*, vol. 7, no. 1 (1936), pp. 1–21

Stewart, J., *The Nestorian Missionary Enterprise: The Story of a Church on Fire* (Edinburgh: T&T Clark, 1928)

Stone, David, 'Medieval farm management and technological mentalities: Hinderclay before the Black Death', *Economic History Review*, vol. 54, no. 4 (2001), pp. 612–38

—, 'The productivity of hired and customary labour: evidence from Wisbech Barton in the fourteenth century', *Economic History Review*, vol. 50, no. 4 (1997), pp. 640–56

Stow, *A Survay of London, Contayning the Originall, Antiquity, Increase, Moderne Estate, and Description of that Citie*, etc. (London: J. Windet, 1603)

Stronach, Simon, 'The evolution of a medieval Scottish Manor at Perceton, near Irvine, North Ayrshire', *Medieval Archaeology*, vol. 48 (2004), pp. 143–66

Sumption, Jonathan, *Trial by Battle. The Hundred Years War, Vol. I* (London: Faber and Faber, 1990)

—, *Trial by Fire. The Hundred Years War, Vol. II* (London: Faber, 1999)

The Survey of London, Vol. XLVI: South and East Clerkenwell (New Haven, Conn./London: Yale University Pres, 2008)

The Survey of London: Charterhouse (in preparation)

Theilmann, John and Frances Cate, 'A plague of plagues: the problem of plague diagnosis in medieval England', *Journal of Interdisciplinary History*, vol. 27, no. 3 (Winter 2007), pp. 371–93

Thomas, Christopher, Barney Sloane and Christopher Phillpotts, *Excavations at the Priory and Hospital of St Mary Spital, London* (London: Museum of London Archaeology Service, 1997)

Thompson, A. Hamilton, 'The pestilences of the fourteenth century in the diocese of York', *The Archaeological Journal*, vol. 71 (1914), pp. 97–154

—, 'Registers of John Gynewell, Bishop of Lincoln, for the years 1347–1350', *The Archaeological Journal*, vol. 68 (1911), pp. 301–60

Thornton, Christopher C., 'The level of arable productivity on the bishopric of Winchester's manor of Taunton, 1283–1348', in Britnell (ed.), *Winchester Pipe Rolls and Medieval English*, pp. 109–37

Thurley, Simon, *Lost Buildings of Britain* (London: Viking, 2004)

Tighe, Robert Richard and James Edward Davis, *Annals of Windsor, being a History of the Castle and Town*, etc., 2 vols. (London: Longman & Co., 1853)

Titow, Jan Zbigniew, 'Lost rents, vacant holdings and the contraction of peasant cultivation after the Black Death', *Agricultural History Review*, vol. 42, no. 2 (1994), pp. 97–114

Toms, Elsie, *The Story of St Albans*, rev. edn (Luton: White Crescent Press, 1975)

Tristram, E. W., *English Wall Painting of the Fourteenth Century* (London: Routledge & Kegan Paul, 1955)

Tuck, J. A., 'The emergence of a northern nobility, 1250–1400', *Northern History*, vol. 22 (1986), pp. 1–17

—, 'Nobles, Commons and the Great Revolt of 1381', in Hilton and Aston (eds.), *English Rising of 1381*, pp. 194–212

—, 'War and society in the medieval North', *Northern History*, vol. 21 (1985), pp. 33–52

Twigg, Graham, *The Black Death: A Biological Reappraisal* (London: Batsford Academic and Educational, 1984)

—, 'The Black Death: a problem of population-wide infection', *Local Population Studies*, vol. 71 (Autumn 2003), pp. 40–52

—, 'Bubonic plague: doubts and diagnoses', *Journal of Medical Microbiology*, vol. 42 (1995), pp. 383–5

Veale, Elspeth M., *The English Fur Trade in the Later Middle Ages*, 2nd edn, London Record Society Publications Vol. XXXVIII (London: London Record Society, 2003)

The Victoria History of the County of Bedfordshire, 3 vols. (1904–14)

The Victoria History of the County of Berkshire, 4 vols. (1906–27)

The Victoria History of the County of Buckinghamshire, 4 vols. (1905–28)

The Victoria History of the County of Cambridgeshire and the Isle of Ely, 10 vols. (1938–2002)

The Victoria History of the County of Cheshire, 4 vols. (1987–2005)

The Victoria History of the County of Cornwall, 1 vol. (1906–24)

The Victoria History of the County of Cumberland, 2 vols. (1901–5)

The Victoria History of the County of Derbyshire, 2 vols. (1905–7)

The Victoria History of the County of Dorset, 2 vols. (1908–68)

The Victoria History of the County of Durham, 4 vols. (1905–2005)

The Victoria History of the County of Essex, 10 vols. (1907–2001)

The Victoria History of the County of Gloucester, 9 vols. (1907–2001)

The Victoria History of the County of Hampshire, 5 vols. (1900–1912)

The Victoria History of the County of Herefordshire, 1 vol. (1908)

The Victoria History of the County of Hertfordshire, 4 vols. (1902–23)

The Victoria History of the County of Huntingdonshire, 3 vols. (1926–38)

The Victoria History of the County of Kent, 3 vols. (1908–32)

The Victoria History of the County of Lancashire, 8 vols. (1906–14)

The Victoria History of the County of Leicestershire, 5 vols. (1907–58)

The Victoria History of the County of Lincolnshire, 1 vol. (1906)

The Victoria History of the County of London, 1 vol. (1909)

The Victoria History of the County of Middlesex, 12 vols. (1911–2004)

The Victoria History of the County of Norfolk, 2 vols. (1901–6)

The Victoria History of the County of Northamptonshire, 6 vols. (1902–2007)

The Victoria History of the County of Nottinghamshire, 2 vols. (1906–10)

The Victoria History of the County of Oxfordshire, 15 vols. (1907–2006)

The Victoria History of the County of Rutland, 2 vols. (1908–35)

The Victoria History of the County of Shropshire, 7 vols. (1908–85)

The Victoria History of the County of Somerset, 9 vols. (1906–2004)

The Victoria History of the County of Staffordshire, 13 vols. (1908–2007)

The Victoria History of the County of Suffolk, 2 vols. (1907–11)

The Victoria History of the County of Surrey, 4 vols. (1902–12)

The Victoria History of the County of Sussex, 8 vols. (1905–97)

The Victoria History of the County of Warwickshire, 8 vols. (1904–69)

The Victoria History of the County of Wiltshire, 17 vols. (1904–2002)

The Victoria History of the County of Worcestershire, 4 vols. (1901–26)

The Victoria History of the County of Yorkshire, 3 vols. (1907–25)

The Victoria History of the County of Yorkshire: The City of York (1961)

The Victoria History of the County of Yorkshire (East Riding), 7 vols. (1969–2002)

The Victoria History of the County of Yorkshire (North Riding), 2 vols. (1914–23)

Vinogradoff, P. (ed.), *Oxford Studies in Social and Legal History*, 9 vols. (Oxford: Clarendon Press, 1909–27), *Vol. V* (1916)

Walsh, K., *A Fourteenth-Century Scholar and Primate: Richard FitzRalph in Oxford, Avignon and Armagh* (Oxford: Clarendon, 1981)

Walter Bynum, Caroline, '"Disease and death in the Middle Ages" – a review of *The Black Death: Natural and Human Disaster in Medieval Europe* by Robert S. Gottfried', *Culture, Medicine and Psychiatry*, vol. 9 (1985), pp. 97–102

Walter, John and Roger Schofield (eds.), *Famine, Disease and Social Order in Early Modern Society* (Cambridge: Cambridge University Press, 1989)

Watt, J. A., 'The Anglo-Irish colony under strain', in Cosgrove (ed.), *New History of Ireland*, pp. 352–96

—, 'Approaches to the history of fourteenth-century Ireland', in ibid., pp. 303–13

—, 'Gaelic polity and cultural identity', in ibid., pp. 314–51

Watts, D. G., 'The Black Death in Dorset and Hampshire, *The Hatcher Review*, vol. 5, no. 46 (1998), pp. 21–8

—, 'Inkpen: a Berkshire manor and the plague', *The Hatcher Review*, vol. 5, no. 46 (1998), pp. 29–31

Wells, Sharon, 'Manners maketh man: living, dining and becoming a man in the later Middle Ages', in McDonald and Ormrod (eds.), *Rites of Passage*, pp. 67–81

Wenzel, Siegfried, 'Pestilence and Middle English literature: Friar John Grimstone's poems on death', in Williman (ed.), *Black Death*, pp. 131–59

Wheelis, Mark, 'Biological warfare at the 1346 siege of Caffa', *Emerging Infectious Diseases*, vol. 8, no. 9 (September 2002), pp. 971–5

Williams, Glanmor, *The Welsh Church from Conquest to Reformation* (Cardiff: University of Wales Press, 1962)

Williamson, Raymond, 'The plague in Cambridge', *Medical History*, vol. 1, no. 1 (January 1957), pp. 51–64

Williman, Daniel (ed.), *The Black Death: The Impact of the Fourteenth Century Plague: Papers of the Eleventh Annual Conference of the Center for Medieval & Early Renaissance Studies* (Binghampton, NY: Center for Renaissance and Early Renaissance Studies, 1982)

Wood, James W., Rebecca J. Ferrel and Sharon N. DeWitte-Aviña, 'The temporal dynamics of the fourteenth-century Black Death: new evidence from English ecclesiastical records', *Human Biology*, vol. 75, no. 4 (August 2003), pp. 427–48

Wrathmell, Stuart, *Wharram: A Study of Settlement on the Yorkshire Wolds, Vol. VI – Domestic Settlement 2: Medieval Peasant Farmsteads*, York University Archaeological Publications No. 8 (York: University of York, 1989)

Yu, Hwa-Lung and George Christakos, 'Spaciotemporal modelling and mapping of the bubonic plague epidemic in India', *International Journal of Health Geographics*, vol. 5, no. 12 (2006) http://www.ij-health geographics.com/content/5/1/12

Ziegler, Philip, *The Black Death*, 2nd rev. edn (Harmondsworth: Penguin, 1998)

Acknowledgements

The anticipated pleasure of acknowledging the many people who have helped me write this book has, on many occasions, spurred me on to its completion.

My first thanks should go to those two people responsible for the genesis of this project – Eleo Gordon and my agent Andrew Lownie. It was Will Sulkin at Random House, however, who bought the idea, and I am fortunate in more than the usual ways that he did so: few authors are privileged to have so supportive, and accommodating, a commissioning editor. Had it not been for the timely advice of Leonie Frieda I may never have had such good fortune, so my thanks go to her as well.

The years of research that followed were made all the more fruitful by the help given freely by many academics and specialists. Dr Paula Arthur generously gave me her unpublished but important work on the bishop of Winchester's pipe rolls, Dr Mark Forrest shared with me the remarkable data he has extracted from the Gillingham court rolls, Professor Phythian-Adams located and sent me a copy of the unpublished paper by Eileen and Arthur Gooder, and Philip Temple gave me sight of the draft for his forthcoming volume on Charterhouse for the Survey of London. I enjoyed the advice of Professor Tom James, whose knowledge on the progress of the epidemic through Hampshire is without parallel, and Nick Millea, the Bodleian Map Librarian, while Dr Susan Scott – who so brilliantly exploded the myth of bubonic plague with her collaborator, Christopher Duncan – was a very useful sounding board. I owe a particular debt of gratitude to Dr Rosemary Horrox and Professor Dafydd Johnston, who both permitted me to use their excellent translations, and Professor George Christakos and Professor Hwa-Lung Yu, who re-visited their extraordinary work on the Black Death for me and have made possible the spread maps included in this volume.

I was privileged to receive the assistance and advice of a number of people during the final drafting of the book. Dr Roger Lovatt, who re-fired my love of medieval history when he supervised me at Cambridge and taught me much else besides, read both my proposal and the raw manuscript, offering invaluable comments on both occasions: I am profoundly grateful for all that he has done. Charlotte Valori aided me when my Latin faltered, while Tom Bishop helped with the reconstruction of the Gough Map. I could not have hoped for a more conscientious and understanding editor than Drummond Moir, who guided me through the editing of the manuscript with a sure hand and great kindness; the book has been considerably improved by his contribution. I would also like to thank Reginald Piggott, who produced such beautiful maps, and Kay Peddle, who transformed the manuscript into a book.

Writing a book is an anti-social business, and I have inconvenienced many by my lengthy absences. My aunt Helen Gardner gave up her cottage for two years so I could use it as retreat; I was lucky to have Rosemary Savage to look after me whilst I was there. My colleagues have been extraordinarily understanding, especially in the months when I went missing from the office. That the writing reached an end was in large part thanks to the sustaining friendship and love of a good number of people, only a few of whom I have the space to mention here. The book would not have taken flight without Olivia Bonner, whose encouragement, generosity and kindness I could not repay. Jordan Frieda not only lent me his house in which to complete the initial proposal but was, as ever, a constant friend through the years that followed. Both Edward Devereux and John Prideaux had an unnerving ability to ring at the right moment: they are stalwart friends indeed. Dakis Hagen tackled a later version of the manuscript and offered typically incisive comments. Like several others William Woodhams allowed the book to intrude on his holidays, reading the manuscript and joining me on a Black Death road trip: at every stage he has shown the kind of unquestioning support that makes him and his friendship exceptional. None was more affected by my absence than Emma Winberg, to whom I apologise, both for being away, and for misjudging how long that 'away' would be. All these people, who through no volition of their own had to live with the Black Death and with – or without – me whilst I wrote, have my deepest gratitude.

Brothers and sisters are expected to show forbearance in the face of tiresome siblings, but the mildness shown by Felix, Leonora and Cordelia has been beyond dutiful. All of them have been eager to help despite so little company being offered in return. My father has been, as ever, a model of patience: I am enormously grateful for his help, his indulgence, and above all his quiet but constant understanding. The real reason this book happened, however, was because my mother emboldened me to do it, and ever since she has assisted, reassured and encouraged. My gratitude is greatest, however, for the considerable insight she has offered in the reading of the many drafts I have imposed on her – a gratitude that is matched only by the delight I have in dedicating this book to her.

Index